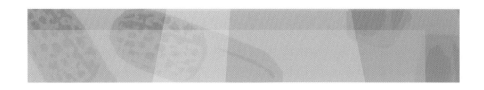

Drugs, Alcohol, and Tobacco

Learning About Addictive Behavior

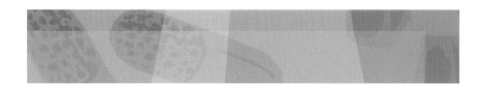

Drugs, Alcohol, and Tobacco

Learning About Addictive Behavior

Volume

Mo to Z
Cumulative Index

Rosalyn Carson-DeWitt, M.D.,
Editor in Chief

MACMILLAN
REFERENCE
USA™

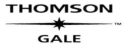

New York • Detroit • San Diego • San Francisco • Cleveland • New Haven, Conn. • Waterville, Maine • London • Munich

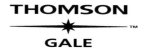

Drugs, Alcohol, and Tobacco: Learning About Addictive Behavior

Rosalyn Carson-DeWitt, M.D.

For permission to use material from this product, submit your request via Web at http://www.gale-edit.com/permissions, or you may download our Permissions Request form and submit your request by fax or mail to:

Permissions Department
The Gale Group, Inc.
27500 Drake Rd.
Farmington Hills, MI 48331-3535
Permissions Hotline:
248-699-8006 or 800-877-4253 ext. 8006
Fax: 248-699-8074 or 800-762-4058

LIBRARY OF CONGRESS CATALOGING-IN-PUBLICATION DATA

Drugs, alcohol, and tobacco: learning about addictive behavior / Rosalyn Carson-DeWitt, editor in chief.
    p. cm.
      Includes bibliographical references and index.
      ISBN 0-02-865756-X (set: hardcover : alk. paper) — ISBN 0-02-865757-8 (v. 1) — ISBN 0-02-865758-6 (v. 2) — ISBN 0-02-865759-4 (v. 3)
      1. Drug abuse—Encyclopedias, Juvenile.   2. Alcoholism—Encyclopedias, Juvenile.   3. Tobacco habit—Encyclopedias, Juvenile. 4. Substance abuse—Encyclopedias, Juvenile.   5. Compulsive behavior—Encyclopedias, Juvenile.   6. Teenagers—Substance use—Encyclopedias, Juvenile. I.

Carson-DeWitt, Rosalyn.
HV5804 .D78 2003
613.8—dc21

2002009270

Printed in Canada
1 2 3 4 5 6 7 8 9 10

Preface

In 1995 Macmillan Reference USA published the outstanding *Encyclopedia of Drugs and Alcohol*, edited by Jerome Jaffe. An extensively revised second edition, entitled *Encyclopedia of Drugs, Alcohol, and Addictive Behavior*, was published in 2001. Now Macmillan Reference USA is drawing from the fine work done for these prior encyclopedias to publish *Drugs, Alcohol, and Tobacco: Learning About Addictive Behavior*, a three-volume set targeted towards general and younger readers.

Alcohol, drugs, and tobacco have myriad ill effects on the lives of children and teenagers. Babies are born addicted to crack or harmed by exposure to alcohol while in the womb. Children live in poverty and chaos, at high risk of neglect, abuse, and homelessness because of their parents' drug and/or alcohol problems. Increased school dropout rates, a high risk of psychiatric problems, and a greater chance of severe injury or death due to violence, motor vehicle accidents, and self-injury endanger the worlds of children and teens raised amid substance abuse. Furthermore, children from substance-abusing homes are more likely to turn to smoking, drugs, or alcohol. Then comes the convergence of the genetic propensity for substance abuse, the availability of alcohol and drugs, and peer pressure, all factors that increase a child's risk of engaging in substance abuse or addictive behaviors.

Drugs, Alcohol, and Tobacco: Learning About Addictive Behavior was the brainchild of Hélène Potter, director of new product development at Macmillan Reference USA. Aware that initiating substance use prior to the age of fifteen carries a greater risk of severe problems, and aware that prevention must begin with thorough education, Ms. Potter conceived of and pushed through this valuable project. Designed to engage, interest, and educate children and teens, this work provides information on specific drugs (such as nicotine, alcohol, marijuana, and ecstasy), risk and protective factors for addiction, diagnosis and treatment of addictions, medical and legal consequences of both casual use and addiction, costs to families and society, drug production and trafficking, policy issues, and other compulsive disorders (including gambling, cutting, and eating disorders).

Although the *Encyclopedia of Drugs, Alcohol, and Addictive Behavior* was used as a structural basis for this present work, the entire table of contents was revised to focus the new work on the needs and interests of young students. An impressive cadre of experts and academics was commissioned to review, revise, rewrite, and refocus every article from the original collection, or to produce new articles pertinent to the project's goals and relevant to children and teenagers. New ancillaries provide additional resources that will be particularly helpful to children and teenagers researching topics for school or for their own personal use.

The result is *Drugs, Alcohol, and Tobacco: Learning About Addictive Behavior*, a collection of over 190 alphabetically arranged articles intended to reach out to an audience of children and teenagers with information that can help them understand issues surrounding addictive behavior on both an academic and a personal level. The thoughtful, visually interesting design of the text includes call-out definitions in the margins of articles (so that young students do not have to flip to a separate glossary, although that is provided as well); lively marginalia that highlights interesting facts or makes reading suggestions for fiction that deals with topically similar issues; and more than 200 full-color illustrations that help young readers to organize and to compare and contrast information. Articles are followed by cross-references. Appendices include a wide-ranging list of organizations (including their addresses, phone numbers, and web sites) from which readers can seek more information or obtain contacts for personal help; a complete glossary of terms; and an annotated bibliography that will point students toward further research, assist teachers with class preparation, and guide individuals who are struggling with the effects of addiction in their personal lives.

Many fine people deserve considerable thanks for contributing to the birth of this new work, beginning with Hélène Potter, whose vision and guidance were essential throughout the production process. Editor Oona Schmid slaved over every aspect of the project and supported everyone else's work with competence and good humor. Jan Gottschalk consulted on the project, sharing her considerable experience with middle-school students, and providing excellent input regarding relevancy of material, fit with middle-school curriculum, and appropriateness for middle-school readers. Copyeditor Jessica Hornik Evans put in countless hours to make entries suitable in length, scope, and reading level for middle-school students. Amy Buttery worked to ensure that data presented were up-to-date and pertinent to young teenagers. And once again, my husband Toby, and our children Anna, Emma, Isabelle, and Sophie, graciously tolerated the presence of a fifth child in the guise of an encyclopedia in our home.

In closing, I would like to acknowledge the efforts of clinicians who are working on the front line to treat families grappling with addiction in their lives; academics who teach about substance abuse and its effects on individuals, society, and the international community; researchers who are studying issues that may lead to better ways to diagnose, treat, and prevent addiction; policymakers who struggle to find ways to protect society from the crime and violence associated with addictions; and the many individuals who awaken each day to face the effects of addiction wreaking havoc on their lives and to try once again to find their way free of addiction's stranglehold.

Rosalyn Carson-DeWitt, M.D.
Editor in Chief

July 2002

Contributors

The text of *Drugs, Alcohol, and Tobacco: Learning About Addictive Behavior* is based on the second edition of Macmillan's *Encyclopedia of Drugs, Alcohol, and Addictive Behavior*, which was published in 2001. We have updated material where necessary and added original entries that are of particular importance to the general public and younger students. Articles have been condensed and made more accessible for a student audience. Please refer to the List of Authors at the back of volume three in this set for the authors and affiliations of all those whose work appears in this reference. Here we wish to acknowledge the writers who revised entries and wrote new articles specifically for this set:

Peter Andreas

Linda Wasmer Andrews

Christopher B. Anthony

Samuel A. Ball

Robert Balster

Amy Buttery

Kate B. Carey

Jonathan Caulkins

Allan Cobb

Roberta Friedman

Jessica Gerson

Frederick K. Grittner

Angela Guarda

Becky Ham

Carl G. Leukefeld

Jill Max

Thomas S. May

Tom Mieczkowski

Cynthia Robbins

Heather Roberto

Ian Rockett

Joseph Spillane

Michele Staton Tindall

Marvin Steinberg

Michael Walsh

Michael Winkelman

Jill Anne Yeagley

Table of Contents

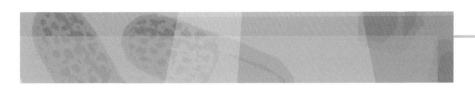

Moonshine

Moonshine is the common name for illegally produced hard liquor—whiskey, rum, brandy, gin, and vodka. (Another name is white lightning.) The term probably was first used in 1785. In that year a British book on vulgar language described "moonshine" as the clear brandy that was smuggled to the coasts of Kent and Sussex in England. In the New World, moonshine was made in homemade stills (apparatus for distilling liquor), usually from corn. It was especially popular in rural areas in the southern United States before, during, and after Prohibition, and it continues to be made today. The alcohol content of moonshine is usually high, often as much as 80 percent (160 proof). First-run moonshine contains a number of impurities, some of which are toxic, so it is necessary to double and triple distill the liquor to purify it for drinking. SEE ALSO ALCOHOL: HISTORY OF DRINKING; PROHIBITION OF ALCOHOL.

Morning Glory Seeds

The seeds of the morning glory (*Ipomoea*) contain substances that are similar to those in lysergic acid diethylamide (LSD), a **hallucinogenic** drug. People who eat morning glory seeds may feel different. However, the experience is not identical to an LSD-type "trip," even though the seeds are sold on the street as an LSD equivalent. Morning glory seeds are easy to purchase legally, but many varieties available in garden-supply stores have been treated with insecticides and other toxic chemicals that will induce vomiting if the seeds are eaten. SEE ALSO HALLUCINOGENS; LYSERGIC ACID DIETHYLAMIDE (LSD) AND PSYCHEDELICS.

hallucinogen
substance that can cause hallucinations, or seeing, hearing, or feeling things that are not there

Morphine

Morphine is a major component of opium, a product of the poppy plant. Named after Morpheus, the Greek god of sleep, morphine is a powerful analgesic (painkiller). Doctors frequently prescribe it to relieve moderate to severe pain, especially in cancer patients. In the 1800s morphine was available in stores to anyone who wanted to buy it. At that time, little was known about physical dependence, and many people became addicted to morphine. Today, morphine is considered a controlled substance and is regulated by law. Because doctors know more about physical dependence, few patients become addicted to it.

Morphine produces a wide variety of actions, some desired and others not. The definition of a desired action and a side effect depends on the reason for using the drug. For example, opiates such as morphine can be used to treat diarrhea. However, a person taking morphine for pain would find constipation an undesirable side effect.

Constriction (narrowing) of the pupils of the eyes is one of the most widely recognized signs of opiate use. In addition, morphine produces **sedation**. At higher doses, morphine depresses respiration, meaning that the patient loses the ability to breathe automatically. Very high doses of morphine stop a person's breathing entirely—a common occurrence in overdoses. Another common side effect of morphine use is nausea.

Morphine is given either by mouth or by injection. Injection has much more potent or powerful effects. Physicians who are experts in the treatment of pain increasingly give morphine through continuous infusion. In order to avoid uneven treatment of pain (total relief when the drug is at its peak in the body; continued pain as the medication wears off), the morphine is diluted and given with fluid directly into the veins, at a very slow but steady rate. This keeps the concentration of morphine in the body at a steady state, so that the patient does not have periods of relief alternating with periods of pain. Another method of administering morphine involves a pump that allows the patient to push a button, releasing a tiny dose of morphine. The pump is set up to allow a specific dose of morphine at a specific time interval (sometimes as frequently as every five minutes). Some studies have shown that these patient-controlled analgesia (PCA) pumps are very effective at keeping a patient's pain to a minimum.

With **chronic** use, the effect of morphine lessens. In other words, a person develops **tolerance** to the drug's effects. To main-

sedation process of calming someone by administering a medication that reduces excitement; often called a tranquilizer

chronic continuing for a long period of time

tolerance condition in which higher and higher doses of a drug or alcohol are needed to produce the effect or "high" experienced from the original dose

tain the effect the person received originally, it is necessary to increase the dose. When a person becomes physically dependent on morphine or other opiates, stopping the drug will bring on the **withdrawal** syndrome. Early symptoms of withdrawal include restlessness, tearing eyes, runny nose, yawning, and sweating. Eventually, further symptoms include dilated pupils, sneezing, elevations in heart rate and blood pressure, cramping, and gooseflesh. (The expression "cold turkey" comes from the look of the skin during withdrawal.) SEE ALSO ADDICTION: CONCEPTS AND DEFINITIONS; OPIATE AND OPIOID DRUG ABUSE.

withdrawal group of physical and psychological symptoms that may occur when a person suddenly stops the use of a substance or reduces the dose of an addictive substance

Mothers Against Drunk Driving (MADD)

Mothers Against Drunk Driving (MADD)☎ is a national organization that works to reduce drunk driving and to help the victims of drunk-driving accidents. Many of MADD's members are volunteers who have personally suffered from the results of drunk driving. MADD was founded by Candy Lightner, whose 13-year old daughter, Cari, was killed by a drunk driver on May 3, 1980. Lightner was outraged to learn that only two days previously the driver had been released from jail, where he had been held for another hit-and-run drunk-driving crash. Although he had been arrested for drunk driving several times before, he was still driving with a valid California license. Lightner decided to begin a campaign to keep drunk drivers off the road, so that other mothers would not have to suffer the anguish that she was experiencing. On September 5, 1980 (Cari's birthday), MADD was incorporated.

☎ See *Organizations of Interest* at the back of Volume 3 for address, telephone, and URL.

Since then, MADD has evolved into an organization with millions of members and hundreds of local chapters across the United States. Chapters have also been started in Canada, Great Britain, New Zealand, and Australia. Membership is not restricted to mothers of victims or to the victims themselves. Everyone who is concerned about the drunk-driving issue is welcome to join. Funding for the organization comes from membership dues and contributions. MADD also applies for and receives grants from federal and state governments and private organizations. Paid staff are employed to provide leadership on the state and national levels. MADD is involved in three major kinds of activity: (1) advocacy for stricter drunk-driving laws and better enforcement, (2) promotion of public awareness and educational programs, and (3) assistance to victims.

The Legislative Agenda

According to MADD, drunk driving is a violent crime. One of its rallying slogans is, "Murder by Car Is Still Murder!" Over the years, MADD members have worked to generate public support for passage of stricter drunk-driving laws, more appropriate punishments, and more consistent enforcement measures aimed at deterring drunk driving. In the 1980s intense **lobbying** efforts were undertaken for the passage of laws making 21 the minimum legal age for drinking (now in force in all fifty states). The group believes that this measure has saved thousands of lives that would have been lost in drunk-driving crashes.

lobbying activities aimed at influencing public officials, especially members of the legislature

MADD has also lobbied for changes in legal procedures that would make the system more responsive to victims of drunk driving. For example, in many states victims had been barred from the courtroom during the trial of the accused in their own drunk-driving cases, because their testimony (or even their presence) might prejudice the jury. As a result of the efforts of MADD and other groups, all fifty states have passed victims' rights bills. These bills ensure that victims will be notified about court hearings and, in most states, allowed to testify about the impact of the crime on their lives. Other lobbying efforts have sought to close legal loopholes that drunk drivers were using to avoid punishment. For example, some drivers refused to take a breath test for **blood alcohol concentration (BAC)** and then were allowed to plead guilty to a lesser charge. In other cases, drivers were allowed to claim that despite their BAC, their driving was not really impaired.

blood alcohol concentration (BAC) amount of alcohol in the bloodstream, expressed as the grams of alcohol per deciliter of blood; as BAC goes up, the drinker experiences more psychological and physical effects

MADD has had a central role in the passage of over 1,000 tougher drunk-driving laws that close these loopholes and establish other deterrence measures, such as mandatory jail sentences for drunk drivers. MADD also supports efforts to require offenders to undergo treatment for alcoholism and/or drug dependency, if this is deemed necessary.

Public Awareness and Education

MADD is involved in various efforts to raise public awareness and concern about drunk driving. The "National Candlelight Vigil of Remembrance and Hope" is held in many locations each December, drawing victims together to give public testimony to the suffering that results from drunk driving. During the "Red Ribbon Tie One On for Safety" campaign, which takes place between Thanksgiving and New Year's Day, MADD encourages citizens to attach a red ribbon to their car as a reminder to themselves and others to drive sober. MADD's well-known public awareness campaign of the past used the slogan

"Think . . . Don't Drink and Drive" in public-service announcements on radio and television and in print materials. Another campaign, "Keep It a Safe Summer" (KISS) emphasized the need for sobriety during recreational activities that involve driving, boating, or other risky activities. MADD also provides curriculum materials for schools and each year sponsors a poster and essay contest for children on the subject of drunk driving.

Assistance to Victims

Programs that provide aid to victims of drunk-driving crashes are at the heart of MADD's mission. Support groups help victims share their pain with others who understand their feelings. MADD members send "We Care" cards to victims of recent crashes. Specially trained victim advocates offer a one-on-one personal relationship with victims, trying to respond to both their emotional and practical needs. Victims are informed about their legal rights and on the judicial procedures relevant to their cases. They can call a toll-free number (1-800-GET MADD) for information and for help in case of crisis. MADD also offers training for police in notifying people about the deaths of their loved ones and specialized training for other community professionals, such as clergy and medical workers, who are called upon to assist victims.

Since the founding of MADD in 1980, the percentage of traffic deaths involving alcohol has steadily decreased from almost 60 percent of all traffic deaths to around 50 percent. MADD's 1990 goal "20 x 2000" aimed to reduce that proportion by an additional 20 percent by 2000. This goal was reached three years early, in 1997. Current goals include reducing alcohol-related traffic fatalities to 11,000 or fewer by the year 2005. In 1999, MADD expanded its mission statement to include prevention of underage drinking. Future efforts will focus on more effective law enforcement, increased punishments, and prevention programs that include education for youth and more responsible practices by establishments that sell alcohol. SEE ALSO BLOOD ALCOHOL CONCENTRATION; BREATHALYZER; DRINKING AGE; DRIVING, ALCOHOL, AND DRUGS; STUDENTS AGAINST DESTRUCTIVE DECISIONS (SADD).

Naltrexone

Naltrexone is a drug used to treat people who are dependent on opiate or opioid drugs such as heroin. Naltrexone has the ability to antagonize, or reverse, virtually all the effects of opiate/opioid drugs. It blocks the pleasurable or rewarding effects of opiate drugs, so that addicts do not feel a craving for the drugs. This antagonist effect is long lasting. In addition, naltrexone does not produce any pleasurable effects on its own. As a result, the patient has little incentive to misuse the medication and will not become **dependent** on it.

Treatment with naltrexone is most successful when combined with a program of counseling and other rehabilitation services. Addicts who are employed and able to manage their lives, and who are highly motivated to beat their addiction, have the best treatment results. This is especially true when addicts face severe economic or legal consequences for failing treatment. For example, health professionals with an addiction problem must get treatment in order to keep their medical licenses. These addicts typically take naltrexone regularly for several years (known as maintenance treatment) and remain **abstinent** from opiates. Some programs have reported five-year success rates as high as 95 percent. In contrast, most street addicts have unstable living situations and support their drug use through criminal activity. Typically, these addicts refuse to take naltrexone. If they do begin treatment, in general they quickly drop out. Naltrexone's ineffectiveness for this type of addict is probably due to the drug's lack of pleasurable effects. Many such addicts prefer maintenance treatment with methadone, an opiate drug that produces some desirable effects.

In the 1990s researchers studied naltrexone as a treatment for alcoholism. Alcoholic men who had gone through detoxification were given naltrexone. Naltrexone reduced the likelihood that these men would return to alcohol use. A 1999 study showed that naltrexone reduces the desire and craving for alcohol. However, it can sometimes increase the negative side effects, including headaches. Naltrexone is especially effective in the treatment of alcoholism when use of the drug is combined with therapy to change the patient's behavior. Naltrexone is also being studied experimentally as a possible treatment for cigarette smoking and eating disorders. SEE ALSO ALCOHOL TREATMENT: MEDICATIONS; HEROIN TREATMENT: MEDICATIONS; OPIATE AND OPIOID DRUG ABUSE; TOBACCO TREATMENT: MEDICATIONS.

Narcotic

The term *narcotic* comes from a Greek word that means "to make numb." Its history as an English word begins in the fourteenth century. At that time and for several more centuries, the term referred to drugs that provide relief from pain and put a person into a **stupor**.

These analgesic (painkilling) drugs were opium and other opiate/opioid substances (which contain opium).

During the nineteenth century, the meaning of narcotics changed to include a wider range of drugs. By the turn of the twentieth century, any drug that can lead to addiction, from heroin to cocaine, was called a narcotic. During the twentieth century, narcotics became an even less exact term. Legally, the term refers to drugs that can lead to abuse and addiction. Many drugs are subject to legal restrictions as "addictive narcotics." However, not all drugs nowadays called narcotics cause addiction. In addition, not all drugs called narcotics have painkilling effects. Although the media and the general public still use the term, scientists no longer use it in their discussions and studies of drugs. SEE ALSO DRUGS OF ABUSE; OPIATE AND OPIOID DRUG ABUSE.

Narcotics Anonymous (NA)

Narcotics Anonymous (NA)☎ is an organization that helps people who are addicted to drugs. NA has adapted the **Twelve Steps** of Alcoholics Anonymous (AA)☎ to form its own unique program for overcoming addiction.

NA grew out of the experiences of two AA members. In 1944 an AA member, known as Houston, recruited a new member who was not only an alcoholic but also an abuser of morphine. The AA program helped the new recruit to overcome his alcohol addiction but not his morphine addiction. The recruit soon wound up as an involuntary patient in a hospital in Lexington, Kentucky. Houston was puzzled that AA could help with alcoholism but not with addiction to other drugs. With the help of a doctor at the Lexington hospital where the recruit was being treated, Houston started a group specifically for drug addicts. Weekly meetings have taken place in that hospital ever since.

In 1948 an addict known as Dan began attending the meetings. Dan recovered from his addiction and went home to New York, hoping to form the first group for drug abusers outside the Lexington hospital. Dan looked up others whom he had known at Lexington and suggested weekly meetings. Narcotics Anonymous began with four members and slowly grew in size. The group decided to encourage addicts to seek treatment in institutions rather than going through withdrawal at home. AA established a policy of "cooperation, but not affiliation" between AA and NA. According to this

☎ See *Organizations of Interest* at the back of Volume 3 for address, telephone, and URL.

Twelve Steps program for remaining sober developed by Alcoholics Anonymous; adopted by many other groups, such as Narcotics Anonymous

Narcotics Anonymous (NA) advises asking these types of questions to see if a person has an addiction. The actual number of "yes" answers is not as important as whether drugs are causing problems or negatively affecting someone's life.

• Do you ever use alone?

• Have you ever used a drug without knowing what it was or what it would do to you?

• Has your job or school performance ever suffered from the effects of your drug use?

• Have you ever thought you could not fit in or have a good time without drugs?

☎ See *Organizations of Interest* at the back of Volume 3 for address, telephone, and URL.

AIDS stands for acquired immunodeficiency syndrome, the disease caused by the human immunodeficiency virus (HIV); in severe cases it is characterized by the profound weakening of the body's immune system

policy, AA freely offered the Twelve Steps and other strategies to NA for adaptation.

NA soon attracted many people who abused a wide variety of drugs—heroin, barbiturates, amphetamines, and marijuana. As a result, NA decided its focus must be on addiction itself rather than on any one drug. They changed the wording of AA's step one from "We admitted we were powerless over drugs" to "We admitted we were powerless over our Addiction." In other words, not every member had a problem with the same drug, but they all shared a belief that they suffered from a disease of addiction. In contrast, Cocaine Anonymous ☎ or Marijuana Anonymous ☎ are groups that focus on specific drugs.

NA members who have quit using drugs pass on their experiences and hopes to new members. In this way they help people still suffering from addiction to become drug-free. SEE ALSO ADDICTION: CONCEPTS AND DEFINITIONS; TREATMENT TYPES: AN OVERVIEW.

Needle Exchange Programs

A common practice among injecting drug users is the sharing of needles and other injection equipment. Sharing needles allows diseases to spread from one user to another. HIV, the virus that causes **AIDS**, has been reported among injecting drug users in sixty countries, from all continents except Antarctica, and from both industrialized and developing nations. The Centers for Disease Control and Prevention (CDC) estimates that injection drug use directly accounts for 25 percent of infections among men and women. This figure does not include cases of HIV infection with an indirect relation to injection drug use, such as those having sexual contact with people who acquired the virus through injection drug use.

Once HIV becomes well established in a population of injecting drug users, their sexual partners are at risk of contracting the virus. In addition, pregnant women can pass the virus on to developing fetuses. Injecting drug users are the main source for both heterosexual transmission of HIV and transmission of HIV to a fetus. According to the CDC, at least 36 percent and possibly as many as one-half of new HIV infections are caused by the sharing of needles and syringes, either directly due to injection drug use, through unprotected sex with someone who acquired HIV infection through injection drug use, or in the case of young children, through birth to a mother who acquired HIV infection through these means. A CDC report

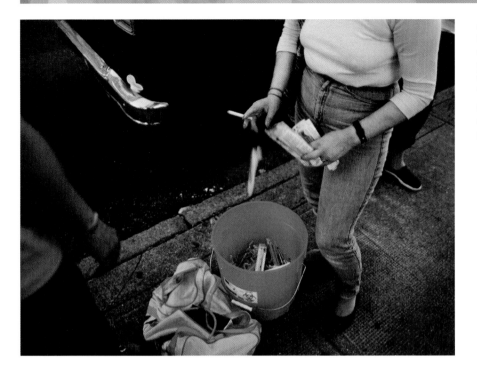

A volunteer collects used syringes as part of a needle exchange program in Vancouver, British Columbia. This program is designed to prevent the spread of infectious diseases.

also estimates that three out of four AIDS cases among women are due to injection drug use or heterosexual contact with someone infected with HIV through injection drug use, and over 75 percent of new infections in children are the result of injection drug use in a parent.

The spread of HIV/AIDS has led many countries to develop needle exchange programs. In these programs, the drug user can turn in used injection equipment (needles and syringes) and receive sterile equipment in exchange. The sterile equipment is provided legally and at no cost. The hope is that providing sterile equipment can slow or stop the spread of disease among people who inject drugs.

Controversy

Needle exchange programs have been the subject of a great deal of controversy in the United States and many other countries. Some opponents of the programs are concerned that increasing legal access to injection equipment will lead to increasing use of illegal drugs. However, research studies show that needle exchange does not lead to an increase in drug use on either a community or an individual level. In fact, some studies show a slight decrease in the frequency of injection among participants in needle exchange programs.

Opponents also argue that increased legal access appears to condone illegal drug use and sends the wrong message about illegal drug use. Supporters of needle exchange programs disagree. They argue that the programs do not send the message that the injection of drugs like heroin and cocaine is acceptable. Instead, needle exchange programs send the message that previous policies on illegal drug use cannot cope with the urgent public-health crisis of HIV infection among injecting drug users, their sexual partners, and their children. Supporters argue that society's ability to treat drug users so that they will never take drugs again is clearly limited. In this view, letting drug injectors, their sexual partners, and their children die of HIV infection is inhumane, and providing needle exchanges is an essential way to prevent further disease and death.

Opponents have also expressed the concern that exchange programs could attract people who had not previously injected drugs. However, the majority of participants in needle exchanges have long histories of drug injection, usually from five to ten years or more. Studies show no evidence of new injectors participating in programs.

State governments are often responsible for decisions about supporting or opposing needle exchange programs. One of the most controversial issues facing states is whether to make possession of needles and syringes legal or criminal. As of 2000, in an effort to reduce the spread of HIV through injection drug use, many states made it illegal to purchase, sell, or possess syringes without prescriptions. In some of these states, syringe prescription laws have been repealed, and pharmacy regulations and practice guidelines restricting the sale of sterile syringes have been changed. Other states (such as New Hampshire) renewed their needle exchange programs.

Unfortunately, the debate over these programs is often a political issue rather than a public-health issue. Political leaders may want to avoid the appearance of approving of drug use by approving of needle exchange programs. As a result, they may concentrate more on the political angle of the issue rather than on determining the best policies for health.

How the Programs Work

Needle exchange programs have had varying degrees of success. Programs that offer sterile needles but do not offer support services to drug users have been ineffective. Simple equipment exchanges are not enough to prevent the spread of HIV. The organization of services offered by needle exchange programs is critical to their success. Programs must be located where drug users will find them, and they must have hours of operation geared toward the population they serve. Even more important is the attitude of the staff toward the participants in the exchange. Participants should be treated with dignity and respect. Staff members should not take a judgmental attitude toward the participants' morality or ability to manage their lives. The participants care enough about their health and the health of others to participate in the program.

Needle exchange programs can also offer other services, such as distribution of condoms without cost to prevent the sexual transmission of HIV. When participants develop trust in the staff members, the staff may be able to determine other health and social-service needs. Staff can then refer participants to drug treatment programs or other social services. Some programs offer a variety of programs on site, including drug treatment, self-help recovery groups, women's support groups, tuberculosis screening and treatment, and Bible study groups.

Effectiveness

The National Institutes of Health in February 1997 concluded that needle exchange programs in general have reduced behavior that poses the risk of spreading HIV by about 80 percent. Virtually every major scientific study since that time confirms the conclusion that needle exchange programs are effective and do not have the unwanted effects which cause concern among opponents. In addition, the CDC, the American Medical Association, the American Public Health Association, and the Joint United Nations Programme on HIV/AIDS (UNAIDS) have all concluded that enough data exist to suggest that needle exchange programs are successful at reducing the number of HIV cases.

Some opponents argue that needle exchange programs should not be funded with public money, such as federal, state, or city taxes. A recent study found that needle exchange programs are in fact cost-effective. Through needle exchange programs, one HIV infection can be prevented for one-third the cost of medical care for an infected person. SEE ALSO COMPLICATIONS FROM INJECTING DRUGS; SUBSTANCE ABUSE AND AIDS.

Neuroleptic

Neuroleptic drugs are medications used to treat **psychoses** such as schizophrenia. Neuroleptics are also called antipsychotics. This group of drugs includes chlorpromazine (Thorazine), haloperidol (Haldol), clozapine (Clozaril), lithium (Lithonate), and thioridazine (Mellaril). Some of the newer drugs include risperidone (Risperdal), quetiapine

psychosis mental disorder in which an individual loses contact with reality and may have delusions (i.e., unshakable false beliefs) or hallucinations (i.e., the experience of seeing, hearing, feeling, smelling, or tasting things that are not actually present)

(Seroquel), and olanzapine (Zyprexa). Some neuroleptics have other medical uses, such as the treatment of nausea, vomiting, and movement disorders (including Huntington's disease and Gilles de la Tourette's syndrome). SEE ALSO ANTIPSYCHOTIC.

Nicotine

Nicotine is a chemical substance found in the tobacco plant and its products, including cigarettes, cigars, pipe tobacco, and smokeless tobacco (such as chewing tobacco and snuff). People who smoke cigarettes or use tobacco in other ways can become addicted to the nicotine contained in these products.

Nicotine can occur in two forms. The active form, called L-nicotine, is found in tobacco plants of the genus *Nicotiana*. These plants belong to the nightshade family (*Solanaceae*). *Nicotiana* plants, especially *Nicotiana tabacum*, were grown for their leaves in South America before the arrival of Christopher Columbus. The inactive form of nicotine, D-nicotine, is not present in tobacco leaves. Instead, a small amount forms when tobacco is burned during smoking. In addition to tobacco plants, small amounts of nicotine are found in foods of the nightshade family, such as tomatoes and eggplants. Nicotine that has been extracted from tobacco leaves is widely used as an insecticide.

The Effects of Nicotine

Nicotine acts in complex ways in the human body. Its effects depend on the amount of the dose, how the dose is taken (for example, by mouth or by injection), the time over which the dose is given, and the individual's history of exposure to nicotine. In high doses, nicotine produces nausea, vomiting, **convulsions**, muscle paralysis, coma, and circulatory collapse, and causes a person to stop breathing. These severe effects can occur if a person accidentally absorbs an insecticide that contains nicotine or takes an overdose of nicotine.

convulsion an involuntary and violent tightening of the muscles

Nicotine's effects are very different in the smaller amounts found in tobacco products. Taking nicotine by smoking a cigarette or other tobacco products can speed up heart rate and blood pressure; increase the force of contraction of the heart; constrict (narrow) blood vessels in the skin, producing cool, pale skin; constrict blood vessels in the heart; relax the skeletal muscles; increase body metabolic rate; and release hormones such as epinephrine (adrenaline), norepinephrine, and cortisol into the bloodstream.

In the brain, nicotine produces effects partly by enhancing the release of neurotransmitters (brain chemicals) that carry information from one neuron (brain cell) to another. Nicotine enhances the release of the following brain chemicals:

- dopamine, which can produce pleasure
- norepinephrine, which can suppress appetite
- acetylcholine, which can produce arousal
- serotonin, which can reduce anxiety
- beta endorphin, which can reduce pain

Because nicotine produces these desirable effects, people who use tobacco products want to do so repeatedly. As a result, people often become addicted to nicotine. SEE ALSO ADDICTION: CONCEPTS AND DEFINITIONS; ADOLESCENTS, DRUG AND ALCOHOL USE; BRAIN CHEMISTRY; NICOTINE WITHDRAWAL; TOBACCO: DEPENDENCE; TOBACCO: MEDICAL COMPLICATIONS; TOBACCO: POLICIES, LAWS, AND REGULATIONS; TOBACCO: SMOKELESS; TOBACCO TREATMENT: AN OVERVIEW; TOBACCO TREATMENT: BEHAVIORAL APPROACHES; TOBACCO TREATMENT: MEDICATIONS; TOLERANCE AND PHYSICAL DEPENDENCE.

Nicotine Withdrawal

Nicotine is one of the most addicting substances known. In fact, the risk of becoming **dependent** on nicotine following any tobacco use is higher than the risk of becoming dependent on alcohol, cocaine, or marijuana. People who use several drugs often say that quitting tobacco is more difficult than giving up alcohol or cocaine.

dependent psychologically compelled to use a substance for emotional and/or physical reasons

Nicotine affects the functioning of the central nervous system, which is made up of the brain and spinal cord. Repeated use of nicotine results in **tolerance**, and the individual must use higher doses of the drug to obtain the same effects that first occurred at lower doses. As the body becomes tolerant to nicotine's effects, it becomes dependent on nicotine for normal functioning. Removal of nicotine from the body results in feelings of **dysphoria**. The individual needs to continue using nicotine to feel well and to function normally.

tolerance a condition in which higher and higher doses of a drug or alcohol are needed to produce the effect or "high" experienced from the original dose

dysphoria depressed and unhappy mood state

Nicotine Tolerance and Dependence

The cigarette is a very fast and effective way to deliver nicotine to the body. Effects occur after a single inhalation of tobacco smoke. Nicotine quickly crosses the blood-brain barrier. Once in the brain, it interacts with brain chemicals and structures involved in making

endocrine system
cells, tissues, and organs of the body that are active in regulating bodily functions, such as growth and metabolism

gastrointestinal tract
entire length of the digestive system, running from the stomach through the small intestine, large intestine, and out the rectum

skeletal system
bones and related parts that serve as a framework for the body

intoxicated state in which a person's whose physical or mental control has been diminished

---

IN THEIR OWN WORDS

"I just quit smoking less than a day ago. It's hard to quit. They say in promotional campaigns that smoking isn't addicting and anyone can quit. That's not it at all. I would say that on a scale of 1 to 10 smoking by far surpasses 10 and is one of life's most challenging tests."

—Amy, 21 years old.

---

abstinence complete avoidance of something, such as the use of drugs or alcoholic beverages

craving powerful, often uncontrollable desire for drugs

the user feel pleasure. Nicotine alters moods, causes blood pressure and heart rate to rise (affecting the cardiovascular system), and harms the entire body, including the **endocrine system**, **gastrointestinal tract**, and **skeletal system**.

A person's first exposure to nicotine is usually not a pleasant experience. The person may feel sick and become **intoxicated**. After a few weeks of daily smoking, the body adapts to nicotine and the unpleasant effects are less noticeable. Once tolerance and dependence develop, smokers use whatever dose of nicotine (or number of cigarettes) they desire. The higher the dose, the greater the level of dependence.

As smokers become dependent on, or addicted to, smoking, they feel normal, comfortable, and effective when taking nicotine. They feel dysphoric, uncomfortable, and ineffective when lacking nicotine. It becomes difficult for smokers to give up nicotine even for very short periods.

Nicotine Withdrawal Symptoms

Nicotine withdrawal symptoms include: depressed mood; insomnia (inability to sleep); irritability, frustration, or anger; anxiety; difficulty concentrating; restlessness; decreased heart rate; and increased appetite or weight gain. The severity of the symptoms will depend on the severity of nicotine dependence. Withdrawal symptoms are strongest in the first few days after a person stops smoking and usually diminish within a month, although some smokers may continue to have withdrawal symptoms for many months.

Stopping smoking has other consequences as well. People may lose the ability to think and reason clearly, learn normally, exercise memory, and make good judgments. These effects begin a few hours after the last cigarette (dose of nicotine), peak during the first few days of **abstinence** (when smokers trying to quit are most likely to start smoking again or relapse), and mostly disappear within a few weeks.

Another symptom associated with withdrawal is **craving** cigarettes. Cravings may last six months—longer than some of the other symptoms of nicotine withdrawal. Cravings present a major difficulty to someone trying to quit smoking. Because of cravings, the majority of smokers who attempt to quit relapse within the first week of quitting.

Individuals with other problems—such as a history of depression, alcoholism, or illegal substance abuse—are likely to have more se-

SYMPTOMS AND DURATION OF NICOTINE WITHDRAWAL

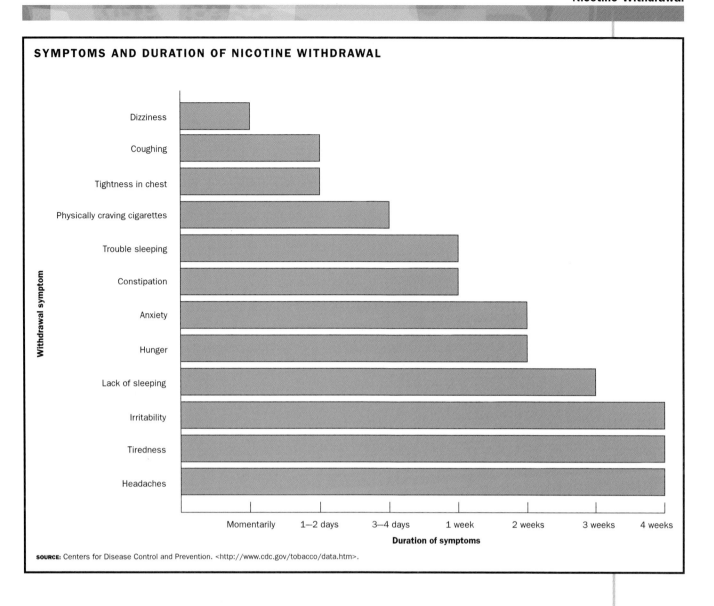

SOURCE: Centers for Disease Control and Prevention. <http://www.cdc.gov/tobacco/data.htm>.

vere nicotine withdrawal symptoms. Biological processes play a major role in nicotine withdrawal, but behavioral factors also have a strong influence on the ability to stop smoking. Cigarette smoking becomes a part of people's daily habits, so that many situations prompt them to smoke. For example, having a cup of coffee, relaxing at the end of a meal, watching television, or spending time with friends or family members who smoke can all create the desire to light a cigarette.

Information from the Centers for Disease Control and Prevention shows that symptoms of nicotine withdrawal, including coughing, anxiety, hunger, and irritability, can last from days to weeks.

Treatment of Nicotine Withdrawal Symptoms

One approach to treating withdrawal symptoms uses medications, either through nicotine replacement therapy or drugs that relieve symptoms. Another approach tries to change the behavior of the smoker so that he or she can quit smoking and avoid relapse.

Nicotine Replacement Therapy. The purpose of nicotine replacement is to substitute the nicotine in tobacco with a safer and more controllable form of nicotine so that the smoker can quit using tobacco. There are various nicotine replacement delivery systems, all of which attempt to reduce the amount of nicotine available during the quitting period so that an individual is weaned gradually from nicotine addiction. Two nicotine replacement therapies are available over the counter (without a prescription): nicotine polacrilex gum and the transdermal nicotine patch. Two other delivery systems are available through prescriptions: an oral nicotine inhalation system and a nasal nicotine spray. Both systems have been proven effective.

Symptom Treatment. A number of drug therapies have been approved to relieve or reduce some of the discomfort of quitting smoking. The best known is an **antidepressant**, bupropion (Zyban). Bupropion is effective regardless of whether smokers have a history of depression. Another antidepressant, nortriptyline, has also been approved to relieve withdrawal symptoms. Clonidine, originally used to treat high blood pressure, appears to be modestly effective in blocking cravings for nicotine, especially in women. Other medications that may lessen withdrawal symptoms are being tested. These include mecamylamine, and anxiolytics and **benzodiazepines**, which generally reduce stress and decrease anxiety.

Behavioral Approaches. Behavioral therapists have long tried to help smokers deal with nicotine withdrawal symptoms. Behavioral strategies may require the smoker to sign a contract to quit, with the smoker agreeing to pay a fee if he or she fails to follow through on the contract. Behavioral approaches may offer group support, with individuals holding meetings to support each other in their attempts to quit. Smokers may be taught to think differently about smoking and cigarettes. They may learn relaxation exercises; ways of coping with stressful situations other than through smoking; ways to deal with withdrawal symptoms (deep breathing, drinking water, doing something else); and controlling elements of their environment (getting rid of ashtrays, having a smoke-free home, avoiding places where others will be smoking). Behavioral programs that combine several strategies have had much success in helping smokers quit. In addition, the use of medications is much more successful when combined with behavioral strategies. SEE ALSO NICOTINE; TOBACCO: DEPENDENCE; TOBACCO: MEDICAL COMPLICATIONS; TOBACCO TREATMENT: BEHAVIORAL APPROACHES; TOBACCO TREATMENT: MEDICATIONS; TOLERANCE AND PHYSICAL DEPENDENCE.

antidepressant medication used for the treatment and prevention of depression

benzodiazepine drug developed in the 1960s as a safer alternative to barbiturates; most frequently used as a sleeping pill or an anti-anxiety medication

Nonabused Drugs Withdrawal

The term "drug withdrawal" makes many people think of issues related to drug abuse. However, a number of drugs that have no **abuse potential** and are prescribed for medical illness can lead to symptoms of withdrawal when a person suddenly stops taking them. These symptoms do not necessarily mean that the person was **dependent** on the drug. Nonabused drugs that can produce a withdrawal syndrome include medications prescribed for cardiovascular problems, mood, and personality disorders.

abuse potential the chance, or likelihood, that a drug will be abused

dependent psychologically compelled to use a substance for emotional and/or physical reasons

Cardiovascular Drugs

Beta Blockers. Many patients receive prescriptions for beta blockers (such as atenolol, labetalol, and propranolol) to treat hypertension (high blood pressure), angina pectoris (chest pain from heart muscle deprived of oxygen), heart arrhythmias (irregular heartbeat) following heart attack, and migraine headache. When a patient abruptly stops taking a beta blocker, particularly when angina pectoris is the symptom being treated, the frequency and/or severity of angina pectoris may increase. This occurs within the first few days of discontinuing the beta blocker. (Similar withdrawal symptoms can occur when angina pectoris patients stop taking other cardiovascular drugs, such as nitroglycerin.) Withdrawal symptoms can be prevented by slowly decreasing the drug dose over several days before completely stopping the drug.

Clonidine. This drug is used for hypertension and to treat withdrawal from opiate drugs (such as heroin). When a person abruptly stops taking clonidine, blood pressure may become dangerously high. This occurs within one to two days after stopping the drug and is prevented by slowly (over several days) decreasing the drug dose before stopping it completely.

Antidepressants

Antidepressant drugs are used to treat major **depression** and related illnesses. They are frequently taken daily for periods of weeks or months. A person who abruptly stops taking any of the major classes of antidepressants (such as tricyclic antidepressants, monoamine oxidase inhibitors, or selective serotonin reuptake inhibitors) may experience symptoms such as nausea, abdominal pain, and diarrhea. In addition, some patients complain of a flulike illness, with weakness, chills, fatigue, headaches, and muscle aches. Patients may have difficulty falling asleep and vivid dreams or nightmares. They may be-

UNINTENDED WITHDRAWAL

A drug prescribed for good medical reasons can still cause a withdrawal syndrome. One woman trying to discontinue her prescribed tranquilizers began to experience terrifying symptoms:

"I lost more than 20 pounds. I lived on milk and bananas almost exclusively for two months, because I was scarcely able to swallow. . . . To make matters worse, I had to go through this harrowing time without professional support or guidance. There was virtually no medical help or information available. In fact, there was widespread denial among the medical profession that the problem of prescription-drug addiction existed."

—Joan Gadsby in *Addicted by Prescription: One Woman's Triumph and Fight for Change* (2001).

depression state in which an individual feels intensely sad and hopeless; may have trouble eating, sleeping, and concentrating, and is no longer able to feel pleasure from previously enjoyable activities

psychosis mental disorder in which an individual loses contact with reality and may have delusions (i.e., unshakable false beliefs) or hallucinations

delirium mental disturbance marked by confusion, disordered speech, and sometimes hallucinations

hallucination seeing, hearing, feeling, tasting, or smelling something that is not actually there; may occur due to mental illness or as a side effect of some drugs

schizophrenia psychotic disorder in which people lose the ability to function normally, experience severe personality changes, and suffer from a variety of symptoms, including confusion, disordered thinking, paranoia, hallucinations, emotional numbness, and speech problems

come anxious, jittery, and irritable. Symptoms usually start a few days after a person stops taking the antidepressant and continue for one day to three weeks.

One class of antidepressants, selective serotonin reuptake inhibitors (SSRIs), can produce withdrawal symptoms that are easily confused with the depression for which the drugs are prescribed. Doctors may mistakenly prescribe more antidepressants to individuals who have these symptoms. This cycle of drug treatment is a significant problem, especially since the treatment of depression with medications has increased. The distinct, recognizable withdrawal symptoms that SSRIs can produce include dizziness, sensations that resemble electric shocks, numbness, and tingling skin. To reduce the risk of withdrawal symptoms, some doctors recommend that antidepressants be gradually reduced over a four-week period rather than abruptly discontinued.

Another class of antidepressants is the monoamine oxidase inhibitor (MAOI) drugs, such as Nardil, Parnate, and Marplan. A person who has taken high doses of these drugs for long periods, and who then suddenly stops taking them, can suffer severe symptoms. These include **psychosis** and **delirium**, with visual **hallucinations** as well as mental confusion. Milder symptoms can include anxiety, vivid dreaming, or nightmares. Withdrawal symptoms usually disappear a few days after the person stops taking the drug.

Other Drugs

Neuroleptics. People who suffer from psychotic disorders such as **schizophrenia** are often prescribed neuroleptic drugs (such as Haldol, Stelazine, Resperidone, Olanzapine, and clozapine). Abruptly stopping this class of drugs results in nausea, vomiting, and headaches.

Baclofen. As a muscle relaxant, this drug is used to treat muscle spasms that occur when people suffer from some form of paralysis. When a patient abruptly stops taking baclofen, he or she may have auditory (hearing) and visual hallucinations, severe anxiety, increased heart rate and blood pressure, and seizures. When the dose of baclofen is gradually reduced before the person stops taking it completely, these symptoms either do not occur or are not as severe.

Corticosteroids. The drug prednisone is probably the best-known corticosteroid. Prednisone is used to decrease inflammation in a wide variety of conditions, such as asthma, severe allergies, skin problems, rheumatoid arthritis, and other autoimmune disorders. When a person abruptly stops prednisone therapy, symptoms may include fatigue, weakness, imbalance of blood chemicals, and the inability of the body to respond appropriately. If an individual remains in this state for more than a few hours, severe illness and death can be expected. Doses of prednisone must be slowly decreased over many weeks to prevent a withdrawal syndrome.

Comparison with Alcohol Withdrawal

Alcohol is one of the most common drugs of abuse. The cardiovascular drugs (beta blockers, clonidine, nitrates) and the muscle relaxant baclofen produce withdrawal symptoms similar to that of alcohol. In alcohol withdrawal, like withdrawal from these medications, a person's systems become overactive: blood pressure may soar, the heart may race, and the person becomes highly excitable, shaky, and confused (called delirium tremens). In the case of corticosteroids, the opposite occurs. In prednisone withdrawal, a person becomes unresponsive.

Conclusion

The human body is a coordinated and finely tuned operation of multiple messaging systems. All the drugs mentioned here interfere with these systems in some way, producing both desired and undesired effects. When these systems adapt to the presence of a drug, stopping that drug suddenly can result in withdrawal symptoms. SEE ALSO ALCOHOL: WITHDRAWAL; BENZODIAZEPINE WITHDRAWAL; PRESCRIPTION DRUG ABUSE.

Opiate and Opioid Drug Abuse

Opiates are substances created from opium that act to depress or slow the action of the central nervous system. Opium is the dried juice of the opium poppy (*Papaver somniferum*), a plant grown since ancient times. The term "opiates" is generally used to refer to morphine, heroin, and codeine. Opioids, a larger category, refers to opiates and synthetic (artificially produced) substances that have morphine-like effects. When used for medical reasons, opioids are unlikely to result in **dependence**. However, as drugs of abuse, opioids lead to the same conditions of dependence and addiction as opiate drugs—conditions from which it is extremely difficult to recover.

dependence psychological need to use a substance for emotional and/or physical reasons

Chemical Background

The juice of the seed pod of the opium poppy is a sticky brown sap. The sap contains 7 to 15 percent morphine, the main active

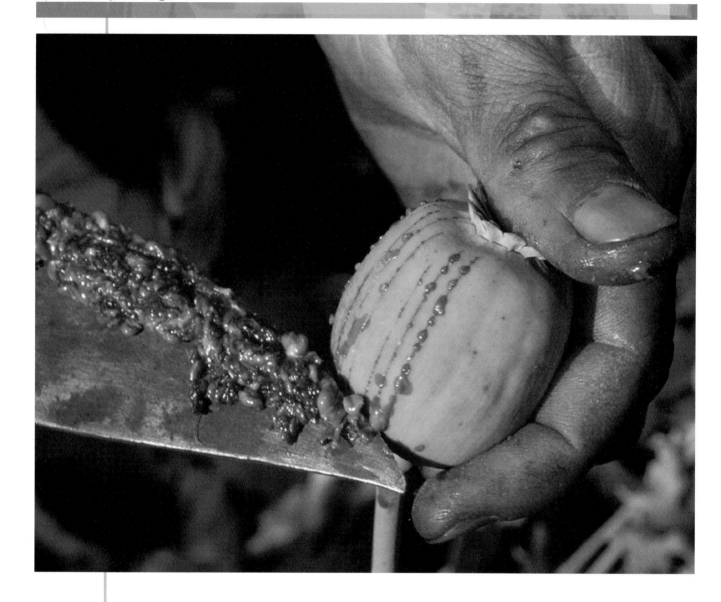

The milky juice of unripe seedpods from the opium poppy plant is used to make opiates.

ingredient. The name morphine is derived from the Greek god Morpheus, the god of dreams and sleep. In 1803 morphine was first isolated from opium. Morphine is a crystal alkaloid (an organic compound containing nitrogen). In 1874 a chemist discovered that morphine could be bonded to a common industrial acid, acetic anhydride. The result was a potent opiate, diacetylmorphine, that could be used as a painkiller. This opiate was introduced to the market in 1898 as heroin. Another active ingredient in opium is codeine. Opium poppy sap usually contains less than 2 percent codeine. Codeine is used as a painkiller, cough suppressant, and for treating diarrhea.

The History of Opiate and Opioid Use

Archaeological records indicate that the earliest use of opium poppies as medicine started more than 5,000 years ago. The first recorded use of opium was in Mesopotamia (an area in modern-day

Iraq). The ancient Egyptians grew opium poppies and used parts of the plant as medicines. Through trade, opium made its way into ancient Greece and Rome. Opium and poppies are often mentioned in the myths and epic tales from that time. Opium was usually taken by eating parts of the plant, taking the dried juices in elixirs (liquid mixtures), or smoking.

During the seventh century, opium spread throughout the Middle East and western Asia. Opium was used as a trade good. The use of opium potions that were either eaten or drunk for the treatment of minor ailments was widespread. By the eleventh century, doctors had noted that the more opium people took, the more opium they needed to have the same effect. By the fourteenth century, doctors had observed that long-term use of opium by a person degenerates, corrupts, and weakens the mind.

In 1803 morphine was isolated from opium. Morphine was seen as a powerful painkiller, and within twenty years it changed medicine. The effects of morphine are strongest when put directly into the bloodstream. This led to the invention and refinement in the 1840s and 1850s of the hypodermic syringe. The advancements in medicine also increased the strength of opium. By 1906 there were more than 50,000 patented medicines that contained opiates.

In the past 150 years, scientists have attempted to change the chemical makeup of morphine and codeine to eliminate unpleasant side effects that caused health problems. One of the first attempts (in the 1890s) produced an agent known as heroin. Unfortunately, heroin is not an improvement when it comes to the problems of **tolerance**, dependence, or abuse. Ironically, it was originally marketed as a cure for opium addiction and alcoholism; yet it led directly to heroin addiction. In fact, since about 1950, heroin has become the principal drug of opioid abusers.

tolerance a condition in which higher and higher doses of a drug or alcohol are needed to produce the effect or "high" experienced from the original dose

In the United States federal and state laws control the production and distribution of opioid drugs. Opioid users must get their drugs from **illicit** sources, and opioid dependence has become closely connected to many kinds of crime. Because illicit opioid drugs are expensive, their users often turn to illegal activities—such as theft, fraud, prostitution, and illicit drug traffic—to make money to pay for their drugs.

illicit something illegal or something used in an illegal manner

Opioids as Pain Medication

Opioid analgesics (painkillers) are extremely useful in controlling both **acute** and **chronic** pain. Morphine is routinely used to combat severe pain. The patient is given a small dose, and patients with severe

acute having a sudden onset and lasting a short time

chronic continuing for a long period of time

euphoria state of intense, giddy happiness and well-being, sometimes occurring baselessly and out of sync with an individual's life situation

toxic something that is poisonous or dangerous to people

pain rarely experience the **euphoria** effect that drug abusers seek. When taken under medical supervision, opioid drugs are unlikely to be **toxic**. The most common side effects of opioids prescribed for pain include nausea, drowsiness, and constipation. In addition to relief of pain, doctors may prescribe opioid drugs to suppress coughing and to stop diarrhea (the drugs decrease activity in the intestines). The most commonly used opioids in medicine for pain relief include:

- morphine sulfate (Duramorph, MS Contin, Roxanol)
- meperidine (Demerol)
- hydromorphone (Dilaudid)
- oxymorphone (Numorphan)
- methadone
- codeine phosphate and codeine sulfate
- oxycodone (Percocet, Percodan)
- hydrocodone (Hycodan, Vicodin)

Opioids are also, however, among the most common drugs of abuse. Health-care providers are very cautious when prescribing opioid drugs because of the risks of dependence and tolerance. Doctors are also concerned about the sale of these drugs to illegal markets. For years, concerns about patients becoming addicted led to pain being under treated and the unnecessary suffering of many patients. In the 1990s the federal government and a number of state organizations undertook initiatives with the aim of setting policy on how to appropriately treat pain. These pain initiatives worked to educate the medical community about how to adequately treat pain, when to worry about potential addiction in a patient, and when not to worry about such addiction.

Addiction to Opioids

Addiction to opioids is both a psychological and physical addiction. Heroin is especially addictive. When the body is exposed to heroin, the brain tells the body that heroin is needed to survive. With limited or one-time use, the effects of addiction are mild and usually not noticed. With extended use, tolerance builds and more opiates are needed. The increased use of opiates intensifies the effects of withdrawal and the user becomes more addicted.

With continued daily use and dependence, the user's life becomes an uncontrolled cycle of seeking the drug, getting high, coming down, and trying to secure more drugs. Young people who become dependent during high school often drop out and never develop regular work habits or job skills. Users may manage to stop taking drugs for

IN THEIR OWN WORDS

"Drugs are destroying more people than poverty ever did."

—John E. Jacob, President, Urban League

extended periods (sometimes because they are in prison), but almost all return to taking drugs within six months.

Complications of Opioid Abuse

Many of the complications of opiate use are related to the unsanitary conditions associated with drug use. Sharing needles often leads to diseases such as hepatitis (a liver disease) and AIDS. Opiate abusers often have other risky behaviors such as unprotected sex with multiple partners, which leads to sexually transmitted diseases. Long-term users often also have scarred veins, cutaneous abscesses (localized areas of pus under the skin), and phlebitis (inflamed veins).

The death rate of opioid users is about three times the rate expected for non-drug-abusers. Many of the deaths are due to overdose, homicide, suicide, accidents, and liver disease. In the 1980s AIDS appeared as an additional hazard for injecting drug users.

Physical Complications. People who take opioids without a prescription often do so to achieve a feeling of relaxation and euphoria, a state of intense well-being. Instead, they sometimes experience the opposite effect, **dysphoria**. Once a person becomes dependent, opioid abuse and addiction can produce a range of physical problems. Abuse of pure forms of opioid drugs can have the following effects:

dysphoria depressed and unhappy mood state

- respiratory depression (loss of the ability to breathe automatically)
- lung infections (a danger to users who inject drugs)
- viral hepatitis (a liver disease; a danger to users who inject drugs)
- osteomyelitis (inflammation of bone and the bone marrow caused by bacterial infection; users who inject drugs are prone to this infection)
- swelling of veins and skin irritations caused by repeated injections
- constriction of pupils
- sweating
- nausea and vomiting
- constipation
- itching
- convulsions (especially with high doses of Demerol and Darvon)

Heroin sold on the street is typically impure. It is diluted by the seller with powdered materials and injected by the user in an unhygienic manner. The size of the dose is also difficult to measure.

Heroin use of this kind results in extremely dangerous complications, including:

- strokes (damage to an area of the brain caused by interruption of oxygen delivery to that area)
- inflammation of brain blood vessels (which can cause brain damage by depriving areas of the brain of oxygen)
- bacterial meningitis (a bacterial infection of the membranes that cover the brain and spinal cord)
- aneurysms (weakness in the walls of arteries, which puts them at risk of bursting)
- brain abscesses (walled-off areas of infection within the brain)
- damage to the spinal cord that could lead to paralysis
- widespread injury to muscle tissue (due to infections and blood vessel problems after years of injections)
- death from overdoses

Treatment of Opioid Dependence

The modern treatment of opioid dependence is often called detoxification. Drug withdrawal is done as an inpatient or outpatient procedure. The patient may live in a treatment center as an inpatient, or live at home, receiving treatment as an outpatient. Self-help groups such as Narcotics Anonymous ☎ are available, as well as special religious programs for drug users. Because the addiction is both physical and psychological, the most effective treatment programs use counseling and group therapy in addition to treatment with drugs.

☎ **See *Organizations of Interest* at the back of Volume 3 for address, telephone, and URL.**

In another treatment, known as methadone maintenance, a heroin user is given methadone, a legally prescribed opioid drug, as a substitute. Once on methadone, the user does not suffer from symptoms of the withdrawal syndrome. This treatment helps chronic heroin users to return to normal activities. Once they stop using heroin, they can also end the criminal activities needed to obtain it. Ending opioid use entirely is a possible, though distant, goal. To become drug free, the user must also gradually end methadone maintenance. Most opioid abusers find it very difficult to maintain abstinence from either illegal opioids or methadone maintenance programs.

Successful treatment of opioid dependence is extremely difficult. Users usually suffer from chronic emotional distress, so that ending drug use is especially challenging. If opioids are easily available, the user typically cannot control his use. The only way the user finds relief from withdrawal symptoms, which persist for six months or longer after the last dose, is to take more of the drug. Finally, in opioid users, drug seeking, and the criminal behavior necessary to obtain drugs, become part of a person's lifestyle. The individual's only friends are likely to be users themselves. The person comes to see himself as a user, with no chance for change. Studies show that only a minority of opioid users remain **abstinent** for long periods.

Withdrawal

Within a day or two of stopping morphine or heroin, a person experiences the following withdrawal symptoms: restlessness, weakness, chills, body and joint pains, muscle spasms, twitching, gastrointestinal cramps, loss of appetite, nausea, vomiting, diarrhea, tearing eyes, runny nose, gooseflesh, rapid breathing, dilated pupils, hypertension (high blood pressure), and tachycardia (rapid heart beat). After a person has been off drugs for several weeks, she enters a long-term phase of withdrawal, lasting at least six months. The symptoms include: hypotension (low blood pressure), bradycardia (low heart rate), hypothermia (lower than normal body temperature). The pupils become small and constricted. Other signs of long-term abstinence may include an inability to concentrate and a decrease in fine-motor control. Patients who stop taking methadone after becoming dependent on it feel tired and weak. They often withdraw from society, with feelings of inefficiency, decreased popularity and competitiveness, and loss of self-control. Patients who withdraw from methadone also have a higher chance of developing **schizophrenia**.

Conclusion

Opioid use in the United States is related to family breakdown, poverty, lack of education, unemployment, and crime. Anything that reduces these problems would likely reduce illicit opioid use. Easy solutions seem unlikely. SEE ALSO COMPLICATIONS FROM INJECTING DRUGS; HEROIN; HEROIN TREATMENT: BEHAVIORAL APPROACHES; HEROIN TREATMENT: MEDICATIONS; MEDICAL EMERGENCIES AND DEATH FROM DRUG ABUSE; METHADONE MAINTENANCE PROGRAMS.

abstinent describing someone who completely avoids something, such as a drug or alcohol

schizophrenia psychotic disorder in which people lose the ability to function normally, experience severe personality changes, and suffer from a variety of symptoms, including confusion, disordered thinking, paranoia, hallucinations, emotional numbness, and speech problems

Opium

The unripe seed capsules of the poppy plant (*Papaver somniferum*) produce a milky juice called opium. The opium poppy has white or blue-purple flowers and is widely grown in Asia, India, and Turkey, which supply much of the world's opium. Opium contains substances known as opioids, many of which are used as medicines to treat pain. The major opioid analgesics (painkillers) are morphine and codeine.

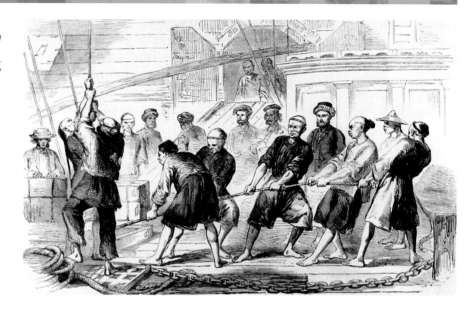

In this drawing from the *Illustrated London News,* July 1857, workers in Hong Kong transfer bales of opium from one ship to another for export to the West.

Another important opioid is thebaine, which is used to make opioid analgesics such as oxymorphone, oxycodone, and naloxone. Morphine extracted from opium can also be used to make heroin, an illegal opioid and a major drug of abuse in the United States.

People have known about and used opium since ancient times. Initially it was used for the treatment of diarrhea and then for the relief of pain. Today, the major medicinal use of opium is to treat extreme diarrhea. Physicians may prescribe paregoric, a preparation made from a concentrated extract of opium.

The opium plant was introduced into India by Arab traders of the thirteenth century. It later spread to China, where the Chinese invented a method of smoking opium in pipes. In the eighteenth century, the British bought tea from China and in return shipped opium to the Chinese. By 1900 about 25 percent of the Chinese smoked opium, although it was banned by the emperor. In the early twentieth century, international conferences placed limits on the traffic in opium and opium products.

People who abuse opium either smoke it or eat it. Opium eating is widely practiced in India, Turkey, Afghanistan, and Southeast Asia. Opium is used as a household remedy for pain and other ailments, much as it has been for hundreds of years. Approximately 50 percent of opium eaters in India, for example, use it for medicinal purposes. Small numbers of immigrants to the United States have brought these customs with them, but opium abuse is rare in this country. SEE ALSO HEROIN; MORPHINE; OPIATE AND OPIOID DRUG ABUSE.

Overdose *See Accidents and Injuries from Drugs*

Pain Medications *See Opiate and Opioid Drug Abuse*

Personality Disorder

People may use, misuse, or abuse substances for a number of reasons. Some possible reasons are the influences of peers, family problems, and the availability of substances in the community. For certain people, personality problems are just as important as these social influences. This article provides information on personality traits and disorders that are often seen in substance abusers.

Personality traits are the stable ways people have of thinking, feeling, perceiving, and relating to others. The social environment does shape personality traits to some extent, but people are also born different in the degree to which they are sociable, emotional, agreeable, impulsive, active, and so on.

Research does not support the idea that a person can have an addictive personality. However, research does show that several traits are common among substance abusers. These traits are thought to be one group of risk factors for tobacco, alcohol, and drug use and abuse:

- sensation seeking, or wanting to try new experiences
- hostility or aggressiveness
- impulsiveness
- disinhibition (poor control over behavior)
- low self-esteem
- social conformity
- being very emotional or consistently having negative emotions

This does not mean that anyone who has these traits will abuse substances. In fact, some or all of these traits and behaviors may be a normal phase of adolescence. However, individuals who show these traits very early in childhood and then throughout life are at higher risk for substance abuse. This risk increases when the individual also has a family history of alcohol or drug abuse, when the individual's peer group is one that engages in troublesome or illegal behaviors, and when drugs are easily available.

When personality traits become extreme and inflexible, they can interfere with day-to-day functioning and cause distress for the individual or those closest to him or her. When the individual has several problematic personality traits for a number of years, has significant problems stemming from these traits, and behaves in ways

---

DSM-IV Personality Disorders and Their Trait Descriptions

Personality Disorder	Common Personality Traits
Antisocial	impulsive; reckless; manipulative; cruel; deceitful; nonconforming; irresponsible; criminal; aggressive; lacking remorse
Avoidant	social inhibition; inadequacy; sensitivity to criticism; fear of rejection, ridicule, or embarrassment; shyness
Borderline	intense and unstable relationships, mood, behavior, and self-image; suicidal behavior; emptiness; angry temper; impulsive
Dependent	indecisiveness; submissiveness; low self-confidence; neediness; helplessness; fear of independence and lack of support; overly compliant
Histrionic	attention-seeking; dramatic emotionality; seductive; provocative; shallow; vague; suggestible
Narcissistic	exaggerated self-importance; craving for admiration; rage when criticized; lack of empathy; entitlement; exploitative; superior; envious; inflated
Obsessive	overly orderly and controlled; perfectionistic; inflexible; stubborn
Compulsive	miserly; workaholism; formality; preoccupied with rules and standards
Paranoid	suspicious; distrustful; unforgiving; personalizing; hostile; withholding; guarded about intimacy
Schizoid	socially detached; emotionally constricted; solitary; lack of pleasure; indifferent; cold; loner
Schizotypal	social discomfort; odd thoughts and speech; unusual perceptions; suspicious; peculiar behavior; eccentric

Personality disorders are diagnosed based on typical trait descriptions, as outlined in the *Diagnostic and Statistical Manual of Mental Disorders.*

norm behavior, custom, or attitude that is considered normal, or expected, within a certain social group

depression state in which an individual feels intensely sad and hopeless; may have trouble eating, sleeping, and concentrating, and is no longer able to feel pleasure from previously enjoyable activities; in extreme cases, may lead an individual to think about or attempt suicide

that are sharply different from the **norms** of his or her culture, the person may be given a psychiatric diagnosis of personality disorder. Often, a personality disorder may be less distressing to the person who has it than it is to others. As a result, people with personality disorders are not motivated to change or seek help unless their behavior causes social problems or they also have another psychiatric disorder that is causing them distress. People with both a substance use disorder and another form of mental illness, such as **depression**, have a dual diagnosis.

Personality disorders are the most common type of psychiatric disorder found in substance abusers. Based on many research studies, personality disorders are found in 50 to 75 percent of substance abusers. The current system for diagnosing personality disorders has sparked significant controversy in the field of mental health. With the current diagnostic system (DSM-IV Axis II), there are ten different personality disorders that can be diagnosed, each with its own grouping of traits. Among substance abusers, Antisocial, Borderline, Avoidant, Dependent, and Paranoid are the more common personality disorders. Histrionic, Narcissistic, Schizoid, Schizotypal, and Obsessive-Compulsive Personality Disorders are less frequent, but still more common among substance abusers than among people who are not substance abusers.

The personality traits that come to define a personality disorder are usually recognizable by adolescence. However, most teenagers will not be diagnosed with a personality disorder until they reach adulthood. By that time, a long-term personality pattern shows consistent evidence of interfering with work or family functioning. Until then, it can be hard to tell the difference between personality problems that are common or limited to adolescence and problems that will become chronic (long-term) characteristics of a personality disorder.

When a person has a personality disorder in addition to a substance abuse problem, he or she has an increased risk for suicide, hospitalization, repeated treatments, and HIV infection due to risky drug use or sexual behaviors. Such an individual may act abusively toward others and have family, employment, and legal problems. The presence of personality problems combined with substance abuse almost always indicates a need for professional treatment of some sort in addition to community interventions provided by school, church, or self-help meetings. Personality disorders are difficult to treat and usually require several years of psychotherapy. Medications are sometimes helpful in controlling extreme moods or behaviors. In some cases personality disorder can improve over time as the person ages. SEE ALSO DIAGNOSIS OF DRUG AND ALCOHOL ABUSE: AN OVERVIEW; RISK FACTORS FOR SUBSTANCE ABUSE; SUICIDE AND SUBSTANCE ABUSE.

Peyote

Peyote (or peyotl) is the common name for the cactus *Lophophra williamsii* or *Anhalonium lewinii*, which is found in the southwestern United States and northern Mexico. Peyote contains mescaline, a **hallucinogenic** substance. People who seek a **psychedelic** drug experience may take peyote or pure mescaline.

Peyote was one of the first psychedelic substances that people tried. The Aztecs of Mexico considered it magical and divine. Its use spread to other Native American groups, who used it to treat various illnesses, to communicate with the spirits, and as part of religious rituals. Peyote is still used by some Native Americans, and there are laws in place to protect its use by certain religious groups (such as the Native American Church and the American Indian Church) in specific religious practices. Some states require that the religious group be registered, and others require that peyote users prove that they are at least one-quarter Native American. Peyote suppliers must register with the state and provide proof that they are selling the substance only for ceremonial use to approved groups.

For religious rituals involving peyote, the dried tops of the cactus—the buttons—are chewed or made into a tea. Since peyote may cause some initial nausea and vomiting, the participant may prepare for the ceremony by fasting prior to eating the buttons. Peyote is usually taken as part of a formal group experience and over an extended period of time. The peyote ceremonies may take place at night and

hallucinogenic of a substance that can cause hallucinations, or seeing, hearing, or feeling things that are not there

psychedelic of a substance that can cause hallucinations and/or make its user lose touch with reality

around a communal fire to increase the hallucinogenic effects and visions. SEE ALSO AYAHUASCA; HALLUCINOGENS.

Phencyclidine (PCP)

Although phencyclidine (PCP) and drugs of similar chemical structure are often called hallucinogens, they rarely produce hallucinations. The sensory distortions or apparent hallucinations that PCP does produce are not the same type as the hallucinations produced by use of **LSD**. Instead, PCP belongs to a unique class of drugs often called the dissociative anesthetics. (These drugs produce a brief period of anesthesia during which individuals feel as if they are dissociated, or separated, from their bodies.) This category includes ketamine, which has recently emerged as a widely abused drug in this class. Other drugs in this class have been manufactured with effects similar to those of PCP and ketamine, and are considered early examples of "designer drugs."

PCP was developed in the 1950s as an anesthetic for veterinary surgery and the capture of wild animals and later was tested in human surgical patients. The negative side effects of PCP (such as unpleasant feelings, disorientation, and psychotic symptoms) did not permit its regular use in medicine. In addition, the drug is no longer permitted for veterinary use because supplies were diverted, often stolen or hijacked, leading to widespread abuse in the 1970s.

One of the reasons for the popularity of PCP in the 1970s was that it was very easy to make from readily available chemicals. Now the government requires distributors of the key ingredients of PCP manufacture to keep track of sales, making it much harder to obtain PCP than it once was. Beginning in the 1980s, PCP abuse began to decrease. Use of the drug has now leveled off to considerably below what it was in the 1980s. Nonetheless, PCP is still around, and young people's use of PCP is about as common as their use of heroin. The popularity of PCP varies greatly among regions of the country, and it is used much more often by males than females.

PCP Abuse

Originally, PCP was commonly abused in tablet form (called the PeaCe Pill). When taken this way, its effects are felt within thirty minutes and usually peak in an hour or so. The **intoxication** lasts about four to six hours, although users may feel strange for a day or more. One reason for this method of use was that, in the early 1970s, drug sellers told people that the pills they were buying were THC

LSD lysergic acid diethylamide is a powerful chemical compound known for its hallucinogenic properties

intoxication loss of physical or mental control because of the effects of a substance

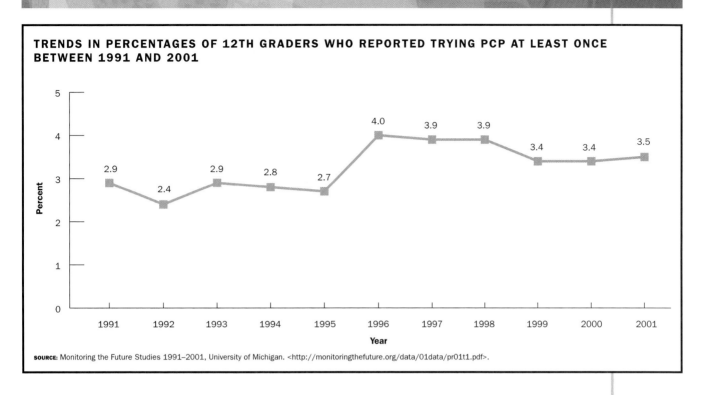

TRENDS IN PERCENTAGES OF 12TH GRADERS WHO REPORTED TRYING PCP AT LEAST ONCE BETWEEN 1991 AND 2001

SOURCE: Monitoring the Future Studies 1991–2001, University of Michigan. <http://monitoringthefuture.org/data/01data/pr01t1.pdf>.

(the active ingredient in marijuana), LSD, or some other hallucinogen. Because the effects of PCP were unexpected and because it was difficult to control the dose, many users experienced bad trips. People who sell PCP still try to make it more attractive by calling it THC or whatever else is currently popular.

PCP abuse increased greatly when people began to smoke and sniff it. When PCP is illegally manufactured, it usually is available in the form of a crystalline white powder. The powder is then dusted onto various kinds of leafy materials, such as parsley, mint, or marijuana. This is why PCP is often called "angel dust," or just "dust." Smoking materials containing PCP are sometimes referred to as "killer weed," "wacky weed," or just "wack." It is also possible to sniff powdered PCP or even dissolve it in water and inject it, although injecting the drug is uncommon. Users also may soak their smoking material in liquid PCP or spray it on and then let it dry before smoking. Liquid forms are sometimes colored. In addition to the ones mentioned, there are many different street names for PCP, and different regions of the country use different names for it. Of all the drugs of abuse, PCP is probably the one that a user is most likely to take without knowing what it is until it is too late.

The Effects of PCP

As with all drugs, the effects of PCP depend on the dose. Users claim that smoking the drug allows them to smoke a little, see if the effects

A study conducted by the University of Michigan in 2001 revealed a slight decline in the number of 12th graders who reported trying PCP, following a sharp increase in 1996.

are as strong as they like, and then smoke more if they wish. By contrast, once users take a pill, sniff it, or give themselves an injection, they are committed to that dose, whatever it is. One of the dangers of PCP, like many other illegal drugs, is the difficulty of determining the dose.

Since PCP was developed as an anesthetic, high doses can produce a kind of dissociative anesthesia in which users have trouble walking or are completely unable to walk, look and feel extremely intoxicated, and are unresponsive when people talk to them. Some people describe this effect as **catatonia**. Others have described this behavior as zombie-like.

catatonia psychomotor disturbance characterized by muscular rigidity, excitement, or stupor

The effects that PCP produces depend on the dose.

1. At low doses, users desire a feeling of dreaminess, uplifting mood, and intense or altered perceptions. Bodily perceptions are particularly affected, with users feeling somewhat numb, a little smaller or larger than usual, and dissociated from the environment. Some have described the effect as looking through the wrong end of binoculars, with everything seeming distant and unreal. Undesirable effects at low doses include impaired judgment, mood swings, panic, and partial amnesia (the inability to remember what has happened).

2. At moderate doses, users desire an increased feeling of intoxication, a feeling of being separated from their own bodies, and greater changes in perception. The undesirable effects of moderate doses include ataxia (the loss of muscle coordination, causing difficulty walking and unsteadiness), confusion, amnesia, a focus on abnormal body sensations, exaggerated mood swings, and panic.

3. At high doses, users become very intoxicated. They will typically show catatonia, blank stare, **delirium**, drooling, severe motor impairment (becoming uncoordinated), muscular rigidity, psychotic behavior, and amnesia. Stroke, coma, suicide, and death, most often through accidental injury, can also occur.

delirium mental disturbance marked by confusion, disordered speech, and sometimes hallucinations

It is important to recognize that PCP's effects on the mind are not at all like those of marijuana or LSD. Another difference from marijuana and LSD is that PCP users will usually appear drunken and disoriented and be uncoordinated. Driving or attempting other demanding activities while under the influence of PCP is very dangerous. Users intoxicated with PCP also show bad judgment and confusion, which may lead to dangerous acts like jumping from buildings, swimming out to sea, and criminal behavior. They can be enjoying themselves and then, with little warning, become terribly

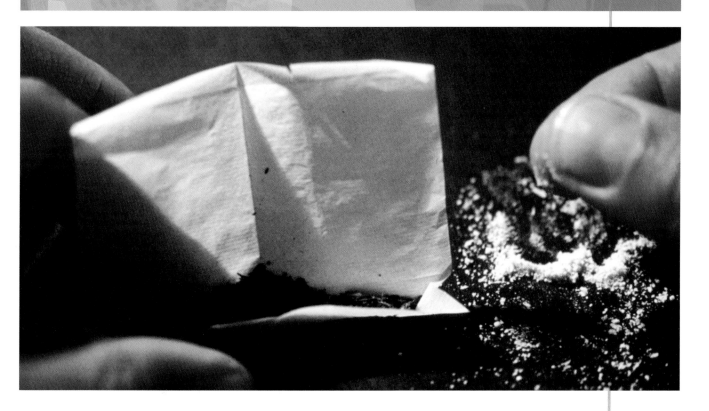

frightened, act bizarrely, and become a danger to themselves and to others around them. Such people often end up in the emergency department of a hospital, with police investigations, parental notification, and other unexpected consequences.

Though PCP may cause sensory distortions, it is not a hallucinogen because it rarely causes users to perceive things that are not there.

PCP is often used with other drugs, such as marijuana, when they are smoked together. PCP users often drink alcohol or use cocaine at the same time as well. A form of PCP mixed with cocaine is sometimes referred to as "space base." The effects of PCP in combination with other drugs are not well understood. Scientists have been unable to test PCP in humans for many years because of safety concerns. People who use PCP, especially in combination with other drugs, are experimenting on themselves, with unpredictable results.

The Effects of Regular Use

PCP abusers will often increase the amount of drug they use over time, but **tolerance** to PCP is not nearly as great as with some other drugs of abuse, such as cocaine, LSD, and heroin. Physical dependence, with users having withdrawal symptoms when steady use of PCP is discontinued, is uncommon. Withdrawal symptoms that are sometimes reported include intense sadness, drug **craving**, increased appetite, and increased need for sleep.

tolerance condition in which higher and higher doses of a drug or alcohol are needed to produce the effect or "high" experienced from the original dose

craving powerful, often uncontrollable desire for drugs

Babies born to PCP-using mothers can be dependent on the drug. Withdrawal signs that have been noted in the newborns include diarrhea, poor feeding, irritability, jerky movements, high-pitched cry, and visual problems. In general, however, most people either do not use PCP frequently enough to become dependent in this way, or the intensity of PCP withdrawal is not severe. Nonetheless, some people develop uncontrolled use of PCP and cannot easily quit without treatment.

By far the most serious danger of PCP abuse is that it can produce long-lasting personality changes and even mental illness in some people. In fact, the effects of both short-term and long-term use of PCP so closely resemble the symptoms of **schizophrenia** that scientists are studying PCP effects on the brain and behavior of animals in order to learn more about this serious mental illness. Psychiatrists and psychologists refer to the serious forms of PCP mental illness as PCP **psychosis**, and people who develop it usually require psychiatric hospitalization and treatment with powerful **antipsychotic drugs**. The PCP psychosis and the milder forms of personality change that can occur in regular users often begins with depression, anxiety, **paranoia**, and confusion. These symptoms are sometimes seen during intoxication, but more serious problems develop if they persist beyond the period of intoxication.

There is little clear evidence of damage to organs of the body other than the brain with repeated use of PCP. In animal studies, PCP and related drugs can produce holes called vacuoles in specific regions of the brain, but it is not known if these occur in people.

Violence and PCP

PCP abuse has been associated with violence, sometimes especially gruesome acts of brutality. Scientists do not know whether PCP alone or PCP in combination with other factors causes normal people to become violent. However, PCP, like methamphetamine, is often made and sold by violent gangs. When criminals and violence-prone individuals use it, the chances of violence are increased.

Scientists do know that PCP cannot make people physically stronger. On the other hand, PCP produces numbness, decreased sensitivity to pain, impaired judgment, and paranoia; as a result of these effects, a person on PCP can become both aggressive and fearless about experiencing pain. Law-enforcement officers are trained to handle arrests of people suspected of PCP use very cautiously.

Studies comparing violence committed by people who took various drugs, such as cocaine, amphetamines, alcohol, and PCP, have generally found that PCP is no more likely than other drugs to be

schizophrenia psychotic disorder in which people lose the ability to function normally, experience severe personality changes, and suffer from a variety of symptoms, including confusion, disordered thinking, paranoia, hallucinations, emotional numbness, and speech problems

psychosis mental disorder in which an individual loses contact with reality and may have delusions (i.e., unshakable false beliefs) or hallucinations (i.e., the experience of seeing, hearing, feeling, smelling, or tasting things that are not actually present)

antipsychotic drugs drugs that reduce psychotic behavior; often have negative long-term side effects

paranoia excessive or irrational suspicion; illogical mistrust

associated with criminal or violent behavior. In fact, the connection between abuse of alcohol, a legal and socially accepted substance, and criminal behavior is one of the most significant public-health problems, far more so than cases of PCP-related violence. Finally, it is important to recognize that PCP has a reputation for being a particularly dangerous drug, with street names like "dead on arrival," "zombie," and "killer weed." People who tend to enjoy risky behavior may try to show how tough they are by taking PCP.

Treatment of PCP Abuse or Overdose

There are currently no drugs available to directly counteract a PCP overdose or bad trips. Treatment may be given for symptoms such as suppressed breathing rates, fever, high blood pressure, increased salivation, or convulsions. PCP may be more easily eliminated from the body by making the urine more acidic and/or pumping stomach contents. Placement of overdose patients in a quiet room has helped to control violent and self-destructive behavior. Psychiatric care is usually needed for people who develop PCP psychosis. Young people who experience problems with PCP abuse can often be helped with substance abuse treatment programs designed for this age group. SEE ALSO DESIGNER DRUGS; HALLUCINOGENS; KETAMINE; RAVE; VIOLENCE AND DRUG AND ALCOHOL USE.

Poverty and Drug Use

Do the poor use drugs more frequently than other economic groups? While many people would answer "yes" to that question, research indicates that a lack of money alone does not increase the chances that a person will use drugs. The relationship between poverty and drug use is more complicated. Beyond the lack of money, poverty leads to certain attitudes, behaviors, and life conditions. These same attitudes and conditions can contribute to drug use.

What Is Poverty?

In the United States, national poverty data are calculated using the official U.S. Bureau of the Census definition of poverty. This definition establishes a poverty threshold. If a family has an income level below that threshold, the family is considered to be poor. The census compares a family's cash income before taxes with that poverty threshold, which adjusts for family size and composition. According to the 2000 U.S. Census, more than 31 million people (11.3%) lived in poverty in the United States. An even higher percentage of these were children and teens: 16.2 percent of people under age 18 lived in poverty.

Poverty is not only a lack of sufficient income or material possessions. It is also a condition in which people lack prestige and have less access to resources. The poor often have different lifestyles and different values from those of people not living in poverty. The conditions that poor people often cope with may include: unemployment or off-and-on employment, low-status and low-skill jobs, unstable family and relationships, low involvement in the community, a sense of being isolated from society, low ambition, and feelings of helplessness. Many people living in poverty are divorced, are single parents, or have unhappy marriages. They tend to have higher rates of dropping out of school, arrest, and mental disorders. Because of limited access to health care, they are more likely to suffer from poor physical health than are people considered middle class or above.

sociologist someone who studies society, social relationships, and social institutions

Many **sociologists** have written about the problem of poverty, and a great deal of their writings focus on the idea of an American underclass. This underclass is thought to be caught in a cycle of poverty affecting several generations of families. Sociologists often describe these families as being isolated from mainstream society, living in urban ghettos, and being at risk for drug use. But other sociologists view poverty from another perspective. They observe that only a small proportion of poor people lead lives fitting this description. Many poor people are poor for only a short time. These people live not only in ghettos but in all regions of the United States, rural as well as urban, and they are of all age and ethnic groups.

Drug Use and Related Problems

Sociologists and others have had difficulties collecting valid information about poverty and drug use. Surveys of drug users do not always present an accurate picture. For example, some individuals will not reveal the severity of their drug problem or the severity of their poverty. Some information on the drug-using population comes from treatment programs or outreach services. But because not all individuals with drug abuse problems make use of such programs or services, they go uncounted. Many studies focus on drugs more likely to be used by the poor, such as crack cocaine and heroin, and not on drugs such as marijuana and cocaine that are more likely to be used by the middle and upper classes. All of these factors contribute to an inaccurate picture of drug use as occurring mainly among the poor.

Despite these obstacles to collecting valid information, researchers have reached some conclusions about drug use among the poor, especially the extreme poor—the homeless. The homeless do appear to be at higher risk for drug abuse, and some findings suggest that drugs may now play a larger role than alcohol in causing homelessness. Researchers have also found that the homeless population is no longer mainly older, white males. Women now make up a large portion of the homeless, and among them are many drug users.

Mental health problems are a related issue in the study of extreme poverty. Studies have found a high rate of mental health problems among homeless substance abusers. Individuals with mental health problems may use illegal drugs to medicate themselves in an attempt to feel better. One reason for this kind of drug use may be that the homeless do not have access to health care, or do not know how to take advantage of available government or charity programs. If drug-abusing homeless individuals received treatment for their mental health problems, some of them might be able to find stable housing and jobs and connect with family. They might also be more likely to stay in drug-treatment programs.

The risk of HIV infection among drug users who live in poverty is also an issue of increasing concern. Youths with mental illness are at particular risk for HIV infection. These youths are more likely to engage in such risky behavior as prostitution and unprotected sex, drug dealing, and drug use by injection. When drug users live in poverty, they often lack access to treatment programs. Private inpatient and outpatient treatment can cost thousands of dollars. Programs funded by the government have long waiting lists for admission. Government policy efforts should try to ensure that lack of money does not bar someone from participating in prevention and treatment programs.

Social-service professionals should also make special efforts to reach homeless youths, who are at high risk of drug abuse. Necessary services include outreach and sheltering services, substance abuse treatment, counseling, and HIV prevention programs. Unfortunately, many youths who engage in risky behavior do not seek traditional services or programs. Consequently, those most in need may receive the least services. SEE ALSO FAMILIES AND DRUG USE; HOMELESSNESS; RISK FACTORS FOR SUBSTANCE ABUSE.

Prescription Drug Abuse

One unfavorable or unintended response of medical treatment is **addiction** to a prescription drug. A number of drugs used as medicines can lead to addiction or abuse in some people. These drugs include

addiction state in which the body requires the presence of a particular substance to function normally; without the substance, predictable withdrawal symptoms are experienced

PRESCRIPTION FOR PROBLEMS

Some people have called prescription drug abuse a hidden epidemic because there is no way to keep accurate tallies. Yet millions of people who begin to take drugs for medical reasons end up addicted to their medications.

Here are some guidelines for avoiding addiction of a prescribed medicine:

- Follow the instructions printed on the drug label.

- Always take only the prescribed dose at the prescribed time interval, and only for the length of time prescribed.

- Ask your doctor or pharmacist about any concerns and questions.

- Know which drugs are most addictive. In general, stimulants, opiates, and painkillers are the most addictive types of drugs. Within these categories, specific drugs have different abuse potentials—or likelihood of someone ending up addicted.

tolerance a condition in which higher and higher doses of a drug or alcohol are needed to produce the effect or "high" experienced from the original dose

opioids, antihistamines, and steroids, among others. The most commonly abused prescription drugs are those used to treat psychological problems. Barbiturates and amphetamines have the highest potential for abuse. Others, such as the antipsychotics, antidepressants, and lithium salts, have a lower abuse potential.

According to the National Household Survey on Drug Abuse, 3.8 million people ages 12 and older were using prescription drugs for nonmedical reasons in 2000. This represents 1.7 percent of the population aged 12 and older, about the same rate as in 1999 (1.8%). Nonmedical use of prescription drugs increased among youths aged 16 and 17 between 1999 and 2000, from 3.4 percent to 4.3 percent. Adolescent girls were somewhat more likely to use prescription drugs nonmedically than boys (3.3% compared to 2.7%). Amphetamines are somewhat more likely to be abused by young people than other prescription drugs.

Barbiturates

Barbiturates have depressant effects. In the past they were commonly prescribed as tranquilizers and sleeping pills. Although barbiturates have been replaced by newer drugs, the problem of addiction to barbiturates has not been eliminated. People who abuse barbiturates may take large quantities by injection into a vein or muscle. Injections often leads to abscesses. Other users take large amounts by mouth, sometimes on a binge. Users quickly develop **tolerance** and **physical dependence**, and stopping the drugs suddenly can result in severe and life-threatening **withdrawal**.

Amphetamines

Amphetamines have stimulant effects. They increase the user's sense of well-being, energy, and alertness, and they also decrease appetite. In the past amphetamines were prescribed in pill form for people with mild **depression** or weight problems. They were also given to people whose jobs required that they stay awake and alert for long periods, such as medical interns or long-distance truck drivers.

Some laboratories illegally manufacture amphetamines, especially methamphetamine, which is relatively easy to create in the lab. The intravenous use of methamphetamine quickly produces tolerance, and the user requires larger and more frequent doses to achieve the desired effect. The user then typically experiences toxic (poisonous) effects, including repetitive face and hand movements and a repeated chain of behaviors—for example, the user may assemble and dismantle mechanical objects. Users may develop **paranoid psychosis**, in which individuals lose touch with reality and feel that other people are persecuting them.

Benzodiazepines

Benzodiazepines have replaced barbiturates for the treatment of anxiety and sleeping disorders. They are very effective and produce few side effects. They are also less likely to produce addiction. When benzodiazepines are used properly, the risk of addiction is extremely small. Nevertheless, some cases of abuse of benzodiazepines such as diazepam (Valium) and lorazepam (Ativan) have occurred. Abusers may take the benzodiazepine alone or in combination with other drugs. The combination of alcohol and benzodiazepines has a particularly powerful effect. Other users may take benzodiazepines to ease the crash from the high of cocaine use. Some benzodiazepine abuse occurs when the person obtains the drug legally from a doctor. About 50 percent of abusers of benzodiazepines were introduced to the drug as a medical treatment. Other users obtain the drug from illegal sources.

Appetite Suppressants

Another type of prescription drug abuse involves appetite suppressants. Most of these drugs are stimulants, but one, fenfluramine, is a **sedative**. Abusers may take them in binges and use large quantities rather than the typical dose of one per day. As a general rule, the more an appetite suppressant resembles an amphetamine, the more likely it is to be abused.

Stopping the use of appetite suppressants may produce withdrawal symptoms such as fatigue, discomfort, or depression. Because of these problems and growing doubts about the drugs' effectiveness at maintaining weight loss, many doctors have stopped prescribing appetite suppressants.

In the early to mid-1990s, two prescription diet drugs, fenfluramine (often taken with phentermine and popularly known as fenphen) and dexfenfluramine (Redux), became popular. These drugs increased the amount of the brain chemical serotonin, creating a feeling of being full or satisfied. Stories in the news media depicted fenphen and Redux as cures for obesity. By 1996 millions of prescriptions had been written for these diet pills.

In 1997 reports of heart valve disease in women taking fen-phen or Redux began to surface. The Food and Drug Administration issued a Public Health Advisory describing the drugs' dangers. By September 1997 the manufacturer withdrew these drugs from the U.S.

physical dependence condition that may occur after prolonged use of a particular drug or alcohol, in which the user's body cannot function normally without the presence of the substance; when the substance is not used or the dose is decreased, the user experiences uncomfortable physical symptoms

withdrawal group of physical and psychological symptoms that may occur when a person suddenly stops the use of a substance or reduces the dose of an addictive substance

depression state in which an individual feels intensely sad and hopeless; may have trouble eating, sleeping, and concentrating, and is no longer able to feel pleasure from previously enjoyable activities; in extreme cases, may lead an individual to think about or attempt suicide

paranoid psychosis symptom of mental illness characterized by changes in personality, a distorted sense of reality, and feelings of excessive and irrational suspicion; may include hallucinations (i.e., seeing, hearing, feeling, smelling, or tasting something that is not truly there)

sedative medication that reduces excitement; often called a tranquilizer

Psychotherapeutic drugs are the most commonly abused prescription drugs in the United States, followed by pain relievers and stimulants.

PERCENTAGES AND NUMBERS OF PEOPLE REPORTING USING PAIN RELIEVERS, TRANQUILIZERS, AND SEDATIVES FOR NON-MEDICAL REASONS IN 1999 AND 2000

Drug	Percentages		Numbers (in thousands)	
	1999	**2000**	**1999**	**2000**
Psychotherapeutics	15.4	14.5	34,076	32,443
Pain Relievers	9.0	8.6	19,888	19,210
Tranquilizers	6.3	5.8	13,860	13,007
Stimulants	7.2	6.6	15,922	14,661
Sedatives	3.5	3.2	7,747	8,843
Methamphetamine	4.3	4.0	9,442	8,843

SOURCE: SAMHSA, Office of Applied Studies, National Household Survey on Drug Abuse, 1999 and 2000. <http://www.samhsa.gov/oas/NHSDA/2kNHSDA/appendixf1.htm#f.1>.

class action suit legal action taken by one or more individuals on their own behalf, as well as on behalf of all others who have an identical interest in the alleged wrongdoing

market. In December 1999 the company agreed to compensate thousands of people who took either drug in a $3.75 billion settlement of a nationwide **class action suit**.

Opioids

Addiction and abuse are extremely rare outcomes when doctors use opioid drugs, such as morphine, to relieve the pain of cancer patients. Most experts agree that the risk of addiction during opioid treatment for cancer pain is so small as to have no influence on the decision to use these drugs.

Treatment for prescription drug abuse often involves a combination of:

- gradual weaning from the abused drug
- antidepressants or sedatives to help decrease withdrawal symptoms
- cognitive-behavioral therapy to work on slowly changing the user's attitudes, feelings, emotions, and behaviors with regard to drug use
- support groups to help the user connect with other substance abusers who have been through similar challenges

SEE ALSO BARBITURATES; BENZODIAZEPINES; DRUGS OF ABUSE; OPIATE AND OPIOID DRUG ABUSE; SEDATIVE AND SEDATIVE-HYPNOTIC DRUGS.

Prevention

The use of alcohol, tobacco, and other drugs—whether legal or illegal—by various age groups and special populations continues to be a

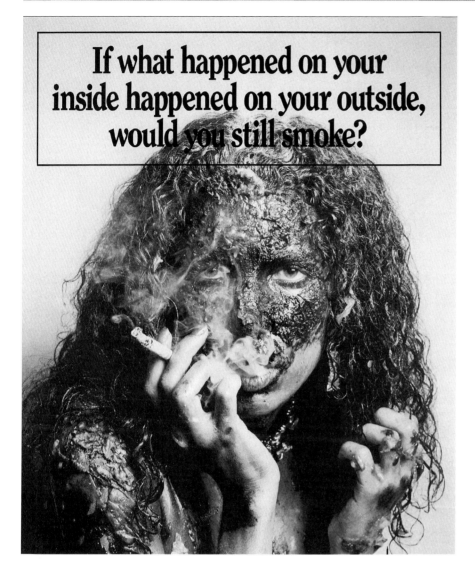

If what happened on your inside happened on your outside, would you still smoke?

This poster by the American Cancer Society is targeted at young people in an attempt to convince them that cigarette smoking is "uncool." This image is a marked contrast to the sleek advertisements used by tobacco companies.

problem in the United States. The use of illegal drugs increased among American adolescents throughout the 1990s, and this increase caused special concern. In response, the American public has become increasingly interested in the concept of prevention. The prevention movement began in the 1970s and has gained in popularity since then. Parents have organized to address the factors that lead to substance abuse, in order to prevent drug use among young people. In many cases, youth groups have also formed to help parents prevent substance abuse among young people and their peers. Supporters of the prevention movement emphasize that preventing substance abuse has a greater chance of success than helping people quit after they have become addicted. They also point out that prevention is less costly than treatment programs.

Parent groups have used several strategies to prevent their children from using drugs. One of these strategies is to change laws they

paraphernalia equipment that enables drug users to take the drugs (e.g., syringes and needles)

☎ See *Organizations of Interest* at the back of Volume 3 for address, telephone, and URL.

AIDS acquired immunodeficiency syndrome, the disease caused by the human immunodeficiency virus (HIV); in severe cases it is characterized by the profound weakening of the body's immune system

see as harmful to children. For example, parent groups mounted an intensive effort to obtain laws to ban the sale of drug **paraphernalia**. In the early twenty-first century, nearly every state had such laws. These groups also battled with supporters of the legalization of marijuana. In general, parent groups focus on ensuring that drug-education materials convey a no-use message, rather than recommending the "responsible use" of drugs that are both illegal and harmful.

Another area of parents' concern is alcohol abuse. Families of young people killed by drunk drivers organized groups such as Mothers Against Drunk Driving ☎ (MADD), Remove Intoxicated Drivers (RID), and Students Against Drunk Driving (SADD)—now Students Against Destructive Decisions ☎—to prevent accidents involving alcohol. As with the parent-led, drug-free movement, parents who led the anti-drunk-driving movement first raised the nation's awareness about the problem and then developed strategies to address it.

Another concern of the prevention movement is the glamorization of drug use on television, in films, in song lyrics, and on the Internet—all influences on young people. Media groups have formed to address public concern about these influences. For example, the Entertainment Industries Council has developed programs to work with film makers to educate them about substance abuse and to encourage them to deglamorize drug use in movies. The National Academy of Television Arts and Sciences has taken steps to increase the industry's awareness of the impact it could have on reducing substance abuse through the power and reach of the mass media. Since the mid-1980s advertising and public relations agencies have worked together in the Partnership for a Drug-Free America. ☎ These agencies volunteer their talent and time to create and produce antidrug commercials targeted at young people.

Since its origins in the 1970s, the prevention movement has spread to the military, the business community, schools, and the religious community. Ethnic and cultural groups, worried about the use of drugs by their members, have created prevention groups as a way to strengthen their communities. Local, state, and national political leaders have created policies and allocated resources to stem the flow of drugs into the country and to help people prevent substance abuse in their families and communities. The **AIDS**-prevention community has joined the substance-abuse prevention community in order to stop the spread of the disease among drug users.

Prevention services and policy changes have reduced the regular use of alcohol, tobacco, and other drugs in the communities they serve. These communities have benefited in several ways: fewer high-

Drug	Age Group	1979	1992	1999	2000
Any Illicit Drug	Young Adults	38.0%	13.1%	18.8%	15.9%
	Seniors	38.9%	14.4%	25.9%	5.5%
	Youth	16.3%	5.3%	9.0%	9.7%
Marijuana	Young Adults	35.6%	10.9%	16.4%	13.6%
	Seniors	36.5%	11.9%	23.1%	3.0%
	Youth	14.2%	3.4%	7.0%	7.7%
Cocaine	Young Adults	9.9%	2.0%	1.9%	1.4%
	Seniors	5.7%	1.3%	2.6%	0.4%
	Youth	1.5%	0.3%	0.7%	0.6%
Alcohol	Young Adults	75.1%	58.6%	60.2%	62.4%
	Seniors	71.8%	51.3%	51.0%	58.3%
	Youth	49.6%	20.9%	19.0%	16.4%
Cigarettes	Young Adults	42.6%*	41.5%	41.0%	38.3%
	Seniors	34.4%	27.8%	34.6%	24.2%
	Youth	12.1%*	18.4%	15.9%	13.4%

*These figures are taken from the Overview of the 1991 National Household Survey on Drug Abuse. Final data were eliminated from later versions of the survey, and no information about cigarette use is available for youth or young adults for 1979.

The significant reductions in drug abuse, drug addiction, and in drug-related deaths that have occurred since the 1980s suggest that prevention efforts should be continued and expanded, and that private sector prevention efforts should be funded to increase positive gains.

way accidents involving alcohol; improved general health because of tobacco prevention; and decreased rates of criminal activity involving illegal substance abuse. Although government policy in the United States still tends to emphasize law enforcement and treatment as a way to control substance abuse, the idea of preventing substance abuse before it starts has gained in public popularity. The prevention movement seeks to create communities in which individuals and families can live healthy lives free of drug abuse and addiction and the problems they cause.

The Principles of Prevention

Over the years, those involved in the prevention movement have developed the following guiding principles for prevention programs:

1. *Reduce or eliminate so-called risk factors—factors that increase a person's risk for substance abuse.* Many factors increase the chances that some individuals will become substance abusers. Prevention programs recognize the following risk factors for substance abuse:

- little commitment to school and education
- academic failure
- early antisocial behavior, **aggression**, and **hyperactivity**
- alienation, rebelliousness, and lack of social bonding to society
- antisocial behavior in early adolescence
- favorable attitudes toward drug use
- early first use of drugs
- family history of alcoholism, antisocial behavior, or criminal behavior

aggression hostile and destructive behavior, especially caused by frustration; may include violence or physical threat or injury directed toward another

hyperactivity overly active behavior

- parental drug use and positive attitudes toward use
- friends (peers) who use drugs

2. Promote and enhance "protective factors"—factors that help a person avoid substance abuse. These include:

- high self-esteem and self-discipline
- advanced social and problem-solving skills
- positive, optimistic outlook on life
- easy-going temperament and affectionate personality
- adequate family income
- structured and nurturing family
- promotion of learning by parents
- warm, close relationship with parents
- little marital conflict between parents
- low prevalence of neighborhood crime

3. Provide services that meet the needs of individuals as well as their families. When families receive training in relationship and parenting skills, the children in these families have fewer substance use problems. Services for individuals at risk of substance abuse or who have already become users include education, intervention, and referral to treatment when necessary. For people in high-risk substance-abuse environments, prevention programs offer further services such as health care, nutrition counseling, and prenatal care.

4. Teach people about substance abuse, guide them to the available services, and teach them how to manage their own lives. When a person becomes knowledgeable about the effects of alcohol, tobacco, and other drugs, this knowledge leads to better decision making. Prevention programs can encourage people to make good decisions and to cope with life's challenges. People with substance-abuse problems learn that they are engaging in risky behaviors, and are given accurate information about the risks of substance abuse. They acquire skills for resisting peer pressure to use drugs and learn how to resist the influence of advertising on their choices. They also learn where to turn when they need help.

One prevention program that is based on the above principles is called Life Skills Training (LST). The main goals of the LST program are: (1) to provide students with the information and skills they need to resist peer pressures to use drugs; (2) to help students develop independence, self-esteem, and self-confidence; (3) to help students cope with feelings of anxiety produced by social situations; (4) to increase students' knowledge of the negative consequences of drug

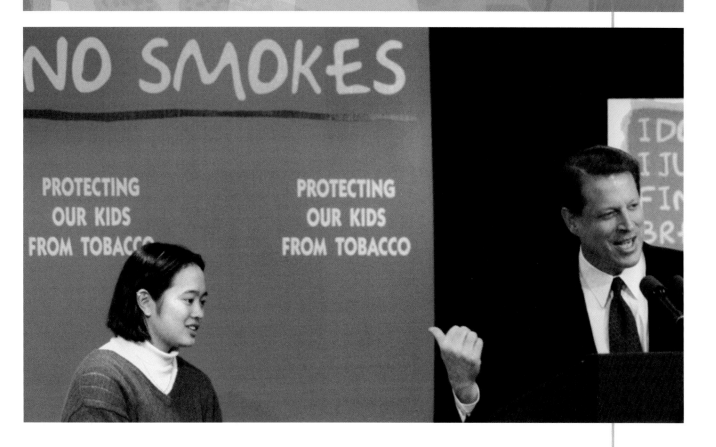

use and of the rates of tobacco, alcohol, and marijuana use; and (5) to promote a lifestyle that excludes drug use.

5. Encourage communities to establish standards of behavior through enforcement of clear policies. Communities that establish positive standards of behavior regarding alcohol, tobacco, and other drug use have been successful in delaying the onset of use. Such communities have taken steps to decrease access to substances by children and adolescents. These steps include setting rules for the location of alcohol advertisements. Community prevention programs can also teach middle-school students how to refuse an invitation to use drugs or other substances. Parents can learn how best to supervise their children in order to prevent the negative influences of peers.

Many communities also face the growing problem of heavy drinking by college students. This problem not only affects campuses and students, but also residents living near college campuses. A 2002 study found that, on an annual basis, drinking by college students between the ages of 18 and 24 contributes to an estimated 1,400 student deaths, 500,000 injuries, and 70,000 cases of sexual assault each year. The study also found that one-fourth of college students in this age group have driven under the influence of alcohol in the past year.

Announcing a government campaign designed to curb youth smoking, then-Vice President Al Gore explains how stiff penalties for retailers who sell to teens will support antismoking efforts.

First-graders participate in an antidrug program at school. A police officer informs the children of the factors that lead to drug abuse and the dangers involved.

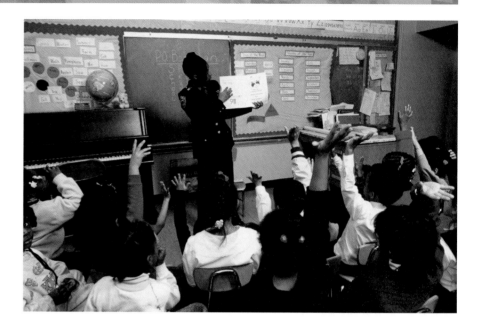

☎ **See *Organizations of Interest* at the back of Volume 3 for address, telephone, and URL.**

The National Institute on Alcohol Abuse and Alcoholism ☎ recommends that college administrators adopt the following policies, in order to reduce excessive alcohol consumption in and around college campuses:

- reinstating Friday classes and exams to reduce Thursday night partying; possibly scheduling Saturday morning classes
- offering alcohol-free, expanded late-night student activities
- eliminating keg parties on campus where underage drinking is common
- establishing alcohol-free dormitories
- employing older, salaried resident assistants or hiring adults to fulfill that role; currently, resident assistants are usually students who serve in a supervisory role in the dormitory in exchange for lower tuition
- further controlling or eliminating alcohol at sports events and prohibiting tailgating parties where heavy alcohol use is standard practice
- refusing sponsorship gifts from the alcohol industry to avoid giving any impression that underage drinking is acceptable
- banning alcohol on campus, including at official faculty and alumni events

Conclusion

Certain misunderstandings about substance abuse have slowed the progress of the prevention movement. Some people believe that substance abuse cannot be prevented because it is a problem passed down through genes. Clearly, genetic and other biological factors contribute to the occurrence of substance abuse. But a person's social environment also has a great impact on whether he or she will turn to drugs. Prevention can address those influences and can play an important role in responding to the problem of drug use and abuse. Federal, state, and local governments need to ensure that the best practices in prevention and education are provided to all ages. SEE ALSO ADOLESCENTS, DRUG AND ALCOHOL USE; BINGE DRINKING; MEDIA REPRESENTATIONS OF DRINKING, DRUG USE, AND SMOKING; PREVENTION PROGRAMS; RISK FACTORS FOR SUBSTANCE ABUSE; SUBSTANCE ABUSE AND AIDS.

Prevention Programs

Prior to the 1980s most schools around the country had courses in health education, tobacco education, alcohol education, or drug education. In these courses, students typically were taught that using tobacco, alcohol, marijuana, or other drugs was bad for their health. Students learned how these substances affected the body, how long the effects lasted, and even how people used them. Many of these education programs tried to scare students by pointing out how many people die each year from drug abuse. The people who designed these programs believed that if students really knew how harmful smoking, drinking, or using drugs is, they would not do it. However, teaching facts or using scare tactics did not work as people expected, and prevention programs had to change. New research showed that, to be effective, prevention programs must deal with the causes of drug abuse.

Most people who use drugs start using them during their early teenage years or slightly before. This is the time when young people are experimenting with many different behaviors, becoming more independent, and discovering their own identity. Contrary to what some adults might think, more than half of all adolescents try at least one substance. Most individuals who try drugs do not use them more than a few times, but those who do run the very real risk of becoming **physically dependent** on them.

Many prevention programs have been developed by organizations established by parents who were concerned about rising rates of drug abuse among young people. These organizations include Partnership for a Drug-Free America, ☎ National Families in Action, the National Federation of Parents for Drug-Free Youth, the American Council on Drug Education, ☎ and Committees of

physically dependent state in which drugs are needed for relief of uncomfortable physical symptoms, rather than for emotional or psychological relief

☎ See *Organizations of Interest* at the back of Volume 3 for address, telephone, and URL.

RELATED READING

Young adults who turn to drugs often see few alternatives, but in *Highs! Over 150 Ways to Feel Really, Really Good—Without Alcohol or Other Drugs* (2000), Dr. Alex Parker gives suggestions for alternatives to drugs and alcohol. Sports, relaxation exercises, and even certain foods are shown as healthy, safe substitutes for drugs.

☎ **See *Organizations of Interest* at the back of Volume 3 for address, telephone, and URL.**

Correspondence, as well as state groups, such as Texans' War on Drugs, Tennessee Families in Action, and Alaskans for Drug-Free Youth, to name a few, and thousands of local groups in cities, towns, and counties across the country.

Many schools and communities throughout the United States have adopted programs aimed at preventing young people from experimenting with alcohol and drugs. Drug Abuse Resistance Education (DARE), an elementary and junior high school program, is the most widely used prevention program in the nation. Other prevention programs include Here's Looking at You, Project STAR, Life Skills Training, and PRIDE.

Dare and Dare Plus

DARE (Drug Abuse Resistance Education) America ☎ is a violence and drug prevention education program designed to equip youths with the skills needed to make healthy decisions about peer pressure, violence prevention, and drug abuse. As the nation's predominant school-based drug abuse and violence prevention program, it is being implemented by more than 8,600 law-enforcement agencies in almost three-fourths of the school systems across the country. DARE is an elementary school program that attempts to teach students that being grown up really means resisting peer pressure. It also means making your own decisions and learning to cope with life's problems in positive ways. The curriculum was developed by educators and is taught by specially trained police officers. It is based on research that indicates that effective prevention strategies offer accurate information, coping and decision-making skills, and positive alternatives to drug abuse.

DARE PLUS (Drug Abuse Resistance Education Play and Learn Under Supervision) is a modified version of the original DARE program. It is an after-school alternative program that seeks to deter and protect youths from drugs, gang activity, and violence by offering a wealth of on-campus activities covering a broad range of interests. Participants are encouraged to improve their academic, vocational, and personal skills, and to get involved in recreational and athletic activities. The program is designed to attract at-risk middle-school youth and offer encouragement and guidance in an effort to keep them in school and out of trouble.

Here's Looking at You

The Here's Looking at You (HLAY) program offers a full alcohol-education curriculum for kindergarten through 12th grade. Students hear fifteen to twenty class presentations each year. HLAY aims to provide information on alcohol and alcoholism, to shape students' attitudes toward drinking, and to help students develop self-esteem and good decision-making skills. Just as doctors give children vaccines to inoculate them against illnesses, the HLAY program tries to inoculate children against alcohol abuse.

HLAY is based on the idea that children will be far less likely to use alcohol or other drugs if they are (1) given full and reliable information about the properties of chemical substances and the consequences of using them; (2) trained in self-control, decision making, and other social skills (including refusal); and (3) assisted in feeling positive about themselves and in bonding with friends, families, schools, and communities.

Project STAR

Project STAR is a program that covers several areas: school, mass media, parents, community, and health policy. For middle schools, the program uses a curriculum that teaches about social influences and is incorporated in classroom instruction by trained teachers over a two-year timetable. Mass media, such as radio, television, and newspapers, are used to promote, reinforce, and help maintain the project. In the parent program, parents work with their children on Project STAR homework, learn family communication skills, and get involved in community action. The community organization component is the essential formal body that organizes and oversees all project-related activities.

The health policy component is a task of the community organization; the aim is to develop and put into place policies that affect alcohol, tobacco, and other drug laws and other local policies, such as establishing and monitoring drug-free sites in the community.

Life Skills Training

Some prevention programs from earlier decades instructed students in facts about drugs and the dangers of drug use. In contrast, the program called Life Skills Training (LST) teaches general skills for living happier and healthier lives. These life skills can help adolescents avoid becoming involved with drugs.

The main goals of the LST program are: (1) to provide students with the information and skills they need to resist peer pressures to use drugs; (2) to help students develop independence, self-esteem, and self-confidence; (3) to help students cope with feelings of anxiety

---

PREVENTION: THE BEST SOLUTION

"Prevention is the best solution to drug use by young people, but it takes time, effort, and resources. Government can only do so much. Prevention has to begin in each community, in whatever ways make sense in that community. We want to support that."

—Elaine M. Johnson, Director, Alcohol, Drug Addiction and Mental Health Administration, U.S. Public Health Service, 1991.

☎ See *Organizations of Interest* at the back of Volume 3 for address, telephone, and URL.

produced by social situations; (4) to increase students' knowledge of the negative consequences of drug use and of the rates of tobacco, alcohol, and marijuana use; and (5) to promote a lifestyle that excludes drug use.

The LST curriculum is a three-year program. It consists of fifteen class periods during the first year, ten booster sessions in the second year, and five booster sessions in the third year. The booster sessions teach students how to put the life skills they learned in the first year into practice. Researchers found that students who had been through the LST program had approximately 50 percent lower incidence of drug abuse than students who had not been through any program.

PRIDE (Parents' Resource Institute for Drug Education)

The purpose of PRIDE ☎ is to help parents form groups to protect their children from using marijuana and other drugs. The organization is based on the following principles: (1) drug abuse is a health issue; (2) the family is the greatest protection against adolescent drug use; (3) families need help from the rest of the community to steer young people safely through the many temptations and dangers that confront them every day.

When it was started in the 1970s, the PRIDE program set up parent peer groups. Parents encouraged each other to get to know and link up with the parents of their children's friends. The peer groups established guidelines for their children's behavior and tried to create positive alternatives to unhealthy and destructive behaviors often begun during adolescence. PRIDE programs later expanded to include larger groups of parents who wanted to work for change throughout their communities to prevent drug abuse among young people. The organization offers training to parents across the nation. PRIDE also added a separate program for youth that trains middle-school and high-school students in how to take a stand against drug use. In both cases, the essence of the PRIDE approach is to help parents and young people resist adolescent peer pressure that encourages negative behavior.

In addition, the PRIDE Drug Use Survey has helped thousands of local school systems determine the extent of alcohol, marijuana, and other drug use among students in elementary, middle, and high school. PRIDE data have also shown that the more involved a student is with drugs, the more likely he or she is to possess a weapon. Efforts to prevent drug use among students may then also help to prevent violence and criminal activity among young people.

Conclusion

Youth drug prevention programs are an essential way to reduce substance abuse in society. Researchers continue to develop new programs and to improve already existing programs to provide the greatest benefit to students, their families, and their communities. However, the prevention of substance abuse requires more than classroom education. The home, peers, and community can also play an enormous role in encouraging kids not to try drugs. SEE ALSO ADOLESCENTS, DRUG AND ALCOHOL USE; ADVERTISING AND THE ALCOHOL INDUSTRY; ADVERTISING AND THE TOBACCO INDUSTRY; MEDIA REPRESENTATIONS OF DRINKING, DRUG USE, AND SMOKING; PREVENTION; U.S. GOVERNMENT AGENCIES.

Prohibition of Alcohol

The Eighteenth Amendment to the Constitution of the United States prohibited the "manufacture, sale and transportation of intoxicating liquors." The amendment, passed by Congress in 1917, was written to become effective one year after its ratification by the states. The amendment outlawed only the manufacture, sale, and transport of liquor, not the possession of alcohol for personal use. It did not make buying liquor from bootleggers (people who produced alcohol illegally) a crime.

To carry out the intent of the amendment, Congress passed the National Prohibition Act, better known as the Volstead Act. The Volstead Act allowed supplies of alcohol to be produced and transported for scientific and other commercial purposes. It also defined an intoxicating liquor as any beverage containing more than 0.5 percent alcohol. It could have set the permissible level higher to allow the production, transportation, and sale of beer, but it did not.

Prohibition took effect in 1920. A Prohibition Bureau was established within the Treasury Department. Under the Volstead Act, Treasury agents could obtain a search warrant only if they could prove that alcohol was being sold. This meant that agents could not search individual homes, no matter how much liquor might be there. Some wealthy people, who had plenty of notice that Prohibition was coming, stored enough alcoholic beverages to last them through most of the following decade. Others began manufacturing alcohol at home. Even people strongly in favor of Prohibition believed that the public would not tolerate any effort to make the act of drinking itself a crime. The Volstead Act, unlike some state laws, per-

In the 1920s illegal bars spread across the United States and were called "speakeasies."

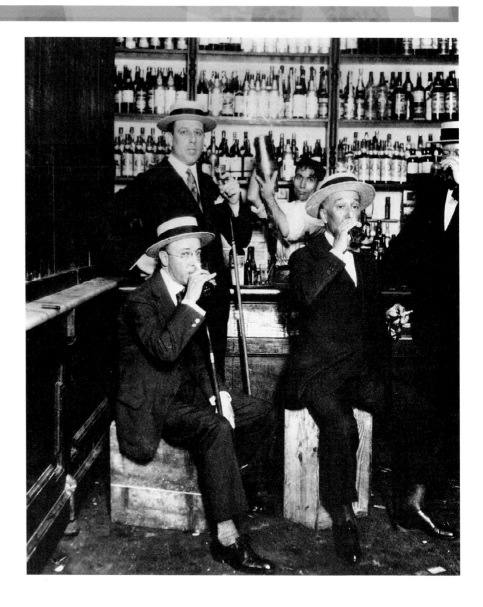

dementia disease characterized by progressive loss of memory and the ability to learn and think

psychosis mental disorder in which an individual loses contact with reality and may have delusions (i.e., unshakable false beliefs) or hallucinations (i.e., the experience of seeing, hearing, feeling, smelling, or tasting things that are not actually present)

mitted the manufacture of beer as long as the beer contained no more than 0.5 percent alcohol (this low-alcohol-content beer was called near beer).

Prohibition did not change the attitudes of most Americans about the morality of drinking. But it did succeed at eliminating 170,000 saloons, and drunkenness during Prohibition decreased. In New York and Massachusetts, two states that had no restrictions on alcohol consumption before 1920, hospital admissions for alcoholism declined sharply. Admissions to state mental institutions for **dementia** and **psychosis** caused by alcoholism also declined. Under Prohibition, deaths from alcohol-related diseases, such as cirrhosis of the liver, fell, and arrests for drunkenness decreased. Commander Evangeline Booth of the Salvation Army observed that there were fewer broken homes because of wages lost to drinking or violence related to drinking during Prohibition.

For the working class, liquor simply became too expensive, and so rates of consumption decreased. The price of a quart of beer or a quart of gin was five to six times higher in 1930 than before Prohibition. However, as bootlegging increased, medical problems linked to alcohol use began to rise again. Still, they did not reach the high levels experienced before 1920.

One unintended consequence of Prohibition was an increase in crime because of bootlegging. Many bootleggers became quite wealthy. Some who were involved in illegal activities before Prohibition directed the wealth flowing in from bootlegging toward organized criminal enterprises. Some of these enterprises later became involved with trafficking illegal drugs. One of the most notorious figures of the era was Al Capone, a central player in Chicago's organized crime racket.

The quality of bootlegged liquor was unreliable, since it was often produced using industrial alcohol. Some industrial alcohol could simply be flavored and sold as scotch, gin, or bourbon. Much of it, however, had been mixed with methanol (methyl alcohol) or other chemicals. These additives made the alcohol undrinkable, or denatured. Bootleggers hired chemists to remove the additives by redistillation ("washing"). Much of the liquor produced in this way was toxic (poisonous) or even lethal. The liquor produced in England and Canada and smuggled in by ship or truck was of a higher quality. One smuggler who brought in such quality liquor, Bill McCoy, provided the basis for a term still used to describe an authentic product—the "real McCoy."

Public criticism of Prohibition grew, and the Volstead Act was difficult to enforce. Many supporters of Prohibition became hostile toward the act's opponents. Supporters believed that Prohibition would eliminate the problem of drunkenness, and that, as a result, treatment of alcoholics would become unnecessary. They were intolerant of drunkards, and some suggested that drinking itself should be a crime. In the nineteenth century, the Temperance Movement had called for the physical and spiritual rehabilitation of alcoholics. In the 1920s a more severe attitude took hold, with some calling for stiffer jail terms, or even exile, for alcoholics.

Despite growing criticism, Prohibition was still alive and well when Herbert C. Hoover was elected president by a large margin in 1928. An overwhelming majority of both houses of Congress and nearly all the state governors supported the Eighteenth Amendment. Even opponents of Prohibition did not expect to see it **repealed**. But the onset of the Great Depression in 1929 dramatically changed the

IN THEIR OWN WORDS

"Politicians are ducking, candidates are hedging, the Anti-Saloon League is prospering, people are being poisoned, bootleggers are being enriched, and government officials are being corrupted."

—Fiorello H. La Guardia, Mayor of New York City, describing Prohibition in 1928.

repeal to revoke or cancel

Many stores post signs that show the year in which you must be born in (or before) to be able to legally purchase alcohol.

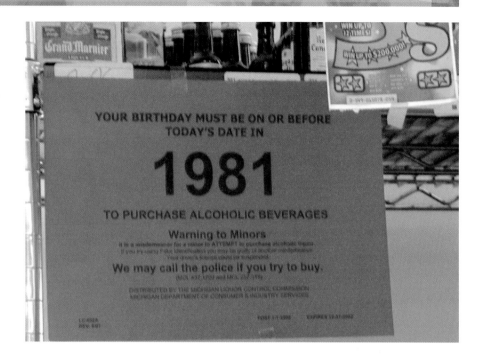

situation. Opponents of Prohibition now argued that the revival of the liquor industry would provide jobs and tax revenue. In the 1932 campaign for the presidency, Franklin D. Roosevelt promised to repeal Prohibition. Almost immediately after his inauguration, he introduced changes in the Volstead Act to legalize the sale of beer.

In 1933 the Twenty-First Amendment to the Constitution was ratified. It was brief and to the point: "Section 1. The Eighteenth Article of Amendment to the Constitution of the United States is hereby repealed." The federal government, however, would still be responsible for regulating and taxing alcoholic beverages. States could continue Prohibition if they wished, and some states did so. New alcoholic beverage control laws restricted the hours when alcohol could be sold (to make taverns and bars less attractive) and banned liquor sales on Sundays and election days. In 1972 a single agency, the Bureau of Alcohol, Tobacco, and Firearms in the Department of the Treasury, took responsibility for overseeing all federal laws concerning alcohol. SEE ALSO ALCOHOL: HISTORY OF DRINKING; TEMPERANCE MOVEMENT; TREATMENT: HISTORY OF, IN THE UNITED STATES.

Psychoactive Drugs

The term "psychoactive" describes a substance that affects the central nervous system (the brain and spinal cord), producing changes in a person's mental activity and/or behavior. Psychoactive drugs may affect the way an individual thinks, behaves, and perceives or experiences his or her environment.

Many popular and widely used substances are psychoactive. These include alcohol, nicotine (tobacco), and caffeine. Dangerous psychoactive drugs that have little or no medical benefit include heroin, **hallucinogens**, and some older **sedative-hypnotics** such as methaqualone. Marijuana has traditionally been placed in this category. However, recent research has shown that marijuana may have some medical benefits in the treatment of glaucoma (an eye disease), nausea, and weight loss associated with cancer or AIDS.

Doctors prescribe psychoactive drugs for many reasons. Among the most important medical uses are as anesthesia for surgery and as analgesics (painkillers). Psychoactive drugs are also drugs of abuse when they are used for nonmedical purposes. These purposes include altering consciousness, improving performance, and improving mood. Some psychoactive substances, such as alcohol and peyote, are used as part of cultural and religious rituals.

Some psychoactive drugs produce an effect in people who suffer from a mental or medical disorder, but produce no effect on normal individuals. Antidepressant drugs, for example, will not affect a person's mood unless he or she is suffering from **depression**. Other psychoactive drugs, such as the sedative-hypnotics, produce similar effects in all individuals.

Psychoactive drugs are used to treat movement disorders, such as Parkinson's disease, and mental illnesses such as anxiety disorders, depression, bipolar disorder (also known as manic-depression), and schizophrenia. In addition, psychoactive drugs used to treat disorders in other parts of the body, such as high blood pressure, arrhythmia (irregular heartbeat), and inflammation, can also affect the central nervous system. In these cases, the psychoactive effects of these drugs are generally considered side effects. SEE ALSO ALCOHOL: CHEMISTRY; HALLUCINOGENS; HEROIN; MARIJUANA; SEDATIVE AND SEDATIVE-HYPNOTIC DRUGS.

hallucinogen a drug, such as LSD, that causes hallucinations, or seeing, hearing, or feeling things that are not there

sedative-hypnotic drug that has a calming and relaxing effect; "hypnotics" induce sleep

depression state in which an individual feels intensely sad and hopeless; may have trouble eating, sleeping, and concentrating, and is no longer able to feel pleasure from previously enjoyable activities; in extreme cases, may lead an individual to think about or attempt suicide

Psychopharmacology

Psychopharmacology is a branch of science that studies the effects that drugs have on the brain, thinking, and behavior. These drugs act on the central nervous system (the brain and spinal cord) and also interact with other body systems, affecting various functions including blood pressure, heart rate and rhythm, breathing rate, and metabolism, the way the body processes and uses nutrients for energy and growth. Drugs studied include medications that are used to treat mental conditions, such as medications to treat depression, anxiety, mania, and **psychosis**. Drugs of abuse may also be studied, including cocaine, marijuana, hallucinogens, and prescription drugs that may be abused for their affects on mood and consciousness.

psychosis mental disorder in which an individual loses contact with reality

Quaaludes

Quaaludes, often called "ludes," are a **sedative-hypnotic** drug, methaqualone, formerly used to treat insomnia. The drug produces a feeling of euphoria (intense well-being) that lasts for a few hours. Fatal overdoses can occur when the drug is used alone, but especially when it is mixed with alcohol and/or **barbiturates**.

A popular drug of abuse among college students in the 1960s and 1970s, Quaaludes are now illegal. In 1975 Quaalude use was about half the level of barbiturate use. In 1981 the annual rate of use was 7.6 percent, and use steadily dropped through 1993, when only 0.2 percent of high-school students reported using it. As with many other drugs of abuse, use of Quaaludes increased somewhat through the early 1990s, reaching 1.1 percent in 1996, where it remained through 1999. Use then dropped to 0.8 percent in 2001. SEE ALSO ACCIDENTS AND INJURIES FROM ALCOHOL; ACCIDENTS AND INJURIES FROM DRUGS; ADDICTION: CONCEPTS AND DEFINITIONS; SEDATIVE AND SEDATIVE-HYPNOTIC DRUGS.

sedative-hypnotic drug that has a calming and relaxing effect; "hypnotics" induce sleep

barbiturate highly addictive sedative drugs that decrease the activity of the central nervous system

Racial Profiling

In law enforcement, a profile is a set of general characteristics and features that are defined as being suspicious. For example, if a series of bank robberies occur involving young men in leather jackets, neighborhood police may profile young men in leather jackets. This means that the police will view people fitting this description as more likely suspects. In turn, the police will be more likely to stop and question young men wearing leather jackets than people meeting other descriptions. Racial profiling is the use of racial generalizations or stereotypes as a basis for stopping, searching, or questioning an individual. In contrast with profiling in general, racial profiling raises serious issues about the civil rights of individuals who are stopped only because they appear to be of a particular race. Some experts prefer the term "racially biased policing" because of difficulties in precisely defining racial profiling.

Racial profiling plays a role in the enforcement of drug laws. For example, the Drug Enforcement Agency uses racial profiling to target people transporting drugs at airports. On the nation's roads and highways, local law-enforcement officers may use a minor traffic violation as an excuse to stop a car and then ask for consent to search the car for drugs. Officers target black drivers more often than white drivers, yet studies show that searches of black drivers are no more likely to turn up drugs than searches of white drivers.

Efforts to halt racial profiling are now in place in many states. In 1999 President Bill Clinton ordered all federal agencies to study their law-enforcement practices in order to end racial profiling where it was found to be in use. During 2000 more than twenty-five states introduced measures dealing with racial profiling by law-enforcement officers, with eighteen states taking significant action. Eight states (California, Kansas, Massachusetts, Missouri, Oklahoma, Rhode Island, Tennessee, and Washington) ultimately passed racial profiling legislation. Efforts to achieve bias-free policing include improving supervision of officers and holding them accountable; improving recruitment and hiring procedures; educating and training police staff; improving outreach to minority communities; and collecting and analyzing data about the race or ethnicity of citizens in their contact with police. Many cities and states are struggling with lawsuits resulting from the heightened awareness of racial profiling. A well-publicized racial profiling suit, brought against the city of Cincinnati and its police department in 2001, was settled in early 2002 after much community involvement. Some fear, however, that in the wake of the September 11, 2001, terrorist attacks on the United States, racial profiling will continue and may be harder to end than was once hoped.

Rave

A rave is a large, typically overnight dance party, with techno usually the preferred form of music. New musical forms and fashion trends often crop up at raves, as do a variety of drugs of abuse known as club drugs. Raves have been a part of youth culture since the late 1980s, when all-night parties and Detroit techno music became a phenomenon in the United Kingdom. Raves are held in a variety of places, from more traditional nightclubs to warehouses to open pastures (sometimes without the knowledge of the owners). Ravers, usually in

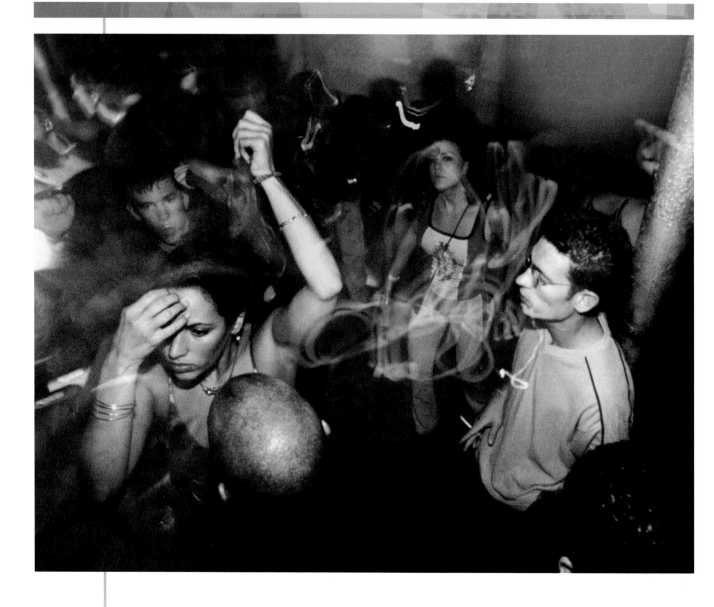

Teens dance in a room filled with pulsating music, smoky air, and whipping lights. Rave venues, known for attracting drugs, often distribute glow sticks to patrons.

their late teens and early 20s, are looking to escape traditional rules and expectations of society and instead to immerse themselves in a much looser underground atmosphere free of adult control.

A central part of rave culture is hedonism, or pleasure seeking. This pleasure seeking often leads to drug use, particularly methamphetamine (often called meth, crank, crystal, speed, or whizz) and MDMA (ecstasy). Other club drugs popular on the rave scene are Rohypnol, GHB, LSD, and ketamine. The abuse of a combination of drugs is so common on the rave scene that it is difficult to come up with a complete list of drugs. Ravers tend to regard the drugs they use as newer and safer than older drugs like heroin and PCP, also referred to as angel dust. But this is rarely true. In fact, deaths have occurred as a result of drug use at raves. Drug problems are common among ravers, making raves a source of public concern. SEE ALSO

Club Drugs; Designer Drugs; Ecstasy; Ketamine; Phencyclidine (PCP); Rohypnol.

Relapse

A relapse is a return of symptoms in an individual who has recovered from an illness or has entered a stable period in a chronic illness. In people with drug addictions, a lapse refers to minor episodes of drug use following a period of **abstinence**, and a relapse refers to major episodes of drug use following abstinence.

Relapse is common among drug addicts. This is true whether substance abusers have quit using drugs as a result of treatment or on their own. For example, up to 60 percent of alcoholics, heroin addicts, and smokers relapse within three months of the end of treatment. Although relapse episodes are common, treatment does help most substance abusers to reduce the frequency and severity of their drug use for long periods after treatment. Health professionals believe that addictions are chronic, or long-term, relapsing disorders. In other words, addicted individuals go through cycles of heavy use, treatment, abstinence or reduced use, and relapse.

Individuals have an increased risk of relapse when they face high-risk situations, or situations that have led to the person's substance use in the past. If the individual believes strongly that he or she can manage the situation without using alcohol or drugs (without relapsing), that person is more likely to avoid relapse. Individuals who lack that strong belief tend to relapse.

Other factors also increase the risk of relapse. Individuals with a family history of substance abuse, who have other psychiatric problems, and whose own histories of substance use are severe are at increased risk for relapse during periods of abstinence. People who go through difficult experiences (such as divorce), who have little support from friends, and who have low motivation for self-improvement are also more likely to relapse. When individuals with these characteristics encounter a high-risk situation, they often return to drug use in an effort to cope.

An important element of relapse is craving. When an individual encounters a situation or experience that has been frequently paired with substance use in the past, this can trigger a craving. For example, a former substance abuser might suddenly experience a craving for cocaine when he sees someone with whom he used to smoke

abstinence complete avoidance of something, such as the use of drugs or alcoholic beverages

cocaine. In other cases, substance abusers appear to have no control over automatic, ingrained processes that led them to use drugs in the first place. These users have very little insight into the factors that led them to relapse.

withdrawal physical and psychological symptoms that may occur when a person suddenly stops the use of a substance or reduces the dose of an addictive substance

Relapses that occur within a few days of a person's becoming abstinent may be due to **withdrawal** symptoms. Users may seek to relieve these symptoms by taking more of the drug they were addicted to. As part of their treatment, substance abusers should be taught to expect a relapse at some point during the recovery phase. Learning to accept relapse as a temporary disruption on the road to recovery, rather than a permanent failure, will increase the likelihood of a long-term, successful recovery. SEE ALSO TREATMENT PROGRAMS, CENTERS, AND ORGANIZATIONS: A HISTORICAL PERSPECTIVE; TREATMENT TYPES: AN OVERVIEW.

Research

Drugs affect the functioning of the brain's chemistry. As a result of these effects, a person who uses drugs can become a slave to them. But the brain has its own processes that set the stage for addiction. Research attempts to identify what those processes are and how they work. Addiction is a uniquely human problem, yet the qualities of addiction can be modeled in animals. Research shows that even rats can be turned into drug addicts.

When it comes to choosing an addicting drug, rats are not all that different from people. Scientists can set up experiments in which rats will give themselves repeated doses of drugs that humans find appealing and addicting. Research into human drug addiction that relies on animals may reveal new ways to treat, and even prevent, human problems with addictive drugs.

Reward Center

Experiments have shown that rats with a tiny wire placed in the pleasure-sensing region of the brain will repeatedly press a bar that sends a slight current out of this probe's microscopic tip. Called an electrode, the wire is designed to deliver the small amount of electricity to a brain region that the researcher selects, based on available maps of the brain.

Self-stimulation experiments in rats have repeatedly demonstrated the presence of a reward center in the brain. Scientists observe the behavior of the rats fitted with electrodes. They count the number of times the rats press the bar, and compare the number of bar presses that results when the electrode is in the reward area, compared to the number that results when the electrode is just outside that area.

To train a rat to press a bar, scientists use food as the reward. Before the experiment begins, electrodes are placed in the rat's brain under surgical anesthesia. Then, for a few days, the rats are given less food than they usually would eat. Next, they are put into a box (called a Skinner box after the behavioral scientist B. F. Skinner, who invented it in the 1930s). The box has a bar that, when pressed, delivers food. The rat does what rats naturally do in a new place—it explores the box by sniffing around and rearing up on its hind legs. The rat can smell that there is food somewhere near, and the rat is hungry. By chance, when coming down from a rearing position, the rat's paw will hit the bar. Suddenly, food appears. The rat learns fairly quickly to repeat this behavior to get more food. It becomes very efficient at pressing that bar to get food, an action called self-administering.

Now, the mechanism that gives food when the rat presses the bar is changed so that no food is delivered, and the electrode is activated. The question is, will the rat continue to press the bar? In other words, will the feeling created by the current inside the brain be rewarding in and of itself, and substitute for food? If the electrode stimulates the reward circuitry inside the brain, the answer is yes. However, if the electrode missed its mark, the rat will soon stop pressing the bar. The bar presses no longer deliver anything of interest to the rat.

How Research Proceeds

Based on this rat model of reward, scientists concluded that the brain has a specific place where rewarding feelings are generated. Researchers were able to determine that any area stimulated by an electrode and giving a sustained rate of bar pressing was in fact a reward area. They could count the number of times that a rat pressed the bar, comparing a weakly rewarding area to a strongly rewarding area. By interpreting the data—the rates of bar pressing—region by region, the researchers were able to map a set of places in the brain that consistently generate reward.

Researchers collected these measurements of reward regions from their rat experiments, and compared the active reward areas to the existing maps of brain functions, including areas where they know which **neurotransmitters** are present. The researchers predicted that

neurotransmitter
chemical messenger used by nerve cells to communicate with other nerve cells

More than half of the proposed 2003 budget of the National Institute on Drug Abuse (NIDA) is dedicated to research project grants.

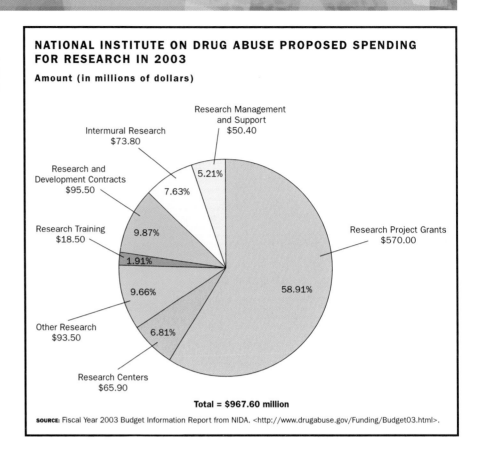

NATIONAL INSTITUTE ON DRUG ABUSE PROPOSED SPENDING FOR RESEARCH IN 2003

Amount (in millions of dollars)

Research Management and Support
$50.40
5.21%

Intermural Research
$73.80
7.63%

Research and Development Contracts
$95.50
9.87%

Research Training
$18.50
1.91%

Other Research
$93.50
9.66%

Research Centers
$65.90
6.81%

Research Project Grants
$570.00
58.91%

Total = $967.60 million

SOURCE: Fiscal Year 2003 Budget Information Report from NIDA. <http://www.drugabuse.gov/Funding/Budget03.html>.

the electrode had to be in regions that are rich in the neurotransmitter dopamine for the rats to press the bar repeatedly.

In another method of experimenting, scientists used a tiny, hollow tube to deliver minute amounts of drugs directly into the reward areas of the brain. The animals pressed a bar until they were exhausted in order to deliver such substances as heroin, cocaine, and other drugs into the specific brain structures making up the reward system. Rats self-administer the most popular drugs of abuse to the point of ignoring food and even sex in some instances—just as people do.

variable something that can change or fluctuate

There are several **variables** in these experiments that must be considered before interpreting the results, or data. These variables include: the location of the electrode inside the brain; the amount of current used; and, in the case of drug delivery directly into the brain, the amount, or dose, of drug given. Checking to see that the electrode is working properly is essential to conducting a good experiment. If it is not, this variable can make it impossible to interpret data correctly. The electrodes are intended to deliver the current only at their tips. The researchers locate just where the tips are placed in the brain in order to make their maps of the reward circuit. They make sure that the insulation placed around the wire up to the tip is not leaky so that current will not leak out along the shaft of the electrode.

If it does leak, some other brain area that the electrode passes through will be stimulated.

Even the sex of the tested animal is important to take into consideration when interpreting results. For some drugs, certain experiments reveal differences between males and females. For instance, female rats appear more sensitive to morphine-like drugs, and continue to self-administer these types of drugs long after male rats stop.

Rat Research and Brain Opiates

Opiates, such as morphine, are drugs made from the opium poppy that have powerful effects on the brain. One of these effects is to stop pain. Opiates are used as analgesia to make a patient more able to tolerate pain after surgery, or for conditions where pain itself is the problem, such as cancer. In the 1970s, the results of a set of experiments showed that the brain is somehow able to control pain on its own. The brain can regulate how it perceives pain by releasing its own painkiller molecules. These simple protein-like materials, produced within an animal's nerve cells, work in much the same way as the molecules of the opium poppy plant. Scientists had discovered the brain's own opiates.

An experiment with rats that had electrodes placed in a core region of the brain showed that they could undergo surgery without any anesthesia if these electrodes were activated. Other scientists then analyzed the region, called the central grey region, using opiate drugs as tracers. These opiate drugs were tagged with a chemical or radioactive label that would show up under the microscope. The opiate drugs stuck to the central grey region in large amounts—in other words, this region was rich in opiate receptors, specific binding sites that take up the drugs. Teams of scientists at Johns Hopkins University in Baltimore, Stanford University in Stanford, California, New York University in New York City, and at a research center in Sweden all helped demonstrate that certain receptors specifically accept morphine and related drugs. The drugs "dock" on these opiate receptors and act to stop pain.

Other researchers examined brain regions that were rich in opiate receptors and found that they also contained a substance that would bind to opiate receptors. In 1973 John Hughes and Hans Kosterlitz in Aberdeen, Scotland, showed that pig brains contained two similar small molecules that acted much like morphine when they were extracted, purified, and injected into lab animals. The shapes of these previously unknown molecules were shown to resemble closely the opiates from poppies and other **narcotic** drugs created by human

narcotic addictive substance that relieves pain and induces sleep or causes sedation; prescription narcotics include morphine and codeine; general and imprecise term referring to a drug of abuse, such as heroin, cocaine, or marijuana

chemistry. Named *enkephalins*, meaning "in the head," they unfortunately proved to be addictive, just like morphine: the effect of the purified enkephalins in animals would lessen unless increasingly higher doses were used.

Years before, Choh Hao Li, at the University of California in San Francisco, had looked at a substance he purified from a gland at the base of the brain. Li believed that this pea-sized gland, called the pituitary gland, might have a substance that aided the body's handling of fat (fat metabolism). Because the gland is so tiny, Li used material from 500 camels to find and purify a single molecule. But this molecule did not do much in his experiments on fat metabolism. Puzzled by his lack of results, he put the molecule in storage.

Sometimes, science involves luck and timing. But it always requires a prepared mind to recognize the significance of a finding and how to fit it in to an existing or developing theory. When Li read of the work on the brain's own opiates, he retested his molecule. He found that it, too, could lessen the perception of pain. This was a bigger messenger molecule, more closely resembling other messenger molecules, called hormones, that come from the pituitary. The small enkephalin molecules are similar in size to many neurotransmitters in neurons. Many hormones come from the pituitary, rather than the small, enkephalin molecules in neurons.

Li's molecule obviously was doing something other than handling fat. Scientists quickly renamed Li's hormone *endorphin*, meaning "the brain's own morphine." Endorphin lasts longer when injected than the much smaller enkephalins, which are nearly instantly broken down by the body. Yet it, too, is addicting. The discovery of the brain's own opiates has not yet led to the design of painkillers that are free from addicting qualities. But it has deepened researchers' understanding of how the brain works, especially at the level of molecular signals.

Experiments throughout the 1970s and 1980s mapped out an opiate-rich circuit within the brain. Many of the areas loaded with the enkephalins or endorphins correspond to regions known to carry pain messages, and to control the brain's ability to acknowledge pain, or to ignore it. And parts of this opiate circuitry overlap with the brain's reward pathways.

Imaging the Living Brain

By 2000 researchers had confirmed that the findings about brain chemistry and addictions in rats apply to brain chemistry and addictions in humans. The same areas mapped in the rats light up when the brains of humans, either using or recovering from addicting drugs, are scanned. Positron emission tomography (PET) is a technique that shows the use of energy by the brain. PET scans can show differences in brain activity in the reward circuitry when cocaine is taken, compared to a normal pattern of brain activity. Also, PET scans suggest that the drug ecstasy can alter the workings of a transmitter called serotonin in the brain of someone who takes the drug repeatedly. In fact, PET scanning reveals that dopamine, the messenger molecule of the reward circuit, is involved in nearly all addictive behaviors that scientists examine. Even alcoholics and obese people have a detectable difference in their dopamine activity on PET scans.

Now that scientists can see inside a living, working human brain, they are trying to uncover the details of addiction. **Craving** for a drug once addiction develops turns out to be a separate phenomenon, and one that may be key to interrupting the process of addiction.

craving powerful, often uncontrollable desire for drugs

Surprisingly, rats that were once addicted to cocaine did not relapse when stimulated in the reward area of the brain. Instead, findings reported in 2001 show that the hippocampus region of the brain, involved in forming memories, was crucial for seeking more drug. The hippocampus, with its rich connections to the reward centers, and the cerebral cortex—the outer region of the brain—may be prompting the drug-seeking behavior.

The brain remains the most complicated frontier for advancing our comprehension of ourselves. Formulating new models, and revising prior ones, will help those who seek release from addictive behavior. SEE ALSO BRAIN CHEMISTRY; BRAIN STRUCTURES; DRUG TESTING IN ANIMALS: STUDYING POTENTIAL FOR ABUSE; DRUG TESTING IN HUMANS: STUDYING POTENTIAL FOR ABUSE; IMAGING TECHNIQUES: VISUALIZING THE LIVING BRAIN.

> **WANT TO KNOW MORE?**
>
> For an illustration of PET scans, check out the National Institute on Drug Abuse's site, at http://www.drugabuse.gov/Teaching3/teaching3.html, slide 10 and 11. Another good web site is Brookhaven Lab's site, at http://www.bnl.gov/pet/studies.htm.

Risk Factors for Substance Abuse

What makes a person abuse drugs? Some people never use drugs, even if drugs are easy for them to obtain. Others use drugs occasionally or regularly for years but never become **dependent**. And some people become addicted and unable to function without drugs. These differences in drug-use patterns are the result of a combination of environmental and genetic factors. Genetic factors refers to a person's genes, which are passed down from parent to child and are shared in part by other family members. Environmental factors include a person's experiences in the family, home, neighborhood, school, work, and other settings.

dependent psychologically compelled to use a substance for emotional and/or physical reasons

RISK FACTORS FOR SUBSTANCE ABUSE

Ecological Environment
Poverty
Living in economically depressed area with:
High unemployment
Inadequate housing
Poor schools
Inadequate health and social services
High prevalence of crime
High prevalence of illegal drug use
Minority status involving:
Racial discrimination
Culture devalued in American society
Differing generational levels of assimilation
Cultural and language barriers to getting adequate health care and
other social services
Low educational levels
Low achievement expectations from society

Family Environment
Alcohol and other drug dependency of parent(s)
Parental abuse and neglect of children
Antisocial, sexually deviant, or mentally ill parents
High levels of family stress, including:
Financial strain
Large, overcrowded family
Unemployed or underemployed parents
Parents with little education
Socially isolated parents
Single female parent without family/other support
Family instability
High level of marital and family conflict and/or family violence
Parental absenteeism due to separation, divorce, or death
Lack of family rituals
Inadequate parenting and little parent/child contact
Frequent family moves

Constitutional Vulnerability of the Child
Child of an abuser of alcohol or other drugs
Less than 2 years between the child and its older/younger siblings
Birth defects, including possible neurological and neurochemical
dysfunctions
Neuropsychological vulnerabilities
Physical handicap
Physical or mental health problems
Learning disability

Early Behavior Problems
Aggressiveness combined with shyness
Aggressiveness
Decreased social inhibition
Emotional problems
Inability to express feelings appropriately
Hypersensitivity
Hyperactivity
Inability to cope with stress
Problems with relationships
Cognitive problems
Low self-esteem
Difficult temperament
Personality characteristics of ego undercontrol:
Rapid tempo, inability to delay gratification, overreacting, etc.

Adolescent problems
School failure and dropping out
At risk of dropping out
Delinquency
Violent acts
Gateway drug use
Other drug use and abuse
Early unprotected sexual activity
Teenage pregnancy/teen parenthood
Unemployment or underemployment
At risk of unemployment
Mental health problems
Suicidal

Negative Adolescent Behavior and Experiences
Lack of bonding to society (family, school, and community)
Rebelliousness and nonconformity
Resistance to authority
Strong need for independence
Cultural alienation
Fragile ego
Feelings of failure
Present versus future orientation
Hopelessness
Lack of self-confidence
Low self-esteem
Inability to form positive close relationships
Vulnerability to negative peer pressure

SOURCE: Adapted from Goplerud, E. N., Ed. (1990). *Breaking New Ground for Youth at Risk: Program Summaries.* (DHHS Publication No. [Adm] 89-1658). Washington, DC: Office for Substance Abuse Prevention.

Risk factors, including genetic and environmental factors, indicate a greater likelihood that a person will abuse drugs, but do not predict or guarantee future drug abuse.

physiology branch of science that focuses on the functions of the body

predisposition condition in which one is vulnerable or prone to something

Genetic Factors

Substance abuse often appears in more than one member of the same family. This is partly—though not entirely—due to the fact that genetic factors play an important role in the development of alcoholism and drug addiction. Identifying purely genetic factors in drug use is an important area of scientific study. **Physiology** is determined directly by genetic inheritance, and scientists have begun to discover that some people may have a **predisposition** to some forms of substance abuse. What this means is that it is much easier for these individuals to become addicted. To put it another way, it is much harder for them to resist becoming addicted.

If an individual's parent, grandparent, or sibling is an alcoholic, that individual's own risk is significantly increased. Studies also show that identical twin males (who have the same genetic makeup) are much more likely to be both alcoholic—if one of them is an alcoholic—than fraternal twins (who share only half of their genes on average). Moreover, adoption studies have found that sons of alcoholic biological parents were more likely to be alcoholics as adults than sons of nonalcoholic biological parents, when both groups were adopted early in life and raised by nonalcoholic adoptive parents. In similar studies of females, evidence of genetic influence was weaker.

As for becoming addicted to drugs other than alcohol, research has not yet been able to confirm the precise role of genetics. However, the rates of drug abuse among relatives of heroin and cocaine addicts tend to be higher than they are in the general population. Genes may also influence an individual's biological response to a drug. For example, genes may increase pleasant sensations (such as relaxation or a good mood) or decrease unpleasant ones, such as nausea or the flushing reaction to alcohol, which can include a high skin temperature and a faster pulse rate.

Genetic differences in brain chemistry may also determine an individual's response to drugs and alcohol. For example, alcohol affects the release of a brain chemical called dopamine. Some severe forms of alcoholism (and possibly addiction to other drugs as well) may occur in people who have nearly 30 percent fewer dopamine **receptors** in their brains than normal. People with this trait may be far less able than others to find enjoyment in everyday activities, and they have much greater difficulty coping with the stresses of life. Because alcohol and many other drugs release a flood of dopamine into the brain, addicts may turn to alcohol and other drugs to feel good.

receptor specialized part of a cell that can bind a specific substance; for example, a neuron has special receptors that receive and bind neurotransmitters

Environmental Factors

Although genetics plays an important role in the development of addiction, this does not mean that addictions are determined only by a person's genes. Environmental influences are also important, because a lot of addictive behaviors are learned by observing others. Watching a parent or another important figure using alcohol and/or other drugs has a major impact on a developing child. It tells the child that this is an acceptable behavior.

The relationship between family members is also important. Research has shown, for example, that teenagers who felt close to their parents and siblings were less likely than others to engage in risky behaviors, including drug abuse. A survey of over 4,000 adolescents has also found that those who had been physically or sexually abused, or had family members with alcohol or drug use problems, were at the greatest risk of developing substance abuse problems. Easy access to drugs is another important factor. If a child grows up in an environment where drugs are common and available, he or she is more likely to try them.

Family Environment. Most people who abuse drugs start in their teenage years, while they are still living with their parents. This gives parents a unique opportunity—and responsibility—to stop the problem before it starts. Several studies have shown that family **interventions** can play a significant role in reducing some of the risk factors associated with drug use. These risk factors include: drug use by family members; lack of a nurturing, supportive family environment; and a lack of clear and consistently enforced rules.

intervention when referring to substance abuse: attempt to help an addict admit to his or her addiction, recognize the ill effects the addiction has had on the addict and on his or her relationships, and get help to conquer the addiction

Experts say that the first thing parents should do is to be very clear about what their standards are, because setting clear standards and establishing limits are crucial for preventing teen drug abuse. Parents should also monitor their children, be consistent and moderate in their discipline, and they should recognize and reward positive behavior by their children. It is also important for teenagers to have the skills to be able to resist peer influences and other social influences to use drugs. It is useful for parents to teach their children so-called refusal skills, so that they know how to say "no" and still keep their friends and have a good time.

Many people believe that allowing older adolescents to drink small amounts of alcohol in the home, with their parents present, may teach them to drink in controlled ways, and that prohibiting it entirely may result in their learning to drink excessively. However, most experts disagree with this position. Studies show that the earlier children begin to drink, the greater the risk that they will abuse alcohol and possibly other drugs as well. Experts also suggest that if parents themselves drink alcohol in the home, they should do so responsibly, only in moderation. Such responsible use by parents does not seem to increase the chances of their children becoming alcoholics. Excessive **binge** drinking by parents, however, is a major risk factor for the development of alcoholism, which may lead to dependence on other drugs as well.

binge relatively brief period of excessive behavior, such as eating an usually large amount of food

Social Environment. More often than not, adolescents begin using drugs by imitating their friends, classmates, or other peers. Teenagers looking for peer acceptance or wanting to appear cool might decide to try taking drugs, beginning a path toward continuing use. Teenagers also want to be seen more like adults, with the freedom to do what adults do. By using tobacco or alcohol—illegal for adoles-

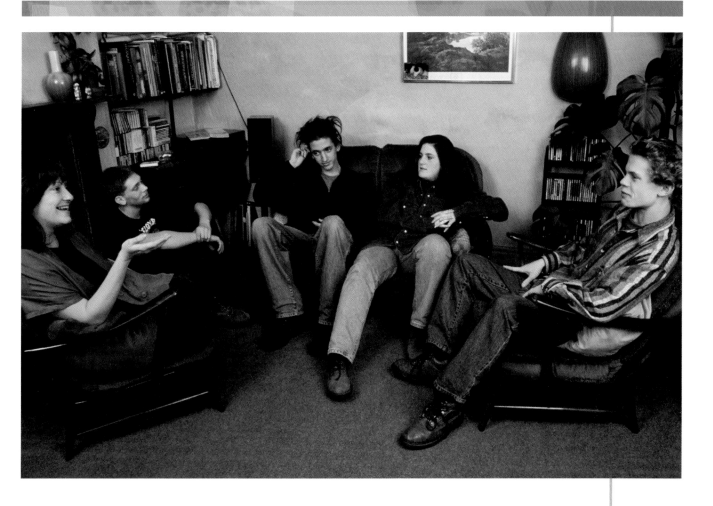

cents, yet both legal and socially acceptable for adults—the adolescent seeks an adult image. Adolescents are exposed to advertising on television and in magazines for beer, wine, and cigarettes that portray drinking and smoking as desirable. They may want to emulate celebrities such as movie or pop stars who are seen smoking or drinking in the media. Once adolescents begin using drugs—for any of these reasons—they may find that they are unable to stop.

Parent intervention is significant in reducing the risk of teenage substance abuse.

Using one drug often leads to the subsequent use of another. Typically, drug use begins with alcohol or cigarettes. These are followed by marijuana, and occasional drinking may develop into problem drinking. Next in the sequence are other illicit drugs. Cocaine use tends to follow marijuana use, with crack-cocaine use occurring after cocaine use. In other words, it is likely that someone who smokes crack has already tried tobacco, alcohol, marijuana, and cocaine. Many adolescents who use drugs in one category, however, do not necessarily progress to drug use in a "higher" category, and many stop before the drug use becomes a habit.

Sexual and Physical Abuse. Researchers are studying the use of illicit drugs by people who were physically or sexually abused as children and adolescents. Some believe that victims of abuse use drugs to help cope with the emotional problems caused by their difficult experiences. Victims of abuse often suffer from a poor self-image, even from self-hatred. They may find that drugs provide an escape from these feelings.

Race. Studies show that black adolescents are less likely to begin using most drugs than their white and Hispanic counterparts. However, with increase in age, rates of drug and alcohol use increase more quickly among blacks than among whites and Hispanics. At age 65 and over, blacks are nearly twice as likely as whites to be dependent on alcohol. Young Hispanic men have about the same level of risk of developing alcoholism as whites. There is growing evidence that racial and ethnic differences in drug use and drug dependence are not due to biological differences. Other factors are far more significant in determining drug use and abuse. These include poverty, the kind of neighborhood people live in, dropping out of school, and the availability of illegal drugs.

Personality Traits

Personality refers to a person's ways of thinking, feeling, and behaving, and it is thought to be shaped by both genetic and environmental factors. Drugs affect not only a person's physical well-being but other aspects of overall well-being as well, including emotional and psychological health. When treating drug abusers, psychologists and psychiatrists try to keep in sight the total picture of the person. Although most experts agree that there is no such psychiatric illness as an "addictive personality disorder," studies indicate that certain personality characteristics do make it easier for some people to become addicted to alcohol or other drugs. These include sensation seeking and **impulsivity**, as well as excessive **aggression** and anxiety.

Sensation Seeking. Sensation seeking is a personality trait of people who seek new and intense sensations and experiences. People with this trait are willing to take physical, legal, and financial risks for the sake of a thrill. Drugs offer one such type of thrill. Among drug users, high sensation seekers are likely to use more than one drug, to use **psychedelic** drugs, and to use stimulants such as cocaine. Sensation seeking is involved in many other activities related to alcohol and drug use, including gambling, smoking, sex, partying, reckless driving, and criminal activities. Taken together, these factors affect the level of risk that an individual will become addicted to alcohol or other drugs.

Impulsivity. Self-regulation is the ability to manage or keep control over one's emotions, behavior, and relationships. People with impul-

impulsivity state in which someone acts before thinking through the consequences of his or her actions

aggression hostile and destructive behavior, especially caused by frustration; may include violence or physical threat or injury directed toward another

psychedelic of a substance that can cause hallucinations and/or make its user lose touch with reality

sive personalities find it difficult to control their own behavior and they often engage in deviant behaviors, including substance abuse. For example, a person who is often angry, tense, and aggressive is unable to control, or regulate, aggressive impulses or hostile feelings toward others. Such a person might use heroin, for instance, in order to feel relaxed and calm.

Aggression. Early problem behavior often leads to drug abuse, and an early history of aggressive social behavior is one of the most important risk factors, according to a large body of research. Young children who engage in high levels of aggressive and disruptive behavior are likely to continue this behavior in the absence of some sort of school-based or family-focused intervention. Such children often do poorly in school and tend to become friends with other young people who engage in disruptive or risky behaviors. It is in this context that young people often begin using tobacco, alcohol, and other drugs.

Anxiety. People who are prone to anxiety and are looking for a chemical way out of it are at increased risk of abusing alcohol and some other drugs. These individuals may discover that alcohol or some other drugs relieve their anxiety or distress. The drug of choice for these self-medicating people is usually some type of **depressant**, such as alcohol, heroin, or a prescription **analgesic** or **tranquilizer**.

Protective Factors

While the above-mentioned risk factors can increase the chances that a person will become addicted to alcohol and/or other drugs, there is also another set of factors, called protective factors, that can help prevent the development of addiction. These include:

- high self-esteem and self-discipline
- advanced social and problem-solving skills
- positive, optimistic outlook on life
- easygoing temperament and affectionate personality
- adequate family income
- structured and nurturing family
- promotion of learning by parents
- warm, close relationship with parents
- little marital conflict between parents
- low prevalence of neighborhood crime

Successful drug abuse prevention programs work by helping to develop and strengthen these protective factors, while at the same

depressant chemical that slows down or decreases functioning; often used to describe agents that slow the functioning of the central nervous system; such agents are sometimes used to relieve insomnia, anxiety, irritability, and tension

analgesic broad drug classification that includes acetaminophen, aspirin, ibuprofen, and addictive agents such as opiates

tranquilizer drug that decreases anxiety and tension

PROTECTIVE FACTORS THAT DECREASE RISK OF SUBSTANCE ABUSE

Ecological Environment
Middle or upper class
Low unemployment
Adequate housing
Pleasant neighborhood
Low prevalence of neighborhood crime
Good schools
School climate that promotes learning, participation, and
  responsibility
High-quality health care
Easy access to adequate social services
Flexible social-service providers who put clients' needs first

Family Environment
Adequate family income
Structured and nurturing family
Promotion of learning by parents
Fewer than four children in family
Two or more years between siblings
Few chronic stressful life events
Multigenerational kinship network
Non-kin support network—e.g., supportive role models, dependable
  substitute child care
Warm, close personal relationship with parent(s) and/or other adult(s)

Family Environment
Little marital conflict
Family stability and cohesiveness
Plenty of attention during first year of life
Sibling as caretaker/confidant

Constitutional Strengths
Adequate early sensorimotor and language development
High intelligence
Physical robustness
No emotional or temperamental impairments

Traits of the Child
Affectionate/endearing personality
Easy temperament
Autonomy
Adaptability and flexibility
Positive outlook
Healthy expectations
Self-esteem
Self-discipline
Internal locus of control
Problem-solving skills
Social adeptness
Tolerance

SOURCE: Adapted from Goplerud, E. N., Ed. (1990). *Breaking New Ground for Youth at Risk: Program Summaries.* (DHHS Publication No. [ADM] 89–1658). Washington, DC: Office for Substance Abuse Prevention.

Factors that decrease a person's risk of abusing drugs include living in a middle- or upper-class household, high self-esteem, and a healthy family environment.

time minimizing risk factors that can contribute to the development of substance abuse and addiction. SEE ALSO CHILD ABUSE AND DRUGS; CHILDHOOD BEHAVIOR AND LATER DRUG USE; CONDUCT DISORDER; ETHNIC, CULTURAL, AND RELIGIOUS ISSUES IN DRUG USE AND TREATMENT; FAMILIES AND DRUG USE; PERSONALITY DISORDER; POVERTY AND DRUG USE.

Ritalin

Ritalin is the prescription brand name of the drug methylphenidate, a **stimulant** of the central nervous system (the brain and spinal cord). Its effects lie somewhere between those of caffeine and those of amphetamine drugs: Ritalin improves concentration, decreases appetite, produces an elevated mood, and can interfere with sleep.

In the mid-1950s Ritalin was first sold as a mood enhancer and was described as having less **abuse potential** than amphetamine. However, within a few years medical journals published a number of dramatic reports of its abuse and **toxicity**. Like the amphetamines and other stimulant drugs, methylphenidate is a controlled substance. This means that, although it has medical uses, Ritalin also has substantial abuse potential.

stimulant drug that increases activity temporarily; often used to describe drugs that excite the brain and central nervous system

abuse potential describes the chance, or likelihood, that a drug will be abused

toxicity condition of being poisonous or dangerous to people

The main medical use of Ritalin is in the treatment of attention deficit/hyperactivity disorder (ADHD). A child may be diagnosed with ADHD if he or she is extremely active and/or has difficulty in maintaining attention. Stimulant medications are often used to treat ADHD, and Ritalin is one such drug. Traditional formulations of Ritalin require a child to take two or three doses each day to control symptoms. A newly available form of Ritalin requires only a single daily dose. Ritalin can help calm children with ADHD, allowing them to focus and concentrate for longer periods of time. It can also help them control their impulsive behavior. Side effects of prescribed Ritalin can include insomnia (the inability to sleep), loss of appetite, and weight loss, all effects of stimulant drugs in general.

Ritalin is abused when it is taken by someone who has not been prescribed the medication, or when it is taken in a higher dose than was prescribed. Furthermore, some high-dose users begin by swallowing pills but often switch to injecting the drug so as to increase its effects and achieve the initial rush that is typical of intravenous drug abuse (injecting drugs directly into the veins). This can be particularly dangerous, because Ritalin pills contain talcum, a substance that does not dissolve in water. When the pills are dissolved in water and injected into the veins or under the skin, the talcum can create abscesses (pockets of infection) at the injection site. Untreated, these sores may lead to serious infection throughout the body. Talcum can also block small blood vessels, causing serious damage to the lungs and the retina of the eye.

Ritalin is frequently prescribed for young people with ADHD, and doses often need to be taken at school. As a result, Ritalin is often readily available at schools and may be sold, stolen, or given to others who use it for its nonmedical effects, which are similar to other amphetamines. Those who abuse Ritalin are usually seeking its stimulant effects, such as appetite suppression, wakefulness, and increased focus/attentiveness (for long nights of studying), and euphoria (a feeling of intense well-being). With continued use, **tolerance** to these effects can develop, so that users will often increase their doses to achieve the desired effects of their initial doses.

Ritalin abuse may result in serious side effects, including rapid heartbeat, increased blood pressure, chest pain, joint pain, and uncontrolled movements of the body. When higher and higher doses are taken, serious side effects may occur, including changes in mood, confusion, delusions (false beliefs), depersonalization (feeling that self or surroundings are not real), and hallucinations (seeing, hearing, or feeling things that are not there). Overdose is also possible; signs of overdose include some of the above symptoms as well as agitation;

tolerance condition in which higher and higher doses of a drug or alcohol are needed to produce the effect or "high" experienced from the original dose

severe confusion; convulsions (seizures); fast, pounding, or irregular heartbeat; fever; and vomiting. Continued use of high doses of Ritalin can result in toxic consequences: anxiety, sleeplessness, and eventually a mental disorder known as toxic paranoid psychosis. Ritalin can also be habit-forming in doses higher than prescribed for ADHD, so that unpleasant withdrawal symptoms occur when the user abruptly stops using it.

Ritalin abuse is still relatively uncommon in many areas, but it is clearly growing. For this reason Ritalin is on the Drug Enforcement Administration's list of Drugs of Concern. Most schools have established policies to keep drugs like Ritalin under control, such as locking cabinets where the drug is kept and carefully monitoring students' use of it as medication. However, such policies and systems are not foolproof and are not always practiced as intended. Those who seek to abuse Ritalin often find it relatively easy to obtain. A grave concern in schools today is that students who need their prescribed Ritalin will sell it, leading to wider abuse—as well as untreated students with ADHD. SEE ALSO ATTENTION-DEFICIT/HYPERACTIVITY DISORDER.

Rohypnol

sedative-hypnotic drug that has a calming and relaxing effect; "hypnotics" induce sleep

Rohypnol is the trade name for flunitrazepam, a **sedative-hypnotic** drug used medically in a number of countries. Its street names include "roofies," "roach," "R-2," "trip and fall," and "rope." Rohypnol has become a widely abused drug in many countries, including the United States, Sweden, Mexico, Italy, the United Kingdom, and South Africa. This trend is troubling because many users regard the drug as relatively safe. When used properly for medical reasons, the drug is not dangerous; but illegal use of Rohypnol has many dangerous and undesirable effects. It can cause violent behavior and accidents as well as coma, memory loss, and death. Because the drug can cause unconsciousness and amnesia (loss of memory), Rohypnol has been used in sexual assaults in the United States. Rohypnol is commonly known as the "date rape drug" for this reason. It has also been used in robberies in a number of countries.

benzodiazepine drug developed in the 1960s as a safer alternative to barbiturates; most frequently used as a sleeping pill or an anti-anxiety medication

Rohypnol has never been approved for use in the United States, where it is illegal. In Europe and elsewhere it is a commonly prescribed **benzodiazepine**. Like other benzodiazepines, such as Valium (diazepam) or Xanax (alprazolam), it can be useful for treating sleep problems and anxiety, though only under supervision by a doctor. Rohypnol, like alcohol and the benzodiazepines in general, acts as a **depressant** on the central nervous system (the brain and spinal cord). At lower doses, the depressant effects of Rohypnol include relaxation, reduction of anxiety, and a loosening of inhibitions. As with many abused drugs, a person who uses Rohypnol for a long period develops tolerance. The person then must take larger doses to produce the same effects. Larger doses mean increased dangers and side effects, especially memory loss and learning problems.

Drinking alcohol in combination with Rohypnol increases dangerous side effects even further. This combined use is a common practice among people who take Rohypnol illegally. The dangerous effects of combined used of Rohypnol and alcohol include:

- incontinence (an inability of the body to control excretion)
- loosening of inhibitions
- violence
- **delirium**, blackouts, and **stupor**
- respiratory depression (a slowed rate of breathing)
- death

Long-term use of Rohypnol can produce physical dependence. The level of dependence is even greater than that of drugs such as heroin and morphine. When individuals stop taking Rohypnol suddenly after regular use, they can experience a range of complications. Mild problems include restlessness and anxiety. More severe complications include tremor (shaking), **hallucinations**, and **convulsions** similar to severe alcohol withdrawal. These complications can be avoided if the withdrawal takes place under medical supervision.

Rohypnol has received a great deal of media attention in the United States because of its use in a number of cases of sexual assault. In these cases, a person dissolved Rohypnol in the unsuspecting victim's drink. The victim became unconscious, and was raped or robbed. Other drugs are also being used in this way, including GHB, barbiturates, opiates, other benzodiazepines, and alcohol. Sexual assault is more likely to involve the use of alcohol than any other drug, including Rohypnol. However, criminals of this kind may use Rohypnol and drugs like it because they produce unconsciousness and memory loss much more quickly.

Rohypnol use remains at a low rate compared to other drugs of abuse. Information about rates of Rohypnol use may not be as accurate as rates for other drugs, since at least some people who have taken it remain unaware of it. Also, those who have used it on others may not be reporting it on surveys that ask about individual use. National surveys began including Rohypnol on questionnaires around

depressant chemical that slows down or decreases functioning; often used to describe agents that slow the functioning of the central nervous system; such agents are sometimes used to relieve insomnia, anxiety, irritability, and tension

delirium mental disturbance marked by confusion, disordered speech, and sometimes hallucinations

stupor state of greatly dulled interest in the surrounding environment; may include relative unconsciousness

hallucination seeing, hearing, feeling, tasting, or smelling something that is not actually there, like a vision of devils, hearing voices, or feeling bugs crawl over the skin; may occur due to mental illness or as a side effect of some drugs

convulsion intense, repetitive muscle contraction

1996, when use among people ages 12 to 17 was around 1 percent. Among 8th grade students, use of Rohypnol fell to 0.5 percent in 2000; 0.7 percent reported using it in 2001. Among 12th grade students, use of Rohypnol increased to 1.8 percent in 1998, then fell again, remaining at about 1 percent for the next few years. Addicted users of Rohypnol need to be weaned gradually off the drug, to avoid the discomfort of withdrawal symptoms. Other sedative medications might be used briefly to help the user withdraw from Rohypnol. SEE ALSO BENZODIAZEPINE WITHDRAWAL; BENZODIAZEPINES; PRESCRIPTION DRUG ABUSE; SEDATIVE AND SEDATIVE-HYPNOTIC DRUGS.

Schools, Drug Use in

Adolescence is the age at which most people first experiment with alcohol, tobacco, and other drugs. Not surprisingly, school, a neutral site away from the watchful eye of parents, is the first place where many young people talk about, have access to, and even begin to use these substances. Alcohol, tobacco, and marijuana are the first drugs students are likely to abuse. Other drugs of concern in schools include inhalants, which are increasingly popular with younger students; so-called club drugs such as ectasy (MDMA); methamphetamines; cocaine; heroin; LSD; phencyclidine (PCP); and prescription drugs used for nonmedical purposes, including pain relievers, tranquilizers, sedatives, and stimulants like amphetamines and Ritalin.

Although the use of alcohol and tobacco by school-age young people is illegal, it is both legal and socially acceptable for adults. As a result, students can generally get alcohol and cigarettes fairly easily. They are also constantly exposed to advertising for beer, wine, and cigarettes that portrays drinking and smoking as desirable. Not surprisingly, alcohol and cigarettes are the most frequently used substances in schools, and the ones most likely to lead to dangerous consequences or serious health risks in the long term. According to the Centers for Disease Control and Prevention ☎, if current tobacco use trends continue, approximately 5 million children in the United States aged 18 years or less in 2000 will die prematurely as adults because they began to smoke cigarettes during adolescence. Even more disturbing is the estimate that alcohol kills 6.5 times more youth than all other illegal drugs combined, according to Ted Miller, a researcher at the Pacific Institute for Research and Evaluation.

Unfortunately, parents, students, and society as a whole may not view alcohol use and smoking as a problem, so students may have the impression that these substances are not really drugs and using them

☎ See *Organizations of Interest* at the back of Volume 3 for address, telephone, and URL.

is not really dangerous. Most schools have education programs designed to deter alcohol abuse and smoking.

Prevention and Education Efforts

The primary effort to prevent drug abuse in schools has been substance abuse education. More than 90 percent of high schools and 85 percent of elementary and middle schools now have alcohol-, tobacco-, or drug use–prevention programs. Such programs inform students about the risks of drug abuse, smoking, and drinking, and give guidance in resisting peer pressure to use substances. From Nancy Reagan's "Just Say No" campaign in the early 1980s to the more recent high-profile antidrug advertising campaigns, young people are hearing the antidrug message in school and at home. Many nationwide programs such as DARE (Drug Abuse Resistance Education) America ☎ and SADD (Students Against Destructive Decisions, originally Students Against Drunk Driving) ☎ have become standard features of the school landscape. DARE is now implemented in over 75 percent of U.S. school districts and in fifty-two countries around the world. Many other excellent drug use prevention programs are developed each year for use in schools.

☎ See *Organizations of Interest* at the back of Volume 3 for address, telephone, and URL.

Detection and Drug Tests

Efforts to detect drugs and drug abusers in schools are essentially efforts to deter drug abuse. School officials hope that good drug detection will discourage students from abusing or possessing drugs on

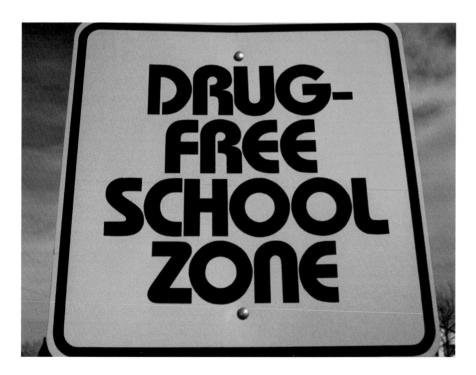

Signs such as this one communicate a community's commitment to keeping drugs away from children.

school grounds for fear of getting caught. However, all forms of drug testing and detection in schools are controversial and raise ethical and legal questions. The effectiveness of such programs is debatable as well.

Drug Testing of Students. Drug testing of students can take several forms. Breath analysis machines can test for recent alcohol use. Urine testing is by far the most common form of drug testing in schools. Hair analysis, not yet common in schools, may be able to accurately test for long-term use of certain drugs. While high-school athletes are somewhat more likely than other students to use anabolic steroids, steroid detection requires very costly tests that few schools purchase.

Breath analysis machines, commonly known as Breathalyzers, detect and measure the alcohol present in air that is breathed out. The Breathalyzer can detect whether a person has been drinking alcohol within the past few hours. Some schools now use the Breathalyzer at school functions such as proms to refuse entrance to students whose test results show that they have **blood alcohol concentration (BAC)** levels above the legal limit. Most states require BAC levels below 0.08 or 0.10 for drivers over 21 and BAC levels from 0.00 to 0.02 for minors. School officials reason that students are more likely to use alcohol before such social events, and are also likely to be driving before and afterward, thus risking their lives and the lives of others. Like other drug testing policies in schools, Breathalyzer use in schools is controversial.

Tests that detect drugs in urine are being used in more and more schools. Urine tests detect the presence of numerous drugs, and can detect use of marijuana, amphetamines, and cocaine within a few days to weeks after use (depending on the type of drug). Because it detects use of marijuana, the most heavily used illegal drug (after alcohol and tobacco, which are illegal for youth), many school officials feel urine testing is a valuable tool in their strategy to deter drug use. However, some students claim they can pass urine tests despite recent drug use by using certain cleansing or masking solutions or by otherwise tampering with the sample. Others claim that urine testing only increases the use of drugs that cannot be detected by means of urine testing, such as alcohol or other drugs that leave the body quickly.

To detect long-term drug use, a few private schools in New Orleans, Louisiana, have begun hair testing for drugs among all students, regardless of any suspicion of drug use (a practice called suspicionless drug testing). Other schools are using hair testing for athletes or other subgroups of students. Analysis of a small hair sample can de-

blood alcohol concentration (BAC) amount of alcohol in the bloodstream, expressed as the grams of alcohol per deciliter of blood; as BAC goes up, the drinker experiences more psychological and physical effects

tect with some accuracy the use of marijuana, heroin, cocaine, amphetamine, and PCP. The American Civil Liberties Union intends to challenge suspicionless hair testing in court on the grounds that its accuracy is not proven and it may be racially biased.

Dogs in Drug Detection. In the late 1990s many school districts began using scent-trained dogs to detect drugs or other contraband material (such as weapons) on school property, including students' lockers, public areas, and cars parked on school grounds. Schools that use detection dogs typically prepare students and staff for the program by explaining how searches will be conducted, what constitutes school property (such as lockers), and what will occur if drugs are detected.

Legal and Ethical Issues of Drug Testing and Detection in Schools

Detection and testing for drugs in schools, whether by use of detection dogs, urine or hair samples, or the Breathalyzer, is controversial. Those in favor argue that such methods are effective, safe ways to help keep schools drug-free, and serve to deter students from using illegal drugs or bringing them onto school grounds. Some students like the fact that drug testing gives them a legitimate excuse to resist peer pressure to use drugs. Those against drug testing claim that these methods violate students' privacy and their Fourth Amendment right (which protects citizens from unreasonable search and seizure), as well as the legal principle that insists that people are innocent until proven guilty. Opponents further believe that it creates an unhealthy climate of mistrust that runs counter to the primary educational mission of schools. Finally, some claim that these programs are not as effective as they might seem, and therefore not worth the expense or the infringements on students' rights.

Who Is to Be Tested? Schools sometimes test students for drugs when there is a reasonable suspicion of drug or alcohol use. In suspicion-based testing, schools should follow criteria to avoid giving the impression that test selection is arbitrary or that certain students may be targeted or picked on. Many schools avoid suspicion-based testing because it is too difficult to carry out in a way that everyone agrees is impartial and fair. The U.S. Supreme Court stated numerous problems with suspicion-based drug testing of students in its 1995 decision, *Veronia School District v. Acton.*

Random or suspicionless drug testing of all students as a condition of attending public school is widely thought to be unconstitutional, because access to education is considered a fundamental right.

DRUG TESTING IN SCHOOLS

Because student drug use was increasing in Veronica, Oregon, the school system began requiring that a drug test–consent form be signed by its athletes. School officials believed that some of the athletes were among the leaders of the school's drug culture. James Acton, a 7th grader, refused to sign the consent form. As a result, he was not allowed to play on the school's football team. In 1995, the U.S. Supreme Court decided that detecting drug use among student athletes was more important than the athletes' privacy and supported the testing.

☎ See *Organizations of Interest* at the back of Volume 3 for address, telephone, and URL.

In 2000 the Lockney, Texas, school district adopted a policy of testing all students in grades 7 to 12 for drugs. The program was struck down by a federal district judge in 2001, and the district did not appeal the ruling. Private schools, which are voluntary, can legally perform random or suspicionless drug tests on all students without threat of a lawsuit. Public schools can, however, exclude students with positive drug tests from extracurricular activities because such activities are voluntary.

Drug testing is more commonly performed as a requirement for participation in sports or other school programs. In the early twenty-first century, about 5 percent of schools nationwide have performed drug tests on student athletes. About 2 percent have tested students involved in other extracurricular activities, according to Lloyd D. Johnston, a researcher at the University of Michigan's Institute for Social Research. ☎ Another trend is to test students who drive to school. The legality of suspicionless drug testing of certain subgroups of the student population is still being decided in the courts.

In 1995 the Supreme Court upheld the right of the school district in Veronia, Oregon, to test student athletes for drugs. In the decision known as *Veronia School District v. Acton*, the court ruled that randomly drug testing school athletes was constitutional. That case relied heavily on evidence that the Vernonia district had a serious drug problem and that athletes were "leaders of the drug culture." The ruling also stated concern that athletes could put themselves and other players at risk of physical harm while under the influence of drugs.

In 2002 the Supreme Court agreed to hear a case from Tecumseh, Oklahoma, where the school district is randomly testing all students involved in interscholastic activities, including band, cheerleading, and after-school clubs. In the Tecumseh case, the crucial legal question involves whether school boards must document a serious drug problem in their schools before adopting random-testing programs. The Supreme Court was expected to rule on this case in 2002.

Those who support testing athletes and extracurricular participants have argued that these students are role models for other students and have a great influence on perceptions of what is acceptable. Some drug test supporters would prefer to test all students but understand that limited testing is the next best thing. Opponents claim that such selective testing is not fair. Most research shows that student athletes and other extracurricular participants are actually less likely to abuse drugs than those who do not participate in sports or other activities. One fear is that drug testing these students may discourage participation among the students who need it most, such as those who have experimented with drugs but have not become regular users, while targeting the most active students for scrutiny. Some drug-free students may avoid participation simply because they are too embarrassed by the urine sample collection process.

Zero-Tolerance Policies

All schools, especially those that perform drug testing, must deal with those students who are caught using drugs or who fail a drug test. Commonly, students identified as drug or alcohol users are expected to enter drug or alcohol abuse prevention programs or, in some cases, treatment programs designed for students in their situation. In the mid-1990s, so-called zero-tolerance policies became the norm for dealing with drug and alcohol use in schools. Zero tolerance means that a school will automatically and severely punish a student for a variety of specific offenses. Punishments usually involve suspension or expulsion, and sometimes referral to law enforcement. In 1998, 88 percent of schools had policies of zero tolerance for alcohol and/or drugs. Like other issues relating to drugs in schools, zero-tolerance policies are controversial.

Conclusion

In addition to concern for the health, safety, and well-being of their students, school officials have good reason to try to prevent drug abuse among students. Drug use interferes with quality education in a number of important ways. Students who use drugs may have problems with learning, motivation, memory, judgment, and school performance. They are also far more likely to cause disruptive behavior in school, thus interfering with the rights of all students to an education. Amid all the controversy and legal debate, schools will continue to struggle with the best ways to keep schools and students safe and drug-free. SEE ALSO ADOLESCENTS, DRUG AND ALCOHOL USE; BREATHALYZER; DOGS IN DRUG DETECTION; DROPOUTS AND SUBSTANCE ABUSE; DRUG TESTING METHODS AND ANALYSIS; PREVENTION; RITALIN; STUDENTS AGAINST DESTRUCTIVE DECISIONS (SADD); ZERO TOLERANCE.

Sedative and Sedative-Hypnotic Drugs

Sedatives are drugs that decrease activity and have a calming, relaxing effect. People use these drugs mainly to reduce anxiety. At higher

anticonvulsant drug that relieves or prevents seizures

dementia disease characterized by progressive loss of memory and the ability to learn and think

dependence psychological need to use a substance for emotional and/or physical reasons

depression state in which an individual feels intensely sad and hopeless; may have trouble eating, sleeping, and concentrating, and is no longer able to feel pleasure from previously enjoyable activities; in extreme cases, may lead an individual to think about or attempt suicide

doses, sedatives usually cause sleep. Drugs used mainly to cause sleep are called hypnotics. The difference between sedatives and hypnotics, then, is usually the amount of the dose—lower doses have a calming effect and higher doses cause sleep.

Currently, the most commonly prescribed sedatives are benzodiazepines, such as Valium. These drugs are also known as minor tranquilizers. Before the development of benzodiazepines in the 1950s and 1960s, doctors most often prescribed barbiturates to cause sleep and sedation. Because barbiturates have a high potential for abuse, doctors today rarely prescribe them. The exception is phenobarbital (Luminal), which is still used as a sedative and as an **anticonvulsant**.

Sedative-hypnotics can produce side effects in some people, especially the elderly and the very young. Elderly patients who need a sedative-hypnotic sometimes take chloral derivatives, which include chloral hydrate. These drugs are less likely to cause restlessness in older patients who suffer from confusion or **dementia**. They are also relatively safe to give to children for sedation before or after surgery. Chloral derivatives can, however, cause stomach irritation and rashes.

Doctors often recommend antihistamines for patients who need only a mild sedative. Drugs such as diphenhydramine (the sedative ingredient in the over-the-counter medicines Benadryl, Nytol, and Sominex) and hydroxyzine (the prescription drugs Atarax and Vistaril) are safe and do not produce **dependence**. However, they should not be used together with alcohol. The most common side effect of these medications is dry mouth.

An advance in the development of sedative-hypnotics occurred with the discovery of the non-benzodiazepine drugs zolpidem (Ambien), zopiclone, and zaleplon. These drugs are short-acting hypnotics that produce fewer side effects, such as a hangover effect (remaining sedation after the person stops taking the drug). Patients who take them for insomnia are less likely to have sleep problems again when they stop taking the drugs. This "rebound insomnia" is a common problem with benzodiazepines. These new drugs are also less likely to be abused than many of the other sedative-hypnotics and cause little respiratory depression.

Buspirone (BuSpar) is the only anti-anxiety medication that is not a sedative. It does not produce depressant effects or dependence. As a result, doctors are increasingly prescribing it to treat **depression** as well as anxiety. Unlike sedative drugs, buspirone does not affect the patient's alertness or motor skills; it does not intensify the effects of alcohol; and it does not produce a withdrawal syndrome.

PERCENTAGE OF STUDENTS WHO REPORTED USING SEDATIVES (OR TRANQUILIZERS) BETWEEN 1997 AND 2001

	8th Graders					10th Graders					12th Graders				
	1997	1998	1999	2000	2001	1997	1998	1999	2000	2001	1997	1998	1999	2000	2001
Tranquilizers															
lifetime	4.8	4.6	4.4	4.4	4.7	7.3	7.8	7.9	8.0	8.1	7.8	8.5	9.3	8.9	9.2
annual	2.9	2.6	2.5	2.6	3.0	4.9	5.1	5.4	5.6	5.9	4.7	5.5	5.8	5.7	6.5
30-day	1.2	1.2	1.1	1.4	1.6	2.2	2.2	2.2	2.5	2.9	1.8	2.4	2.5	2.6	3.0

SOURCE: 2001 Monitoring the Future Study (MTF). The MTF survey is conducted by the University of Michigan's Institute for Social Research and is funded by the National Institute on Drug Abuse, National Institutes of Health. <http://www.nida.nih.gov/Infofax/HSYouthtrends.html>.

The Medical Use of Hypnotics

Approximately 10 percent of young adults complain of serious sleep problems. By the age of 70 or older, 30 to 50 percent of adults will have sleep problems. For many, a prescription for a sedative-hypnotic drug is an effective treatment. Sleep problems in adults are of three main types: (1) Having trouble getting to sleep. This type of sleep problem varies little with age. (2) Having trouble staying asleep. This type of sleep problem worsens with age. (3) Waking up very early in the morning. Early-morning wakening is often a symptom of depression.

Because sleep problems occur more frequently in older adults, use of sedative-hypnotic drugs is more common in older age groups. For example, in the United States 2.6 percent of all adults take a benzodiazepine as a sleeping pill during a year. Among the elderly, 16 percent take sedative-hypnotics during a year. Of that 16 percent, 73 percent take the drug regularly for a year or more. Across all age groups, roughly twice as many women as men take sedative-hypnotic drugs. The most commonly prescribed hypnotics include several benzodiazepines: flurazepam (Dalmane), quazepam (Doral), temazepam (Restoril), and triazolam (Halcion). Other hypnotics not related to the benzodiazepines are hydroxyzine (Vistaril), an antihistamine, and chloral hydrate (Noctec).

Some people take sedative-hypnotics only occasionally for specific sleep problems. These problems may be caused by grief, stress over a limited period of time, or long-distance flights. Many more people take them over months and even years to cause nightly sleep. However, medical advice is to use sedative-hypnotics for only about two weeks. Most sedatives are taken by mouth, but some can be taken by injection.

Benzodiazepines. Benzodiazepines remain by far the most frequently used sedative-hypnotic drugs. There are three main concerns

Sedatives are often prescribed to reduce anxiety or help with sleeping problems; a 2001 survey found that nearly one out of ten 12th graders has taken sedatives at some point in his or her life.

withdrawal physical and psychological symptoms that may occur when a person suddenly stops the use of a substance or reduces the dose of an addictive substance

about the use of the benzodiazepines as hypnotics: (1) side effects experienced while the patient is taking the drug; (2) the possibility that the patient may become physically and psychologically dependent on or addicted to the drug; and (3) rebound insomnia and **withdrawal** symptoms when the patient stops taking the drug.

Benzodiazepines can be grouped in three ways according to how long their effects last. Long-acting drugs include flurazepam, diazepam (Valium), and chlordiazepoxide (Librium). Medium-acting drugs include temazepam. Short-acting drugs include triazolam, oxazepam (Serax), and lorazepam (Ativan). All of these drugs have proven effective when used for short periods. Improvements in sleep correspond closely with the actions of each particular drug. For example, temazepam is absorbed into the bloodstream relatively slowly and does not have the effect of helping someone fall asleep more quickly. A person who has trouble falling asleep will have more success with triazolam, which is absorbed quickly.

The Effects of Sedative-Hypnotic Drugs

Very high doses of most sedative-hypnotic drugs produce general anesthesia and can depress, or slow, a person's respiration so much that breathing must be maintained artificially or the person will die. The benzodiazepines are an exception to this. Higher doses of these drugs typically produce sleep and are far less likely to severely depress respiration.

In some people, sedative-hypnotics produce effects opposite to the calming, soothing feelings the drugs usually produce. Instead, these people experience excitement and confusion. This tends to occur more frequently in the very young and in older people.

Each sedative-hypnotic has a minimum dose at which it will produce effects. Doctors may prescribe a dose that is twice as high as the minimum to be effective at solving a patient's sleep problems. Further increases may, however, cause side effects.

Benzodiazepine sedatives have three major side effects:

- cumulative effects: when a person takes a second or third dose before the previous doses have been degraded or destroyed by the body

- additive effects: when a person takes a benzodiazepine together with another sedative or alcohol, causing the effects to be greater than with any single dose alone

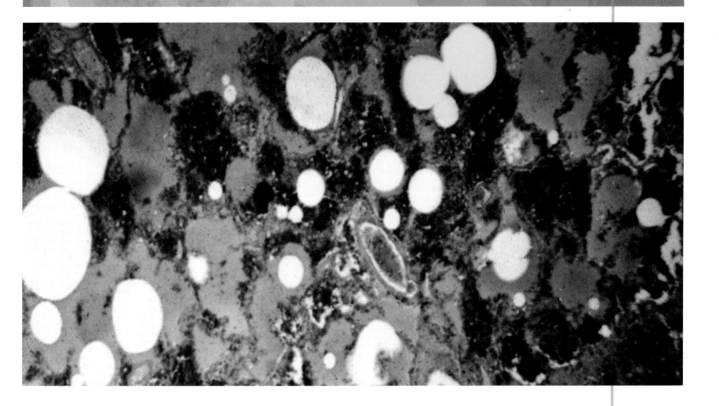

Lung showing the effects of Pentobarbitol, a sedative.

- residual effects: when a person continues to experience the effects of a medication after he or she has stopped taking it

Patients taking benzodiazepines may experience drowsiness, reduced speed of reaction and muscle response, and impaired concentration. These effects can impair a person's ability to function. Doctors should caution patients about driving and operating machinery. When a person takes the drug repeatedly, he or she can develop tolerance to these sedative effects.

All benzodiazepines can impair the ability to learn and remember new information. This effect on memory is strongest a few hours after a person takes the drug. Such effects may be greatly reduced by the time the person wakes the next morning. Rarer side effects include loss of inhibitions and aggressive behavior. These have been reported for some benzodiazepines (such as triazolam and flunitrazepam) more than others.

Rebound Insomnia. When a patient takes a benzodiazepine to treat insomnia and then stops taking the drug, the sleep problem may actually be worse than it was before the medication. The size of the dose can determine whether a patient will suffer from rebound insomnia. For this reason, doctors should prescribe the lowest effective dose. They should also warn patients not to take a higher dose to fall asleep more quickly or to have better sleep.

Dependence and Withdrawal

Some argue that rebound insomnia is a sign of physiological dependence on benzodiazepine hypnotics. Others disagree, arguing that dependence occurs only when withdrawal from a drug leads to symptoms other than a return of the original problems.

Psychological dependence on benzodiazepines can develop rather quickly. After only a few weeks, patients who attempt to stop the medication may experience the following:

paranoid feeling excessively or irrationally suspicious

- restlessness or difficulty settling down to complete a task
- disturbing dreams
- **paranoid** ideas, including groundless feelings that people do not like you or do not want you to do well, as well as **delusions**
- feelings of tension or anxiety in the early morning

delusion unshakable false belief that a person holds onto even when facts should convince the individual otherwise

Withdrawal symptoms following moderate-dose usage may include dizziness, increased sensitivity to light and sound, and muscle cramps. Withdrawal following high-dose usage may result in seizures and delirium.

The withdrawal syndrome for benzodiazepines may appear slowly because these drugs remain in the body for relatively long periods after the user has stopped taking the medication. Withdrawal appears to be most severe in patients who use benzodiazepines that are absorbed rapidly (alprazolam, lorazepam, and triazolam). In patients who abuse both benzodiazepines and alcohol, a delayed benzodiazepine withdrawal syndrome may produce complications as the person undergoes withdrawal from alcohol. Patients who are high-dose abusers of benzodiazepines usually require **detoxification** at a hospital as an inpatient.

detoxification process of removing a poisonous, intoxicating, or addictive substance from the body

The Abuse of Sedatives and Sedative-Hypnotic Drugs

Abuse of benzodiazepines by themselves is relatively unusual, but it does sometimes occur among users who seek a high from massive amounts of these drugs. Abuse of tranquilizers and sedatives follows the same basic trend in use as that of many other drugs: It peaked in the 1970s, fell from the 1970s until the mid 1990s, and then began to rise again gradually. Among 8th graders, abuse leveled off in 2001; among 10th and 12th graders, abuse continued to rise slightly in 2001. Street dealers sell benzodiazepines at a relatively low cost in most major cities. Some abusers combine benzodiazepines with other drugs to enhance the effects. For example, alcoholics and heroin addicts will at times use benzodiazepines to supplement the supply of their drugs, since the benzodiazepines have similar depressant effects. Many people who abuse sedatives are or have been heavy drinkers. Patients with a history of alcoholism or other drug abuse problems should not be treated with benzodiazepine sedatives on a long-term basis because they are at high risk of abusing benzodiazepines. Overdosing on benzodiazepines is a medical emergency. Signs of overdose include slowed or shallow breathing and low blood pressure causing dizziness, shock, coma, and eventually death. SEE ALSO ACCIDENTS AND INJURIES FROM DRUGS; ADDICTION: CONCEPTS AND DEFINITIONS; BARBITURATES; BENZODIAZEPINE WITHDRAWAL; BENZODIAZEPINES; DRUG AND ALCOHOL USE AMONG THE ELDERLY; PRESCRIPTION DRUG ABUSE; SUICIDE AND SUBSTANCE ABUSE.

Slang and Jargon

Slang terms in the drug world change constantly. Old terms drop out of the language and new ones take their place as various drugs fall in and out of use. Slang also reflects changes in the groups who sell and use drugs—their geographical location, their ethnicity, and their social status. Yet certain terms last for a remarkably long time, such as some of those for heroin. Other drug-related terms have become a permanent part of the English language, such as "hooked," "spaced out," "high," and "hip." The words listed below have been in use over the last hundred years. Some developed recently. Also included are the origins of these words, if known. SEE ALSO ENTRIES ON SPECIFIC DRUGS SUCH AS INHALANTS OR MARIJUANA; ADOLESCENTS, DRUG AND ALCOHOL USE; USERS.

SLANG AND JARGON IN THE DRUG WORLD

STREET	TERM DEFINITION
Adam	originally named to connote a primordial man in a state of innocence; MDMA, a mild hallucinogen
amp	from "ampule"; the drug is sold in small glass ampules, which are broken open and the contents inhaled
amps	amphetamines
angel dust	since the 1970s, phencyclidine (PCP), an anesthetic used on animals but originally on humans; discontinued because of bizarre mental effects
bagging	taking an inhalant by breathing it from a bag
beamed up	from "Beam me up, Scotty," an expression used in the television series *Star Trek*; "Scotty" is also a term for crack cocaine; intoxicated by crack
beamer	a crack smoker or addict
beans	dextroamphetamines
big C	cocaine
big H	heroin
black beauties	amphetamines

[continued]

SLANG AND JARGON IN THE DRUG WORLD

STREET	TERM DEFINITION
black tar	heroin
blotter	doses of the drug are dripped on a sheet of blotter paper for sale; LSD
blow	(1) to sniff a drug; (2) cocaine; (3) to smoke marijuana ("blow a stick")
breakfast cereal	ketamine
brown	heroin from Mexico diluted with brown milk sugar (lactose), which is less pure than China white; also called "Mexican mud" or "brown sugar"
candy	cocaine, amphetamine, or depressant
caps	(from the appearance) hallucinogenic mushrooms chalk crystal methamphetamine or cocaine
chasing the dragon	(from a Chinese expression for inhaling fumes of heroin after heating it; the melting drug resembles a wriggling snake or dragon) (1) inhaling heroin fumes after the substance is heated on a piece of tinfoil. (2) smoking a mixture of crack and heroin
cola	(a word play on "coke," "cocaine," and Coca-Cola, cocaine is derived from the coca plant); cocaine
cold turkey	(from the gooseflesh that is part of abrupt withdrawal) by extension, ending a drug habit without medicinal or professional help, "going cold turkey"
coming down	(from a high) losing the effects of a drug, all the way down to crashing
cop	(from British slang of the 1700s; to obtain, to steal, to buy; since the 1890s) to get or purchase illicit drugs
crank	crystal methamphetamine
crash, crashing	to come all the way down from a drug high
crystal	(in powder form) methamphetamine or cocaine
cut	to add adulterants to a drug—extending it to make more money in selling it (some adulterants are relatively harmless, some toxic)
dexies	dextroamphetamines or amphetamines
doobie	a marijuana cigarette; a joint
drop	to swallow LSD or a pill
dugie, doojee	(phonetic) heroin
dust	PCP
ecstasy, extacy	(from the euphoria, heightened sensuality, intensified sexual desire attributed to the drug experience) MDMA (methylen-edioxymethamphetamine), a mildly hallucinogenic drug synthesized from methamphetamine and resembling mescaline and LSD in chemical structure
elephant tranquilizer	PCP
Eve	(variant of Adam, MDMA or ecstasy) MDE, a mild hallucinogen derived from amphetamine. "Adam" and "Eve" is a compound of MDMA + MDE = MDEA (n-ethyl-MDA or 3,4,methylene + dioxy-N-ethylamphetamine)
forget pill	Rohypnol. See roofies below
freebase	(the psychoactive alkaloid, the base, has been "freed" or extracted from the cocaine hydrochloride) (1) crystals of pure cocaine; (2) to prepare the base; to smoke it
frost freak	one who inhales the fumes of Freon, a coolant gas, to get high
GHB	gamma-hydroxybutyrate; clear liquid, white powder, tablet, or capsule often combined with alcohol; used mainly by adolescents and young adults, often at nightclubs and raves
ganja	(from *gaja*, Hindi word for India's potent marijuana, consisting of the flowering tops and leaves of the hemp plant, where most of the psychoactive resin is concentrated) marijuana
glading	using inhalants
gluey	one who inhales glue fumes
grass	marijuana chopped up for smoking, which looks like dried grass
grievous bodily harm	gamma-hydroxybutyrate (GHB)
hash, hashish	the concentrated resin of the marijuana plant, containing a high percentage of the active principle, tetrahydrocannabinol (THC)
herb	(used to connote a benign natural substance) marijuana
hit	(1) an injection of a narcotic; (2) a snort of cocaine; (3) a drag from a crack pipe; (4) a toke of marijuana; (5) to cut a drug; (6) a dose of LSD
hog	(from its original use as a veterinary anesthetic) phencyclidine (PCP)

[continued]

SLANG AND JARGON IN THE DRUG WORLD

STREET	TERM DEFINITION
huff	to inhale ordinary household products to get high
ice	extremely pure and addictive smokable form of crystalline methamphetamine
jelly baby or bean	amphetamine pill
joint	(from "joint" as part of paraphernalia for injecting narcotics—particularly the needle; since the 1920s) a marijuana cigarette
jonesing	(after John Jones, the British physician who first described opiate withdrawal in 1700) withdrawal from addiction; by extension, craving any drug
juice	steroids
K, super K, special K, Vitamin K	ketamine, an anesthetic similar in structure to PCP
laughing gas	nitrous oxide
line	(1) a thin stream of cocaine on a mirror or other smooth surface, which is sniffed through a "quill"—a rolled matchbook cover, tube, straw, or tightly rolled dollar bill, etc.; (2) a measure of cocaine for sale.
luding out	(from "ludes," short for Quaaludes—a brand name for methaqualone, an addictive sedative—taking methaqualone
magic mushrooms	hallucinogenic mushrooms
mainline	(from "main line," a major rail route; since the 1920s) (1) the large vein in the arm; the most accessible vein; (2) to inject morphine, heroin, or cocaine into any vein
meth	methamphetamine
Mexican brown	marijuana from Mexico
Mexican mud	brown heroin from Mexico
mud	heroin
mule	(1) a low-level drug smuggler from Latin America; mules often swallow a condom filled with cocaine to be delivered at a destination—a dangerous practice called bodypacking; (2) heroin
nose candy	cocaine
piece	hashish, a form of marijuana
pill popping	(from "popping" something into one's mouth) frequent use of amphetamine and barbiturate pills or capsules
pit	veins on the inside of the arm at the elbow, a main site for injecting heroin and the place to look for tracks
pop	to inject
pot	(from *potaguaya*, a Mexican-Indian word for marijuana) marijuana
quas, quacks	(from Quaalude, a brand name of methaqualone) methaqualone pills, an addictive sedative
reefer	(from *grifa*, a Mexican-Spanish word for marijuana) (1) a marijuana cigarette; (2) marijuana
roach	(from its resemblance to a cockroach) the butt (end) of a marijuana cigarette
rock	(from the appearance) (1) large crystals or a chunk of pure cocaine hydrochloride; (2) crack
roids	steroids
roofies, rophies, ruffies, roach, R2, roofenol	Rohypnol, the brand name for the powerful sedative flunitrazepam; the pills are often used in combination with alcohol and other drugs
shabu	crystalline methamphetamine or crack
sheet	acid (from decorated blotter paper containing doses of the drug); LSD
shoot the breeze	inhale nitrous oxide, or "laughing gas"
shrooming	high on hallucinogenic mushrooms
smack	(perhaps from *shmek*, Yiddish word for sniff, whiff, pinch of snuff; since the 1910s, when heroin users sniffed the drug; in the 1920s and 1930s, some Jewish mobsters were involved in heroin trafficking) heroin
snappers	(the ampule containing the drug is "snapped" open) amyl nitrite capsules; also known as poppers
snow	(from the appearance; also, the drug is a topical anesthetic and numbs the mucous membranes) cocaine hydrochloride
speed	(1) amphetamines; (2) caffeine pills; (3) diet pills
stick	a marijuana cigarette
sugar cubes	LSD

[continued]

Sleeping Pills

sedative-hypnotic drug that has a calming and relaxing effect; "hypnotics" induce sleep

The term "sleeping pills" applies to a number of different drugs in pill form that help a person fall asleep and stay asleep. These drugs are also known as **sedative-hypnotics**. Among the wide range of sleeping pills, many require a doctor's prescription, but some can be purchased as over-the-counter drugs at a pharmacy. Over-the-counter preparations generally contain an antihistamine such as the active ingredient in the allergy medication Benadryl.

depressant chemical that slows down or decreases functioning; often used to describe agents that slow the functioning of the central nervous system; such agents are sometimes used to relieve insomnia, anxiety, irritability, and tension

Prescription sleeping medications are much stronger. They include barbiturates, benzodiazepines, and a number of other compounds. Barbiturates are no longer widely prescribed because of the risk for fatal overdose, especially when these drugs are combined with alcohol or other **depressants**. Benzodiazepines and other sedative-hypnotics can be short-acting or long-acting. In general, doctors prescribe shorter-acting sleeping pills to help a person relax enough to get to sleep. They prescribe longer-acting sleeping pills to help prevent frequent awakenings during the night. Long-term or inappropriate use can cause tolerance and physical dependence. SEE ALSO BARBITURATES; BENZODIAZEPINES; SEDATIVE AND SEDATIVE-HYPNOTIC DRUGS.

Speed

stimulant drug that increases activity temporarily; often used to describe drugs that excite the brain and central nervous system

Speed is the popular name for methamphetamine (also called methedrine), a drug that has strong **stimulant** effects on the central nervous system (the brain and spinal cord). Speed is similar to am-

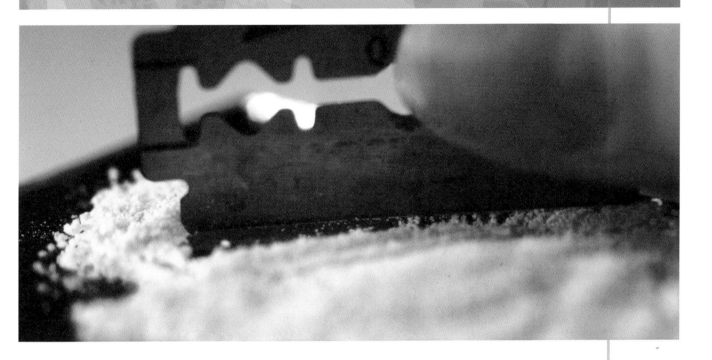

phetamine, but it has greater effects on the central nervous system and lesser effects on the cardiovascular and gastrointestinal systems. In other words, like amphetamine, speed causes increased activity, increased talkativeness, more energy and less fatigue, decreased food intake, and a general sense of well-being. Because speed dissolves more easily in water than amphetamine, drug abusers generally choose to inject speed. Injecting the drug into the veins results in the production of a rush. Some users describe the rush as the most desirable effect of the drug.

A razor blade is used to cut "speed" into lines for snorting. Methamphetamines stimulate the central nervous system and suppress appetite. Prolonged use can lead to addiction and psychotic mental illness.

Japan was the first nation to experience a major epidemic of methamphetamine use. During World War II, the militaries of both Japan and the United States produced large quantities of methamphetamines to keep combat troops alert. In Japan immediately after the war, the drugs were released for sale to the Japanese public. Within a short time there was widespread use and abuse of the drug, much of it by injection. At the peak of the epidemic, more than a million Japanese were using methamphetamines.

Despite the experience of the Japanese, many in the United States continued to believe that amphetamines did not lead to abuse. At the time, these drugs were not subject to any special controls or regulations by the state or federal government. In contrast, government laws control the availability of other drugs, such as codeine, so that these substances are available only with the prescription of a physician and in strictly limited quantities. The first speed epidemic in the United States began in the 1960s in the San Francisco, California area. A number of doctors there were prescribing the drug to people addicted to heroin. These drug abusers self-injected speed as a substitute for heroin. The drug became widely popular, and increasing numbers of people claimed to be heroin abusers just so that they could obtain prescriptions for speed. In the mid-1960s the government began to limit the sale of intravenous speed to pharmacies. As a result, speed that was produced illegally began to appear on the street. By the late 1960s a large number of users throughout the United States were injecting high doses of this illegal speed on a regular basis. Many experienced the drug's toxic (poisonous) effects, including **paranoid psychosis** (amphetamine psychosis).

Speed never completely disappeared from street use, but by the 1970s its availability greatly decreased. This trend began to reverse during the 1980s, with pockets of speed abuse occurring in the United States. One outbreak of speed use occurred in Hawaii, where users were taking the drug in a smokable form. This form of speed is called "ice" or "crystal."

Ice is a large, usually clear crystal of high purity (greater than 90 percent). Users smoke it using a glass pipe with two openings, much like a crack-cocaine pipe. Because it is a large crystal, it is difficult to mix the drug with additives. This purity makes the drug extremely desirable to buyers of illegal drugs. The smoke is odorless and, unlike crack, the residue of the drug stays in the pipe and can be smoked again. Users report that the effects last for as long as twelve hours,

paranoid psychosis symptom of mental illness characterized by changes in personality, a distorted sense of reality, and feelings of excessive and irrational suspicion; may include hallucinations (i.e., seeing, hearing, feeling, smelling, or tasting something that is not truly there)

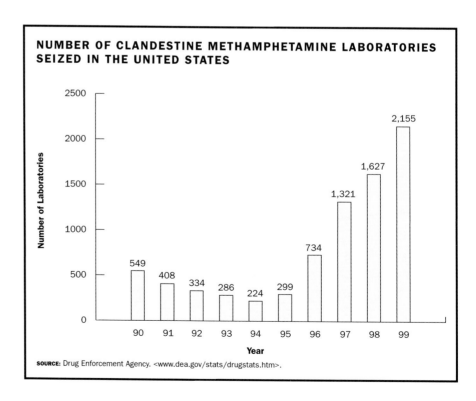

NUMBER OF CLANDESTINE METHAMPHETAMINE LABORATORIES SEIZED IN THE UNITED STATES

SOURCE: Drug Enforcement Agency. <www.dea.gov/stats/drugstats.htm>.

The number of illegal methamphetamine laboratories seized in the United States increased dramatically in the latter half of the 1990s.

although it is likely that this prolonged effect is due to the use of several doses.

Speed users, like cocaine users, often take the drug in binges that last from several hours to several days. During this time the user takes repeated doses of the drug and does not eat or sleep. Ending a speed binge results in a crash, in which the user becomes tired and **depressed**. The most severe toxic effect of repeated speed use is paranoid psychosis, which may last for several months. After a period in which the user remains drug-free, this psychosis generally resolves. However, it can reappear if the user returns to speed abuse.

depressed experiencing feelings of intense sadness and hopelessness

There are no medications to help speed users break their habit. Addicted users may need supportive treatment to help them get through the period of time during which they are stopping drug use. Antiseizure medications may be given to help the user avoid convulsions. Antidepressants may help improve symptoms of depression that occur after stopping speed use.

Treatment of speed abuse usually involves cognitive behavioral psychotherapy. This is a form of talk therapy that helps the user learn new patterns of thinking, feeling, and behaving, to help the user avoid returning to drug use. Information on finding treatment programs in local communities can be found at http://www.jointogether.org/sa/help/treatment/. SEE ALSO AMPHETAMINE; DESIGNER DRUGS.

Street Value

When illegal drugs are seized by police or a drug law-enforcement agency, the officers or agents determine the street value of the drugs. Street value is the total income that drug traffickers would make if each gram were sold at the price currently being offered on the street. The street value then determines the significance of the seizure. In other words, a major drug seizure is one that has a very high street value.

However, the street value of drugs that have been seized is not always equal to the actual amount of income drug traffickers have lost. This is because the price of drugs rises sharply as they move down the distribution chain from the point of entry into the country. The following example shows how street value can be calculated:

- When cocaine comes into the United States, it could be sold at a pure-gram price of about $20 per gram. A 100-kilogram unit contains 100,000 pure grams—thus its costs (to the drug trafficker) could represent $2 million.

- In 2001 a gram of cocaine could sell on the streets directly to cocaine users for about $100.

- One gram equals 1,000 milligrams. Of these 1,000 milligrams of cocaine sold on the streets, about 250 milligrams are "filler" substances. In other words, only 750 milligrams are actually pure cocaine.

- The price of a true "pure gram" of cocaine—1,000 milligrams of pure cocaine with no filler added—would be $133.

- 100 kilograms of cocaine, then, has a street value of $133 times 100,000 grams. In other words, the street value of 100 kilograms of cocaine equals $13.3 million, more than six times as much as its initial cost ($2 million).

SEE ALSO COSTS OF SUBSTANCE ABUSE AND DEPENDENCE, ECONOMIC; LAW AND POLICY: MODERN ENFORCEMENT, PROSECUTION, AND SENTENCING.

Students Against Destructive Decisions (SADD)

In 1981 Robert Anastas, a health educator and hockey coach in Wayland, Massachusetts, watched helplessly as two of his students died of injuries sustained in two separate alcohol-related traffic crashes. Anastas decided to fight back and developed a fifteen-session high school course on driving while impaired. Rather than a class focusing solely on the effects of alcohol while driving, he taught strategies for preventing driving after drinking, and he emphasized the legal consequences of getting caught. In this sense, his curriculum was quite different from traditional driver-education approaches.

Students who took Anastas's course reacted enthusiastically and formed an organization to reduce alcohol-related traffic deaths among their peers. They initially called the organization Students Against Driving Drunk (SADD) in order to focus attention on the act of drunk driving, not on the drivers themselves. One anecdote captures SADD's approach and philosophy: When a student jokingly suggested that SADD involve the governor, Anastas replied, "I believe that if you dream it, it can be done." When the governor became the honorary chairman of SADD, its motto became "If You Dream It, It Can Be Done." Within a year, chapters had been formed throughout Massachusetts and the program was gaining national attention.

Members of the early SADD chapters had a number of goals. They sought to raise awareness of impaired driving among students

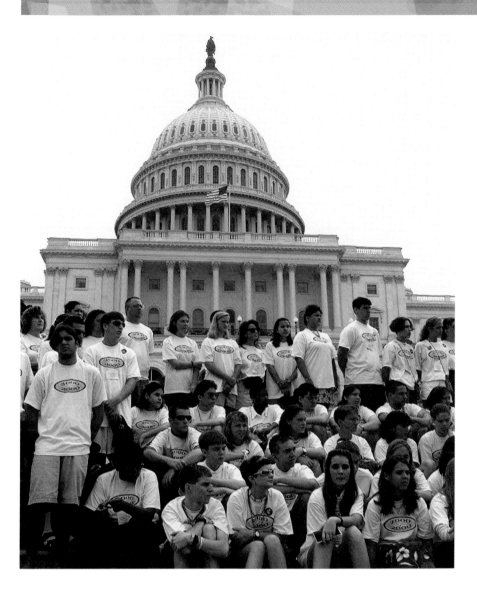

Members of Students Against Destructive Decisions (SADD) demonstrate on the steps of Capitol Hill in Washington, D.C.

through the curriculum developed by Anastas. They also sought to make impaired driving a behavior that kids would no longer accept as normal. Most of their peers did not think of drinking and driving as wrong or risky. The SADD chapters realized that kids needed to see drinking and driving as being outside the limits of normal behavior in order to reduce impaired driving problems. As the students put it, they wanted to change the "drinking and driving is cool" image to another image: "Drinking and driving is dumb." Finally, students in the SADD chapters tried to get high-school students to talk to their parents about drinking and driving. To meet this goal, they developed a "Contract for Life." The contract stated that a student would call a parent if he or she had been drinking or if the person responsible for driving had been drinking, and the parent, in turn, agreed to provide a ride or taxi fare.

SADD was significant in three ways:

1. SADD was among the earliest prevention programs to emphasize student leadership. Other programs had used peer educators or peer counselors trained and supervised by adults, but SADD chapters were run by students who planned activities and took responsibility for making them happen.

2. SADD was among the first youth programs to recognize the importance of changing what kids see as "normal" in order to prevent impaired driving. Earlier programs had emphasized education, attitude change, or scare tactics.

3. SADD was one of the first school-based prevention programs to venture outside the classroom. Although SADD had a curriculum, it also entailed extracurricular, community, and family involvement. In this sense, SADD was the first of the so-called comprehensive school-based prevention programs.

SADD's early growth was rapid. By the mid-1980s there were SADD chapters in every state in the United States and chapters in Europe. SADD received considerable media attention and was the only alcohol-prevention program ever to be the subject of a nationally broadcast made-for-television movie (*Contract for Life: The Bob Anastas Story*).

SADD was also controversial. Some vocal critics argued that SADD's emphasis on preventing drinking and driving in a way approved of drinking by young people. Critics were particularly concerned about the Contract for Life, arguing that by ensuring safe transportation, parents were communicating the message that drinking itself was not a problem. Anastas and others countered that although drinking itself was in fact a problem, young people were dying from traffic crashes, not just from drinking. This debate raged throughout the 1980s. Some funding agencies refused to allow grant money to be used to support SADD chapters. SADD was also criticized for accepting funding from the alcoholic beverage industry. In 1989 SADD divorced itself from this source of funds. It also adopted a strong "No Use" message and changed its Contract for Life to emphasize its commitment to a drug- and alcohol-free lifestyle. The organization specifically separates itself from "safe rides" and "designated driver" programs. However, it continues to describe itself as an "inclusive, not exclusive" organization, recognizing that teenagers make mistakes and should not be punished for them.

☎ **See *Organizations of Interest* at the back of Volume 3 for address, telephone, and URL.**

Over the years, SADD has evolved. Junior high school and college programs have been added, as has an emphasis on seat-belt use. In 1997, in response to calls from its chapters, the organization changed its name to Students Against Destructive Decisions. ☎ This name change signaled an inclusion of other potentially destructive behaviors such as underage drinking and drug use, teen suicide, violence, and unsafe sex or drug use that puts people at risk of HIV/AIDS. Today, SADD chapters focus on education, awareness, and peer support activities on a range of issues around risky behaviors. In recent years, several student safety clubs with very similar approaches to that of SADD have emerged. Members of these clubs, like SADD members, encourage students reaching out to other students to reduce highway deaths.

As is the case with many widespread, visible prevention efforts, few data can be summoned to show whether or not SADD is effective in reducing drinking and driving among youth. In 1995 the Preusser Research Group, with funding from the National Highway Traffic Safety Administration, evaluated SADD's effectiveness and concluded that students attending a SADD school were exposed to substantially more activities and information about the risks of underage drinking and drinking and driving. The survey also found that students at SADD schools were more likely to hold attitudes against drinking and driving. SEE ALSO ACCIDENTS AND INJURIES FROM ALCOHOL; ACCIDENTS AND INJURIES FROM DRUGS; ADOLESCENTS, DRUG AND ALCOHOL USE; DRIVING, ALCOHOL, AND DRUGS; MOTHERS AGAINST DRUNK DRIVING (MADD); PREVENTION.

Substance Abuse and AIDS

AIDS (acquired immunodeficiency syndrome) is a life-threatening disease that results from severe damage to part of the body's immune system. This system serves as a defense against infections and some cancers. AIDS is caused by infection with the human immunodeficiency virus (HIV). HIV gradually destroys certain white blood cells. The loss of these cells results in the body's inability to control microbial organisms that the normal immune system would resist easily. As a result, a person with HIV cannot fight infections. These infections are called opportunistic because they take advantage of damage to the immune system. For example, pneumocystis pneumonia is a type of lung infection that does not sicken people with normal immune systems, but that nearly all people with AIDS will get unless they take medicines to prevent it. Patients with HIV also frequently have certain cancers, such as Kaposi's sarcoma, a cancer of blood vessels.

AIDS was first identified in 1981 among homosexual men in California and New York, and among injecting drug abusers in New

---

RAISE YOUR SELF-ESTEEM

Low self-esteem is dangerous. It can lead to destructive decisions, allow a person to put him- or herself in dangerous situations, and allow peers to have more influence over decisions.

Here are some suggestions for ways to improve self-image:

- realize that each person is unique
- silence the inner critic
- recognize strengths
- take safe risks to improve confidence, such as volunteering, playing a new sport, trying a new hobby
- value the opinion of those who care

This needle may look clean after its use, but a magnified view reveals deposits of bacteria. Unless sterilized with a disinfectant, a needle may transmit viruses (such as HIV) and bacteria that can cause infections.

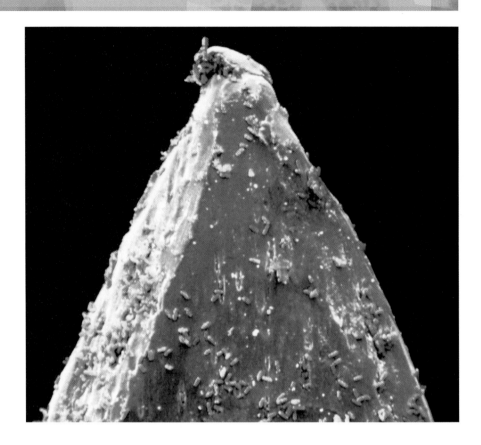

York City. After 1981 the numbers and types of AIDS patients increased rapidly, with millions infected throughout the world. An epidemic like AIDS that spans the continents is appropriately called a pandemic. In the United States alone in 1999, the Centers for Disease Control and Prevention (CDC) estimated that between 800,000 and 900,000 people were living with HIV or AIDS. The CDC estimated that about 339,000 persons were living with AIDS as of December 2000. In 2000, 1,688 young people (ages 13 to 24) were reported as having AIDS, bringing the cumulative total to 31,293 cases of AIDS in this age group.

AIDS has been diagnosed among people who inject various illegal drugs, including opiates (heroin), cocaine, amphetamines, and anabolic steroids. AIDS as a result of injected drug use accounts for a larger proportion of cases among adolescent and adult women than among men. Since the epidemic began, 57 percent of all AIDS cases among women have been transmitted by injection drug use or sex with partners who inject drugs, compared with 31 percent of cases among men. Of the 42,156 new cases of AIDS reported in 2000, more than one-quarter of the cases were transmitted through the use of injected drugs. Children born to mothers who contracted HIV through sharing needles or having sex with someone who injects drugs may become infected as well. AIDS has also been reported among nonin-

---

THE DISTRIBUTION OF REPORTED AIDS CASES AMONG PEOPLE BY CATEGORY OF EXPOSURE (OR POSSIBLE MEANS OF INFECTION)

Exposure Category	Male	Female	Total	Percentage of total
Men who have sex with men	361,867	-	361,867	46.15%
Injecting drug use	142,888	54,203	197,091	25.14%
Men who have sex with men and inject drugs	50,066	-	50,066	6.39%
Hemophilia/coagulation disorder	4,949	285	5,234	0.67%
Heterosexual contact	30,956	54,782	85,738	10.94%
Recipient of blood transfusion, blood components, or tissue	5,031	3,863	8,894	1.13%
Risk not reported or identified	53,429	21,712	75,142	9.58%
			784,032	

SOURCE: Centers for Disease Control and Prevention (CDC) semiannual HIV/AIDS Surveillance Report. Numbers are based on AIDS cases reported to CDC through June 2001. <http://www.cdc.gov/hiv/stats.htm>.

More than one in four people who contract AIDS may have gotten the virus through drug injections with contaminated needles.

jecting drug abusers, such as alcoholics, cocaine snorters, and crack-cocaine smokers, who have been infected through sexual contact.

HIV Transmission

HIV can be transmitted from person to person in three ways: (1) by contact with infected blood or blood components; (2) through intimate sexual contact; and (3) from an infected pregnant mother to her fetus. Drug abusers commonly become infected by sharing needles, syringes, and other injecting **paraphernalia**. Using any paraphernalia contaminated with blood (even in amounts too small to see) can result in transmission of HIV or hepatitis B virus. Sexual contact is a common route of transmission from drug abusers to their sex partners (who can transmit the virus to other sex partners, other drug abusers, or to unborn children). Health-care workers have also been exposed to HIV through unprotected or accidental direct contact with blood of infected patients in health-care settings.

paraphernalia equipment that enables drug users to take the drugs (e.g., syringes and needles)

Drug abuse may also affect the development of AIDS. For example, some research has suggested that HIV-infected individuals who continue to inject drugs and/or continue tobacco use may not survive as long as those who do not abuse those substances. The abuse of nitrite inhalants ("poppers") among HIV-infected homosexual men may lead to development of Kaposi's sarcoma.

Based on estimates from the United Nations AIDS program (UNAIDS), at the end of 2001 an estimated 40 million people were living with HIV infection or AIDS. UNAIDS estimated that 5 million new HIV infections occurred in 2001. This means there were about 14,000 new cases per day. An estimated 3 million adults and children died of HIV/AIDS in 2001. Most of these cases were in the developing countries of Asia and Africa. Numerous HIV surveys have been conducted among injecting drug abusers in several parts of the world. As those currently infected with HIV progress to AIDS, the epidemic will severely challenge the health-care systems, as well as the social and economic well-being, of many nations during the years to come.

HIV does not appear to be contagious by other means. No known cases of AIDS have been linked to transmission from kissing, in nonsexual social or household situations, through air, food, or water, or by mosquito bites.

Signs and Symptoms

The course of HIV infection varies greatly from individual to individual. In general, exposure to the HIV virus leads to infection. Within a few weeks or months of infection, evidence of the virus can be detected in the blood. Some patients develop flulike symptoms resembling **mononucleosis**, but most have no symptoms at this early stage of infection.

mononucleosis
illness caused by Epstein-Barr virus; characterized by extreme tiredness and sore muscles and throat

The second stage of AIDS (from one to fifteen years after becoming infected) is called the latency period. Patients may develop such signs and symptoms as enlarged lymph glands, fatigue, unexplained fever, weight loss, diarrhea, and night sweats. Patients may also develop opportunistic infections or cancers. The diagnosis of one of the opportunistic infections or cancers indicates that the patient has developed AIDS. The most common infection is a type of pneumonia in which the patient develops a fungal infection of the lung. Tuberculosis is another serious infection that has become increasingly common because of the AIDS pandemic.

In late-stage AIDS, the number of opportunistic infections and cancers rises. Kaposi's sarcoma, the most common cancer among AIDS patients, usually shows up on the skin and looks like a bruise or an area of bruises. The cancer grows and spreads to the internal organs. Another common type of cancer in late-stage AIDS is a form of lymphoma, or a tumor of the lymphatic system. Patients with late-stage AIDS may also develop inflammations of the muscles, arthritis-like pain in the joints, and AIDS dementia complex. A patient with AIDS dementia complex loses the ability to reason, becomes apathetic (spiritless and indifferent), has trouble with memory, and becomes unsteady or weak when walking.

AIDS Treatment

Although a cure or vaccine for AIDS has not been discovered as of 2002, a variety of antiviral drugs are used to treat HIV infection.

These drugs are often given in various combinations with each other. Groups of these drugs that are given together are sometimes called AIDS cocktails. Some of the antiviral drugs used to combat HIV include: zidovudine (ZDV, AZT), didanosine (ddI), zalcitabine (ddC), stavudine (d4T), lamivudine (3TC), nevirapine, delavirdine, saquinavir, ritonavir, indinavir, and nelfinavir.

It is important to understand that these medications do not cure AIDS; they simply restrain the virus by stopping it from reproducing or by interfering with its actions within the cells of the human body. It can be difficult to keep up with complicated medication schedules that require taking multiple pills several times throughout every day. Some of the medications have restrictions regarding whether to take with or without food or water, and what foods to avoid while on the medications. Furthermore, the drugs may cause unpleasant side effects. So even though these medications have increased the life spans of people living with AIDS, and have prevented complications that interfere with quality of life, the medication regimens themselves can be frustrating.

Prevention Among Drug Abusers

Because no cure or vaccine for HIV infection exists now (or probably in the near future), the hope for slowing the spread of HIV infection is through education and strategies to change behavior. Among injecting drug abusers, the most effective way to avoid HIV infection is to stop sharing infected needles. (Better yet, drug abusers should stop injecting drugs altogether.) They should also avoid sexual contact with individuals who may be HIV-infected. The rate of HIV infection in former drug abusers in treatment is lower than the rate of infection in drug abusers on the street. **Methadone** maintenance therapy is an effective therapy for heroin addicts and has decreased HIV transmission among patients.

methadone potent synthetic narcotic, used in heroin recovery programs as a non-intoxicating opiate that blunts symptoms of withdrawal

HIV Counseling. Some drug treatment programs offer counseling about HIV infection and partner notification (alerting sexual partners of people with HIV). So far, this counseling has had only limited success. A 2000 report noted that men who have sex with men and also abuse drugs still pose unique challenges to slowing the AIDS epidemic because they have multiple risks for HIV infection and transmission.

Safe Equipment. Some investigators recommend that injecting drug abusers use safer needles and syringes. One approach to reduce HIV transmission among injecting drug abusers is to educate addicts about cleaning and disinfecting needles and syringes between each use. Household bleach appears to be the most effective disinfectant against HIV. Another approach has been the establishment of needle exchange programs. In these programs, addicts can turn in their used needles and syringes and receive new, clean equipment at no cost and without risking criminal drug charges.

Newer Strategies. In a more recent proposal for preventing HIV transmission, treatment facilities would evaluate the mental health of injecting drug abusers. This evaluation would look specifically for major **depression** and **antisocial personality disorder**. Drug abusers with these disorders are at higher risk of HIV infection. Another proposal is to extend HIV prevention efforts to abusers of other drugs, especially cocaine and amphetamines. Finally, some experts in the field stress the need for prevention efforts among Native Americans and Spanish-speaking drug injectors born outside the United States. These two groups have high rates of HIV infection.

For additional information or answers to questions about AIDS and drug use, contact the AIDS Hotline or AIDS National Information Clearinghouse. Telephone numbers, e-mail addresses, and other details are found at the end of this volume. SEE ALSO COMPLICATIONS FROM INJECTING DRUGS; NEEDLE EXCHANGE PROGRAMS.

depression state in which an individual feels intensely sad and hopeless; may have trouble eating, sleeping, and concentrating, and is no longer able to feel pleasure from previously enjoyable activities

antisocial personality disorder condition in which people disregard the rights of others and violate these rights by acting in immoral, unethical, aggressive, or even criminal ways

Suicide and Substance Abuse

Suicide is the eighth-leading cause of death in the United States. Each year 29,000 people take their own lives. About 50 percent of all suicide attempts involve alcohol and illegal drugs (including those who use alcohol or drugs in their attempt or test positively for alcohol or drugs at the time of the attempt). About 25 percent of **completed suicides** occur among drug abusers and those with alcohol abuse problems. The suicide rate of people under age 30 is increasing, largely because of substance abuse among young adults.

completed suicide suicide attempt that ends in death

Suicides among young people nationwide increased dramatically in recent years. Each year in the United States, thousands of teenagers commit suicide. Suicide is the third-leading cause of death for 15-to-24-year-olds, and the sixth-leading cause of death for 5-to-14-year-olds. More than 50 percent of teens who commit suicide have a history of alcohol and drug use. Many teens who are considering suicide suffer from depression.

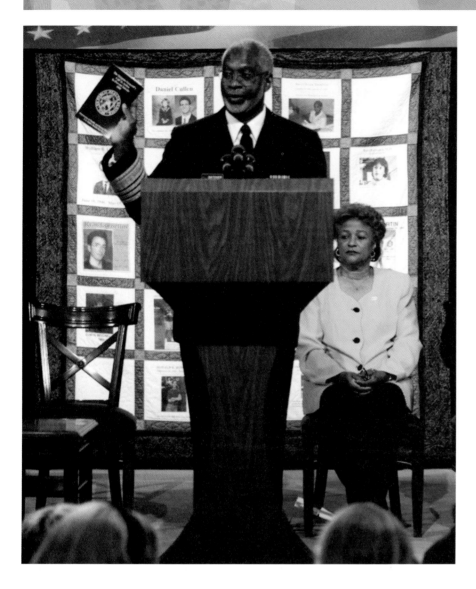

Bringing attention to suicide as a public health threat, Surgeon General David Satcher introduces his report, "Call to Action to Prevent Suicide." The plan's purpose is to encourage people to recognize symptoms and seek assistance.

Substance Abuse and Increased Suicide Risk

Suicides are not random. Each one occurs for particular reasons, such as depression or abuse of alcohol or drugs. Studying such high-risk groups is an important way to prevent suicides.

Researchers studying suicide try to discover what factors in a person's life contributed to his or her suicide. They interview the suicide victim's relatives, friends, and others and study the victim's medical records. They also consider suicide notes and coroner reports. Researchers then compare cases of completed suicide, cases of attempts at suicide, and cases of substance abusers who have never attempted suicide. The differences among these groups may help experts to identify those at particular risk of attempted or completed suicide.

Studies have shown that young adults who drink heavily have an increased risk of suicide in middle adulthood. People who are dependent on alcohol or drugs have an increased risk of death from accidents, disease, and suicide. In fact, suicide is among the most significant causes of death in both male and female substance abusers.

Risk Factors for Suicide Attempts

The strongest risk factors for attempted suicide in adults are depression, alcohol abuse, cocaine use, and separation or divorce. The strongest risk factors for attempted suicide in youth are depression, alcohol or other drug use disorder (including binge drinking and substance abuse), and aggressive or disruptive behaviors. The frequency of suicide attempts among substance abusers is five times greater than the frequency among people who do not abuse substances. This is particularly true for alcoholics, because major depression is 50 percent more common among alcoholics than nonalcoholics. Many people drink alcohol or use drugs such as cocaine to reduce feelings of depression. However, drinking and drug use can actually lead to greater anxiety, depression, and thoughts of suicide. Many people recovering from heroin addiction make suicide attempts.

antisocial personality disorder condition in which people disregard the rights of others and violate these rights by acting in immoral, unethical, aggressive, or even criminal ways

Another psychological disorder that increases the risk for suicide attempts is **antisocial personality disorder** (ASP). This disorder typically affects males who have a genetic **predisposition** for alcoholism. Many males with ASP also abuse drugs.

predisposition condition in which one is vulnerable or prone to something

Drug abusers often have feelings of being unwell or unhappy. Although these feelings may not last long enough to qualify as major depression, they may nonetheless increase drug abusers' risk of attempting suicide. In addition, there is a relationship between injecting drugs and suicide attempts. Addicts who inject drugs are aware that they are engaging in high-risk behaviors and may be less concerned about their well-being overall. Alcoholics and drug addicts often lose their jobs and have troubled relationships. These problems increase their risk of making a suicide attempt.

Risk Factors for Completed Suicide

schizophrenia psychotic disorder in which people lose the ability to function normally, experience severe personality changes, and suffer from a variety of symptoms, including confusion, disordered thinking, paranoia, hallucinations, emotional numbness, and speech problems

The major risk factors for completed suicide among alcoholics are: (1) current drinking, (2) major depression, (3) suicidal thoughts, (4) loss of support from family and friends, (5) living alone, and (6) unemployment. Less is known about how these risk factors affect other substance abusers.

Depression and Other Psychiatric Conditions. Psychiatric conditions such as depression, **schizophrenia**, and ASP play an important role in the suicide of alcoholics and drug abusers. The vast majority of suicide victims have symptoms of depression at the time of their death. At least 50 percent of alcoholics and drug abusers who commit suicide also had depression. Depression is just as likely to affect young people as adults.

Long-Term Use. Long-term substance use makes suicide more likely. Nearly all alcoholic suicides occur among active drinkers, and the person often drinks alcohol immediately before the suicide. An alcoholic who remains **abstinent** has a lower risk of suicide.

Major Life Disruption. The strongest indicator of suicide risk in substance abusers is a major interpersonal loss such as separation or divorce. Among young people, parents' divorce, family violence, a breakup with a boyfriend or girlfriend, stress to perform and achieve, and school failure may trigger suicides. Many suicidal teens report feelings of inner turmoil, chaos, and low self-worth. Also, hopelessness and anger often contribute to adolescent suicide. Most of these problems are associated with both substance abuse and suicide. In other words, troubled or depressed young people may turn first to alcohol or drugs as a means of coping, and later attempt or commit suicide. Other personal problems a substance abuser may face are being unemployed, living alone, and/or lacking the support of family and friends at the time of this final and most severe upset. The individual's expectations of the future may also increase the risk of suicide. For example, a substance abuser may be worried that an overwhelming problem, such as legal or financial trouble, is about to happen. Alcoholics who develop serious medical problems, such as liver disease, pancreatitis, or peptic ulcers, are also at higher risk of suicide.

Prevention

In the months prior to their suicides, substance abusers often see a doctor or are hospitalized for psychiatric problems. Those who talk of suicide may have mixed or confused feelings about their wish to die. Treating the substance abuse problems as well as the mental health problems of these individuals can help them to conquer their wish to die.

Predicting who will complete suicide remains difficult, even among high-risk groups such as substance abusers. Doctors and other health-care professionals often fail to recognize alcoholism and drug abuse in patients and the signs of depression that can lead to suicide. The substance abuser who has active suicide plans or has recently attempted suicide may need hospitalization, **detoxification**, or rehabilitation designed to encourage abstinence from alcohol and drugs

RELATED READING

In *The Power to Prevent Suicide: A Guide for Teens Helping Teens* (1994), authors Richard E. Nelson and Judith C. Galas share insight into the warning signs for suicide, and encourage young adults to reach out to their friends in danger. The book describes how a student can help other teenagers, and it lists organizations such as crisis centers as well.

abstinent describing someone who completely avoids something, such as a drug or alcohol

detoxification process of removing a poisonous, intoxicating, or addictive substance from the body

of abuse. Firearms should be removed from the homes of substance abusers who talk about suicide, especially adolescents and young adults.

Making sure that a person at risk of suicide finds treatment for mental health and substance use problems, as well as increasing social support from family, friends, and health-care professionals, can reduce the risk of suicide. SEE ALSO ACCIDENTS AND INJURIES FROM ALCOHOL; ACCIDENTS AND INJURIES FROM DRUGS; USERS.

Tax Laws and Alcohol

excise tax tax that a government puts on the manufacture, sale, or use of a domestic product

Americans contribute to the income of state and federal government through taxes. Some taxes are sales taxes on everything from gasoline to CDs. Other taxes come out of people's paychecks. The very first tax the U.S. Congress required its citizens to pay was an **excise tax** on domestic whiskey. When that tax was increased from 9 to 25 cents per gallon, farmers of western Pennsylvania staged an armed revolt during the summer of 1794. This revolt is known as the Whiskey Rebellion. Taxing alcoholic beverages has remained a controversial issue to this day. Most policy makers agree that alcoholic beverages should be subject to higher taxes than other items. However, many disagree about the appropriate level for such taxes.

The main reason the government imposes taxes is to gain revenue, or income. Alcoholic beverage taxes have been a major source of funds for the federal government throughout much of U.S. history. In 1907 these taxes accounted for 80 percent of federal internal tax collections. Just before World War II, taxes on alcohol accounted for 10 percent of internal tax collections. Today, taxes on alcoholic beverages continue to affect the prices of alcoholic beverages, but they account for only a small portion (less than 1%) of federal tax collections.

The states also require special excise taxes on alcoholic beverages, as do some local governments. In addition, alcoholic beverages are generally subject to state and local sales taxes. As of 2000 less than 10 percent of revenues for state and local governments came from alcoholic beverage taxes. But revenue is not the only reason that the government imposes taxes. Since the 1970s public officials have supported higher taxes on alcohol as a way to protect public health. Research has shown that the number of traffic fatalities and other costly consequences of alcohol abuse declines as the tax rate on alcohol, and therefore its price, increases.

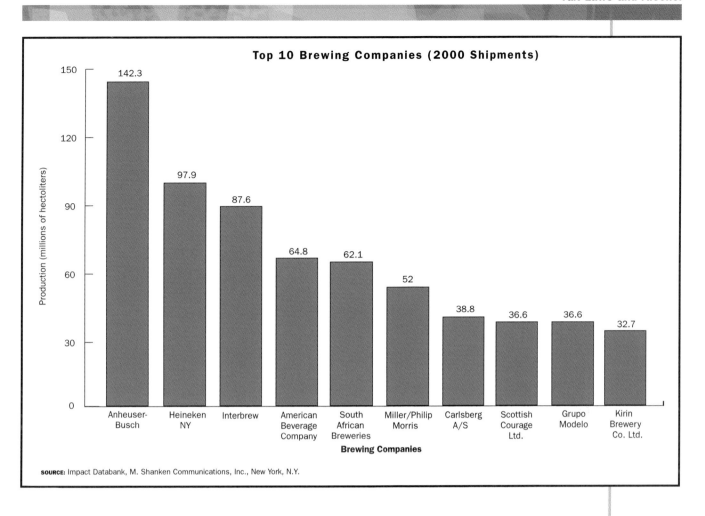

Top 10 Brewing Companies (2000 Shipments)

SOURCE: Impact Databank, M. Shanken Communications, Inc., New York, N.Y.

The Effects of Alcohol Taxes

When a legislature raises tax rates on liquor, wine, and beer, the resulting cost to distributors is passed along to consumers in the form of higher prices. The sales of alcoholic beverages tend to fall when prices increase. Studies show that when the average price of liquor increases by a certain percentage, the quantity of liquor sold generally decreases by the same percentage. Price is a less important factor in the sales of beer and wine.

Price is not the only factor that determines sales. For example, in the 1980s sales and consumption of alcohol declined steadily. This decline cannot be explained by increased prices, since the prices of alcoholic beverages remained more or less constant during this period. Instead, the increasing average age of the population and increasing public concern with healthy lifestyles probably caused this downward trend in alcohol consumption.

Aside from increasing prices and reducing sales, higher taxes on alcohol can have other effects. Evidence suggests that higher alcoholic beverage taxes can prevent public health hazards caused by

Anheuser-Busch, maker of Budweiser, Michelob, Busch, Tequiza, Bacardi, and other alcoholic beverages, was the world's top brewing company in 2000.

productivity quality of yielding results or benefits

drinking. These hazards include injuries from accidents and violent crime, as well as poor health and reduced **productivity** caused by long-term heavy drinking.

One study examined thirty-nine instances in which states increased their liquor tax over a fifteen-year period. Traffic fatalities in those states fell. Increased taxes on beer also produced reductions in state traffic fatality rates. Another study found a close link between alcohol consumption and violent crime rates. An increase in the beer tax helped reduce the number of rapes and robberies in the states that were studied. In other research, a study claimed that higher taxes on beer also reduce sexually transmitted diseases. Higher alcohol prices may also reduce rates of chronic heavy drinking. In one study, researchers found that state liquor taxes could be linked with the death rate from **cirrhosis** of the liver, a disease caused by years of heavy drinking. An inverse relationship exists: As the liquor tax rate increases, the death rate from cirrhosis of the liver decreases.

cirrhosis condition in which the liver is scarred from long term–liver disease; symptoms include weakness, nausea, and confusion

Some critics question the results of the various studies showing a link between higher alcohol taxes and lower rates of accidents, crime, and disease. However, results of these studies support the conclusion that raising alcohol taxes can reduce inebriation (drunkenness) and improve health and safety. These results may play an important role in the public debate over whether to raise alcohol taxes.

Fairness

Although alcohol taxes can reduce consumption and save some lives that would otherwise be lost to alcohol-related accidents, some still question whether these taxes are fair. For example, is it fair that alcohol taxes force drinkers to pay more taxes than nondrinkers of similar incomes? Most alcohol taxes are paid by heavy drinkers, a small minority of the population. One response is that it is fair for drinkers to pay more, because they and no one else are consuming the alcohol. Also, when accidents do occur as a result of drinking, victims share in the cost as they cope with injuries and loss.

IN THEIR OWN WORDS

"[Congress should] impose such heavy duties upon distilled spirits as shall be effective to restrain their intemperate use in the country."

—Benjamin Rush (1745–1813), American physician and member of Continental Congress, petitioning U.S. Congress in 1790.

Another debated issue is that of uniform taxation. A 12-ounce can of beer, a 4-ounce glass of wine, and a 1.25-ounce shot of spirits all contain approximately the same amount of alcohol, but each is taxed differently. The federal tax on a shot of spirits is about twice as high as the tax on a can of beer and about three times as high as the tax on a glass of wine. These differences may be due to the widespread belief that spirits are more intoxicating than beer or wine, and therefore more subject to abuse. Many people think of beer as a drink of moderation and wine as an elegant drink for connoisseurs. But much of the evidence works against this view. In fact, statistics show that beer consumption may be more costly to society (per drink) than spirits. Young men, a group that consumes most of their alcohol in the form of beer, have by far the highest rate of alcohol-related traffic accidents and violent crimes.

Taxes on alcohol have come to serve two purposes. The tax on alcohol, considered a user tax, provides a steady stream of income to the government. In addition, this tax is also sometimes referred to as a sin tax because it represents an attitude toward the consumption of alcohol. Because the tax increases the price of beer, wine, or spirits, some people are discouraged from drinking, while others may moderate their use of alcohol.

Tea

Tea is the most widely consumed beverage in the world, except for water. Over 40 percent of the world's caffeine intake comes from tea. In the United States, caffeine from tea accounts for about 17 percent of caffeine consumed. On average, a 6-ounce cup of leaf or bag tea contains about 48 milligrams of caffeine, a little less than half the caffeine in the same amount of ground roasted coffee, and only slightly more than the amount found in 12 ounces of a cola soft drink. Single servings of tea contain amounts of caffeine that can affect people's moods and performance. SEE ALSO CAFFEINE; CHOCOLATE; COLA DRINKS.

Temperance Movement

In the United States in the 1800s, many organized groups spoke out against drinking. Together, these groups are known as the temperance movement. Temperance means moderation, but in fact many of the reformers in the movement pressed for abstinence, or drinking no alcohol at all. The influence of the temperance movement culminated in 1920 in Prohibition, a period during which the sale of alcohol was illegal.

Many temperance movements that emerged in the United States included men and women from varying ethnic, religious, social, economic, and political groups. They focused on temperance as the solution to problems in their own lives and in those of others. Over the course of the 1800s the strategies used by temperance proponents

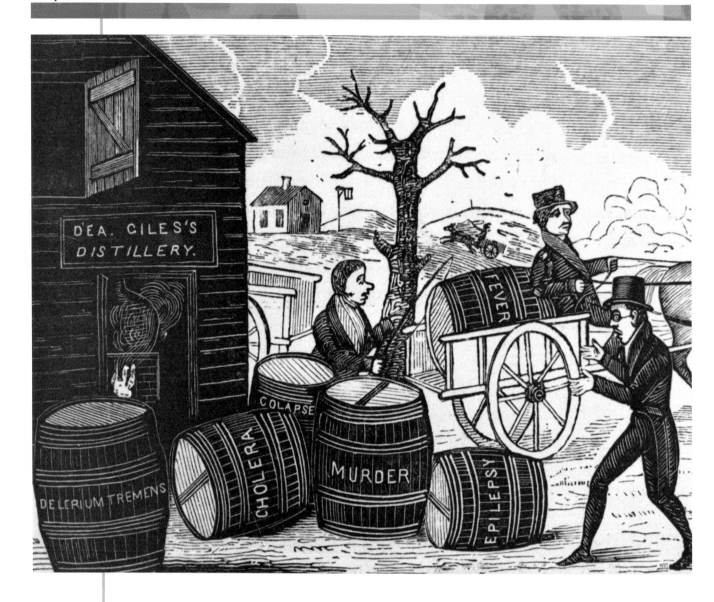

In early nineteenth-century United States, organized groups began a movement against the drinking of alcohol. This political cartoon from 1820 attempts to dramatize the ills of alcohol by placing negative labels such as "murder" and "fever" on alcohol barrels.

changed. They began by trying to persuade people to drink only moderate amounts of alcoholic beverages. By the end of the century, their efforts became more coercive, with proponents pushing for laws to bring about the end of drinking.

Early Phase: 1800–1840

In colonial America and during the early 1800s, alcoholic beverages (brewed, fermented, and distilled) were an important part of the American diet. Many of these beverages were homemade, and people viewed them as "the good creature of God." Among the colonists, all social groups and age groups drank alcoholic beverages, and the consumption rate was very high. Alcohol was also traded, sold, and given to Native Americans. These peoples did not have a history of daily drinking, and for them alcohol had almost immediate negative consequences.

By 1840 a revolution in American social attitudes had occurred. Alcohol came to be seen as "the root of all evil" and the cause of the major problems of the young nation, such as crime, poverty, immorality, and insanity. Important figures such as Thomas Jefferson; Anthony Benezet, a popular Quaker reformer; and Benjamin Rush, the surgeon general of the Continental Army and a signer of the Declaration of Independence, called for temperance as the solution. Temperance advocates formed organizations such as the American Temperance Society to eliminate these social problems.

The American Temperance Society, founded in Boston in 1826, was the first national (as opposed to local) temperance organization. The people who developed the movement wanted to bring about economic and social change. They believed in educating Americans to value sobriety and hard work, in order to create a society with flourishing industry and commerce. Entrepreneurs who were developing businesses supported the movement, because they needed a disciplined and sober workforce.

In a period called the Great Awakening, many religious leaders of the Evangelical and other Protestant churches supported temperance as a way to promote the morality needed for building a "Christian nation." These religious groups helped to make drinking a public and political issue. Also, in the 1820s and 1830s, small-scale farmers and rural groups actively supported the temperance movement. They saw temperance as a way to bring about social progress as the country changed from a rural economy based on small farms to an urban-industrial economy based on larger agricultural networks.

By 1836 the American Temperance Society had become an abstinence society, and ideas about problems associated with alcohol had begun to change. Members began to call constant drunkenness a disease. They believed that alcohol was an addictive substance, a finding supported by the research of Rush. The American Temperance Society tried to persuade people who already were temperate to become abstinent. They did not try to persuade people whom they called "drunkards"—the modern term "alcoholics" came into use later—to reform their drinking behavior. (Attempts to reform and save drunkards was the focus of another temperance movement, the Washingtonians.) In response to the temperance movement, the public began to view the industrious, steady American worker as someone who never took a drink.

Middle Phase: 1840–1860

Well-to-do groups and Protestant evangelical clergy dominated the early phase of temperance reform. In the middle phase, artisans

> ### THE COST OF A LIVING
>
> "I do not say a dollar a day is enough to support a working man, but it is enough to support a man. Not enough to support a man and five children if a man insists on smoking and drinking beer."
>
> —Henry Ward Beecher, American clergyman and writer. Quoted in *Harper's Weekly,* May 8, 1886.

(craftsmen) and women of the lower and lower-middle classes joined the effort. They formed self-help groups among largely working-class drunkards trying to give up drinking. These artisans organized into the Washingtonian societies (named for George Washington), dedicated to helping working-class drunkards who were trying to reform.

In 1840 the first Washingtonian Temperance Society was established in Baltimore. Members took a pledge against the use of all alcoholic beverages and attempted to convert drunkards to the pledge of teetotalism (a word first used in 1834, formed from the "t" in "total" and the word "total" to mean abstinence). By the end of 1841, Washingtonian societies were active in Baltimore, Boston, New York, and other areas in the Northeast.

Washingtonian members remained with the mainstream temperance movement. The wage earners and reformed drunkards stayed with their own societies, and they opposed early efforts at controlling drinking through the law. Beginning in 1851, many local laws were passed that attempted to limit the use of alcohol. However, throughout the rest of the century, some of these laws were repealed, some were made less strict, and many simply were not enforced.

Late Phase: 1860–1920

During the last phase of the temperance movement, American society went through many changes as a result of the Civil War, World War I, and immigration. In expanding urban areas and in factory towns, there was more socializing at the end of the workday as well as at the end of the workweek. There was also more alcohol being produced and consumed. Several temperance societies that emerged during this period included the active participation of women and children, because wives and children were often neglected or abused by drunken husbands and fathers. Irish-American Catholics formed the Catholic Total Abstention Union in 1872; the Woman's Christian Temperance Union (WCTU) was formed in 1874; and the Anti-Saloon League (ASL) emerged in 1896. These societies were able to build tremendous support for abstinence rather than mere moderation or decrease in drinking. The temperance movements emphasized the evil effects of all alcohol and named alcohol as the central problem in American life. They insisted that abstinence was the only solution for this problem.

The WCTU was the first mainstream temperance organization to involve women and children. Its creative and dynamic leaders were Annie Wittenmyer, Frances Willard, and Carry Nation, who also supported the feminist movement, a radical move at the time. The

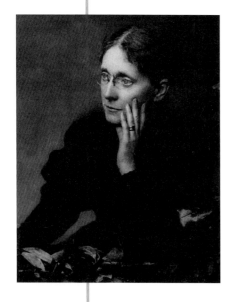

Frances Willard was a leader in the Woman's Christian Temperance Union, which was the first mainstream temperance organization to involve women and children.

WCTU began a crusade to shut down saloons and promote morality. By the late 1800s, the major theme of the temperance movement was the push for legal controls on drinking. The ASL was at the forefront of this effort, raising tremendous support for abstinence instead of just temperance. The ASL always stressed prohibition as its main goal and was very successful at working peacefully with the major political parties. By 1912 local prohibition laws had been passed making most of the South legally dry, or free from alcohol.

In 1917 the United States's entry into World War I boosted the cause of national prohibition. The ASL pushed for a halt to industrial distilling of alcohol (ethanol). Very shortly after the United States joined the war, the selling of liquor near military bases and to servicemen in uniform was prohibited. By 1918 the Eighteenth Amendment to the U.S. Constitution had been proposed, and the ASL had pushed prohibition through thirty-three state legislatures. Consequently, the Volstead Act—called Prohibition—was ratified on January 16, 1919. It went into effect one year later, on January 16, 1920, prohibiting the manufacture, sale, or transportation of alcoholic beverages.

Conclusion

The temperance movement stressed the theme of self-control. This theme appealed mainly to the American middle class but also to some members of the working class. Middle-class people saw the rich as greedy, the working class as restless, and the poor as uneducated immigrants. They felt the need to restore a strong moral foundation, and abstinence was the policy they thought would best bring about morality. Other reform groups, such as the Progressive political party, joined the prohibitionists in their effort to rid cities of saloons so that the United States could move toward becoming a virtuous and moral nation. At the end of the nineteenth century, the American public was receptive to moral arguments for temperance reform and abstinence from alcohol. SEE ALSO ALCOHOL TREATMENT: BEHAVIORAL APPROACHES; ALCOHOL TREATMENT: MEDICATIONS; LAW AND POLICY: DRUG LEGALIZATION DEBATE.

Terrorism and Drugs

Narcoterrorism is shorthand for the close ties that exist between illegal **narcotics** and terrorists. The U.S. Drug Enforcement Administration (DEA) uses the term to refer to situations in which terrorist groups or their members have some part in growing, producing,

> Liquor traffic is un-American, pro-German, crime-procuring, food-wasting, youth-corrupting, home-wrecking, reasonable.
>
> —Anti-Saloon League, statement, 1918.

narcotic addictive substance that relieves pain and induces sleep or causes sedation; prescription narcotics includes morphine and codeine; general and imprecise term referring to a drug of abuse, such as heroin, cocaine, or marijuana

transporting, or selling illegal drugs. However, the specific role that different terrorist groups play can take many forms.

Traffickers in Terror

drug traffickers people or groups who transport illegal drugs

The relationship between **drug traffickers** and terrorists is reciprocal, meaning that they influence each other. The traffickers can benefit from the military skills, weapons, and underground networks of the terrorists. Where the terrorists control large chunks of territory, the traffickers gain by being able to move around freely as well. In return, the terrorists get a steady stream of income from drug money. They also may learn useful tricks of the criminal trade, such as smuggling and **money laundering**.

money laundering activity in which a person or group hides the source of money that has been illegally obtained

The two groups are natural allies, because they have a lot in common. Terrorists and drug producers both tend to thrive in rugged, remote areas where government control is weak and economic conditions are poor. Both groups also make use of countries where banking regulations are lax. In addition, they often team up with corrupt officials, who can provide fake passports, customs papers, and other documents.

Many terrorists involved in the drug trade are guerrillas, self-styled soldiers who are not members of any regular army, but who wage war through unconventional means. These guerrillas often make money by forcing drug growers and traffickers to pay "war taxes." In such cases, the relationship between the two groups may be rooted in conflict rather than cooperation. Still, the groups may be brought together for a time by local family or personal ties. At other times, they may band together to fight the government when it tries to regain control of an area.

Guerrilla Groups

Colombia has been particularly hard hit by the terrorist acts of guerrilla groups linked to the drug trade. These groups include the Revolutionary Armed Forces of Colombia (FARC) and the National Liberation Army (ELN). The FARC—the largest, best-trained, and best-equipped guerrilla group in the country—operates in the eastern lowlands and rain forest. This is the area where coca, the plant from which cocaine comes, is grown. The ELN operates in the northern and central parts of Colombia. These are growing areas for the hemp plant, from which marijuana and hashish are derived, and the opium poppy, from which morphine and heroin are derived.

In the 1980s and early 1990s, a Colombian drug trafficking group led by Pablo Escobar staged a series of vicious terrorist attacks. Among

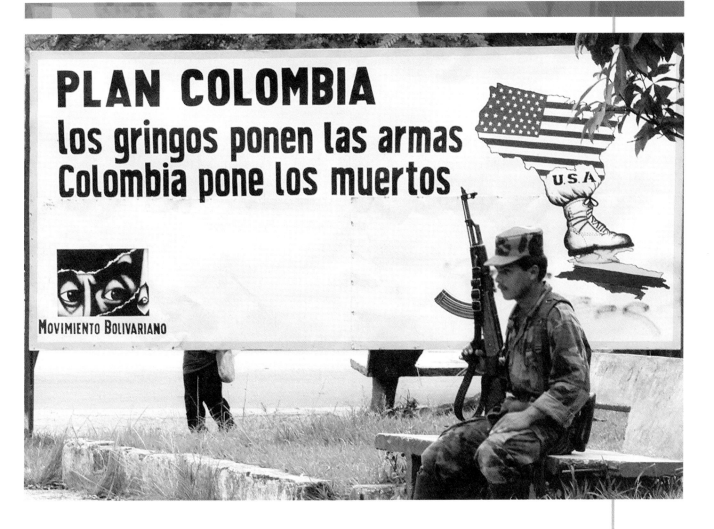

PLAN COLOMBIA
los gringos ponen las armas
Colombia pone los muertos

U.S.A

MOVIMIENTO BOLIVARIANO

the victims and targets were a justice minister, an attorney general, the editor of a leading newspaper, several presidential candidates, and a commercial airliner. Escobar died in 1993, but this did not bring an end to Colombia's troubles. By the dawn of the twenty-first century, violent terrorist acts were still a daily fact of life in that country. In 2000 the U.S. government gave Colombia $1.3 billion in emergency funds to help fight the threat. However, it remains to be seen whether these funds, plus additional military aid, will stop narco-terrorism.

Around the world, several other guerrilla groups have used the potent mix of terror and drugs to advance their aims. In Peru, the Sendero Luminoso (Shining Path) is an extremely violent group that tried to overthrow the government in the 1980s and 1990s. The group is based in remote areas where coca is grown, and it is thought that a source of income for them has been taxes paid by cocaine producers. In the Middle East, the Kurdistan Workers Party (PKK) also has forced drug traffickers to pay taxes in return for protection. In Southeast Asia, guerrillas have long been involved in every stage of the

Colombia has been particularly hard hit by the terrorist acts of guerrilla groups, such as the Revolutionary Armed Forces of Colombia (FARC). A FARC soldier is pictured here with his weapon.

opium/heroin pipeline. And on the Indian peninsula, groups such as the Tamil Tigers (LTTE) and the Sikhs have called on community members living abroad to help them smuggle heroin.

A Global Problem

One disturbing trend is the ease with which terrorist groups from one part of the world may move into another, where they can go about their business in relative safety. For example, two Islamic extremist groups from the Middle East—Hezbollah and the Islamic Resistance Movement (HAMAS)—have set up camp in the border region of Paraguay, Argentina, and Brazil. It is suspected that their illegal activities there include drug smuggling.

In Mexico, government crackdowns against the drug trade also have been met with terrorism. For example, in 2000 the police chief of Tijuana was killed as he drove to his office, two days after the government announced a tough new antidrug policy. However, these attacks seem to have been committed by drug traffickers rather than guerrilla groups. Italy, too, has seen its share of drug violence. During the 1980s and early 1990s, the Sicilian Mafia reacted to tighter government control by killing several leading prosecutors and law enforcement officers. In the early twenty-first century there is also growing concern about the dangerous mix of drugs, violence, and organized crime in parts of the former Soviet Union.

Terrorism Strikes Home

Perhaps the most notorious example of the drug-terror link, however, involves the former Taliban government in Afghanistan. In 2000 this country produced 70 percent of the world's illegal opium supply. Heroin, morphine base, and hashish produced there were sold worldwide. In fact, this flourishing drug trade was the war-torn nation's biggest moneymaker. At the same time, Afghanistan served as home base for terrorist Osama bin Laden and his Al Qaeda network, believed to be behind the September 11, 2001, attacks on the World Trade Center and the Pentagon. According to the DEA, bin Laden himself is suspected of being involved in the trafficking of heroin.

The relationship between the Taliban, drugs, and terrorism is complex, however. Before the attack in 2001, Taliban leaders declared heroin to be anti-Islam. They vowed to ban opium growing and to steer farmers toward crops to help feed the nation's poor. The U.S. government estimated that opium production in Afghanistan in 2001 was only about 2 percent of the amount produced there in 2000. Yet

U.S. officials also say the ban may have been largely a ploy to drive up opium prices by limiting the supply. In fact, the Taliban had long relied on drug trafficking as its major source of income.

Since the September 11 terrorist attacks, government officials and antidrug groups in the United States have been sending a new message to teens: Drugs and terrorism go hand in hand. When you choose one, you support the other. The message seems to be having an impact. In two polls taken in late 2001, young people said they would be less likely to use illegal drugs if they knew that the drug trade helps pay for terrorism. SEE ALSO CRIME AND DRUGS; DRUG PRODUCERS; DRUG TRAFFICKERS; LAW AND POLICY: FOREIGN POLICY AND DRUGS.

Tobacco: Dependence

Just under a quarter of all adults in the United States were current cigarette smokers as of 1999. Although it is illegal in every state to sell cigarettes to people under age 18, about 28 percent of high-school students and 9 percent of middle-school students were smokers as well. In addition, about 6 percent of adult males and 12 percent of high-school boys used smokeless tobacco. No matter what their age, most tobacco users say they want to quit. The reason they have such a tough time doing so is because of nicotine, a naturally occurring, colorless liquid that is the addictive substance in tobacco. Nicotine can be as addictive as heroin or cocaine. Because it has such powerful effects, many tobacco users have to try to quit several times before they succeed.

Nicotine Addiction

Nicotine's effects on the brain are similar to those of other drugs of abuse. Nicotine activates the brain's pleasure center, where it raises levels of dopamine, a brain chemical that plays a key role in controlling the desire to use a drug. Several properties of nicotine increase its addictive nature. When a person smokes a cigarette, nicotine gets to the brain within seconds after every puff. A typical smoker takes ten puffs on a cigarette, delivering nicotine to the brain ten times. Yet the immediate effects wear off within a few minutes, which makes the person want to smoke again and again throughout the day. This not only keeps up the pleasant feelings, but also wards off withdrawal, the unpleasant symptoms that arise soon after a person stops or cuts back on using an addictive substance. The symptoms of nicotine withdrawal include anxiety, irritability, difficulty

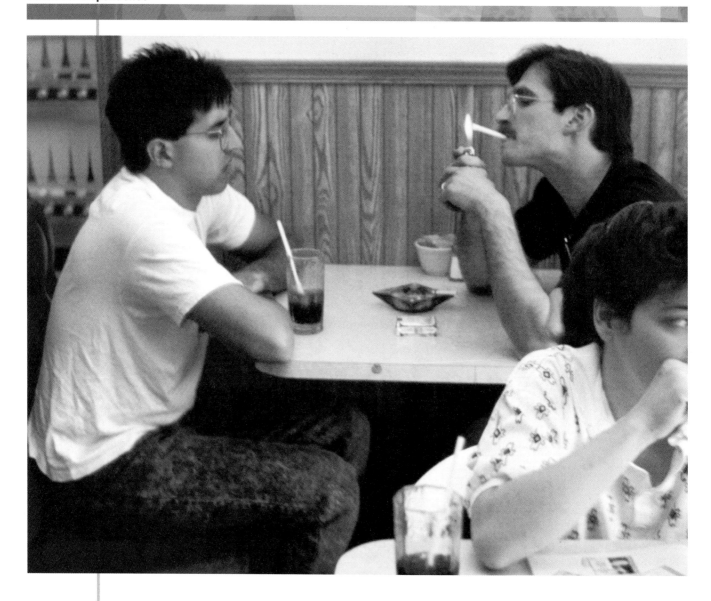

In 1999 just under 25 percent of Americans were current cigarette smokers. Although many smokers say they would like to quit, nicotine—an addictive drug found in cigarettes—makes quitting challenging.

withdrawal physical and psychological symptoms that may occur when a person suddenly stops the use of a substance or reduces the dose of an addictive substance

concentrating, restlessness, hunger, depression, insomnia (having trouble sleeping), and craving for tobacco.

In addition to its direct effects on the body, nicotine also acts indirectly on the mind, through a learning process called conditioning. This process occurs when the physical effects of nicotine occur repeatedly in the presence of specific environmental factors. Over time, these factors can become cues for using tobacco. For example, many nonsmokers find the smell of cigarette smoke a turnoff. After repeatedly pairing this smell with the effects of nicotine, though, smokers often learn to like it. In much the same way, smokers may learn to associate lighting up a cigarette with eating a snack, talking on the phone, or hanging out with friends who also smoke. When they stop smoking, they face not only physical **withdrawal**, but also a psychological challenge: dealing with experiences that, through learning, have become cues to use tobacco.

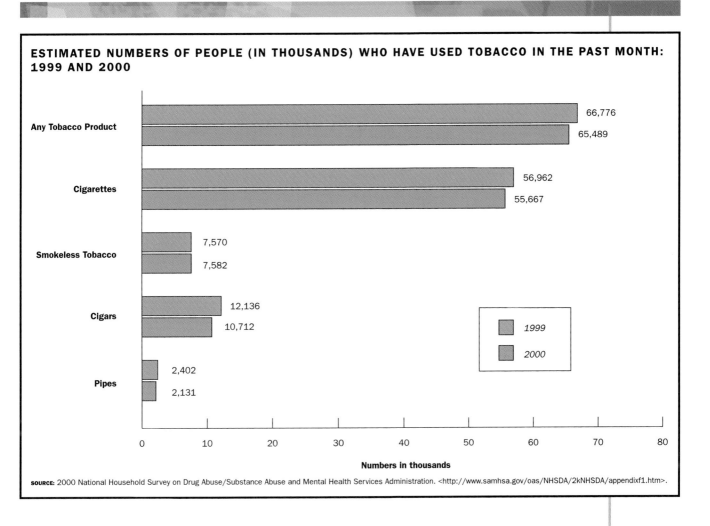

ESTIMATED NUMBERS OF PEOPLE (IN THOUSANDS) WHO HAVE USED TOBACCO IN THE PAST MONTH: 1999 AND 2000

Numbers in thousands

SOURCE: 2000 National Household Survey on Drug Abuse/Substance Abuse and Mental Health Services Administration. <http://www.samhsa.gov/oas/NHSDA/2kNHSDA/appendixf1.htm>.

Quitting the Tobacco Habit

The physical and psychological effects of nicotine explain why tobacco use is such a tough habit to quit. Of all addictions, this is the one most likely to become established during the teen years. About three-quarters of young people who use tobacco daily say the reason they keep doing so is because they find it hard to quit. Similarly, almost half of adult smokers try to stop each year, but most need at least two or three tries before they are successful. Among the common reasons people of all ages give for wanting to quit are to take care of their own health, to protect the health of those around them, to fit into nonsmoking situations, and to save money.

People trying to give up tobacco typically go through a series of stages:

1. Precontemplation—During this stage, the person is using tobacco and is not motivated to stop. He or she is not yet contemplating, or thinking about, quitting.

Tobacco use experienced a slight decline between 1999 and 2000; cigarettes remain the most popular form of tobacco product among users.

2. Contemplation—The person is motivated to stop but has not yet picked a firm quit date in the near future.

3. Action—The person has a quit date along with a plan that has already been put into action or soon will be.

4. Maintenance—The person has stopped the regular, daily use of tobacco for at least one month.

Even after they reach the maintenance stage, however, people still face the risk of relapse, or a return to the old, undesirable behavior (in this case, smoking). Many probably agree with author Mark Twain, who said, "To cease smoking is the easiest thing I ever did; I ought to know because I've done it a thousand times." The hard truth is that 66 percent of smokers who try to quit on their own or with little outside help relapse within two days, and up to 97 percent relapse within one year. Common reasons for backsliding include withdrawal symptoms, environmental cues that make the person want to smoke, and emotional factors, such as stress or **depression**.

depression state in which an individual feels intensely sad and hopeless; may have trouble eating, sleeping, and concentrating, and is no longer able to feel pleasure from previously enjoyable activities; in extreme cases, may lead an individual to think about or attempt suicide

Managing the Urge to Smoke

Giving up smoking means more than just quitting cigarettes. It also means adopting a new, tobacco-free lifestyle. One key is learning to handle the environmental cues that trigger smoking. For example, it may help for people to throw away their cigarettes, lighters, and ashtrays and spend more time in places where smoking is not allowed, such as shopping malls or movie theaters. It also may help to stay busy, as a way to keep from focusing on the urge to smoke. In addition, it can be encouraging to seek support from friends and family members who have been through the same thing. Some people miss having something to put in their mouth. For them, it may help to carry substitutes, such as chewing gum, sunflower seeds, or carrot sticks. Since weight gain is common after giving up smoking, any snacks should be low calorie.

One useful strategy is setting realistic, short-term goals, such as making it through a whole day without smoking. When a goal is met, people can give themselves a little reward, such as spending time on a favorite hobby or buying a treat with the money saved by not buying cigarettes. It helps to maintain a positive attitude, too. Instead of thinking about the pleasures of smoking, people can substitute thoughts about the risks of tobacco, the benefits of quitting, or the pleasures of the reward for not smoking. Finally, many smokers get into the habit of reaching for a cigarette whenever they are under stress. Since giving up smoking can be stressful in itself, they need to find new ways to relax, such as taking deep breaths, meditating, or exercising.

Most people who try to make such a big lifestyle change will have a slip or two. Smoking one cigarette does not mean that all is lost. It simply means that the person needs to refocus on the effort to stop. When it comes to giving up tobacco, persistence pays off. Quitting is difficult, but it is not impossible, as more than 44 million ex-smokers in the United States have discovered.

Getting Help with Quitting

Most people who give up smoking do so on their own. People who want to quit can get guidance from their doctor; a local hospital; nonprofit organizations, such as the American Lung Association or the American Cancer Society; and government agencies, such as the state health department or the Centers for Disease Control and Prevention. ☎ In addition, many communities have self-help groups for people trying to stop smoking. People who take part in such groups can share practical tips on quitting and get moral support from others.

☎ See *Organizations of Interest* at the back of Volume 3 for address, telephone, and URL.

Antismoking medications can be very helpful as well. Research shows that the use of such medications can almost double a person's chances of quitting for good. Some are sold only by prescription, while others are available over the counter. However, certain people should talk to a doctor before trying a medication. These include young people under age 18, women who are pregnant or trying to become pregnant, new mothers who are breast-feeding, people who have a medical condition, and those who smoke fewer than ten cigarettes per day.

One form of medication is replacement nicotine, given in the form of gum, a patch, an inhaler, or a nasal spray. The idea behind nicotine-replacement therapy is that it can reduce the severity of nicotine withdrawal. Yet the amount of nicotine taken in is less than with cigarettes, and it does not come with the other toxins found in cigarette smoke, such as carbon monoxide and tar. Another option is bupropion SR (Zyban), a non-nicotine medication that can reduce withdrawal symptoms and the weight gain that often goes along with quitting smoking.

Other approaches have been tried as well. Professional counseling can be quite effective, especially if it involves specific training in how to identify and cope with smoking cues. Hypnosis is a technique that brings on a state of focused concentration in which people are highly responsive to suggestion. While under hypnosis, a person might be given suggestions such as "smoking is a poison to your body" or "you owe your body respect and protection." This can be useful for some people, particularly when combined with other counseling methods. Acupuncture is a traditional Chinese medical technique in which thin needles or staples are placed at certain points on the body. For people trying to give up smoking, these points are often placed on the ears. However, there is little hard evidence that acupuncture works for this purpose.

Giving up Smokeless Tobacco

People who use smokeless tobacco typically have blood levels of nicotine throughout the day that are comparable to those of cigarette smokers. When they try to stop, they go through nicotine withdrawal, too. Less research has been done on treatment for people trying to give up smokeless tobacco. However, the U.S. Public Health Service (PHS) says guidance and counseling may help these people beat their addiction as well. The general approach is similar to that used for cigarettes, but the specific cues involved may differ. For example, there may be a stronger need for gum or snacks to take the place of the chew or snuff. On the other hand, the PHS says there is not enough evidence that medications increase long-term quit rates in this group.

Conclusion

Getting outside help may make it easier to overcome any form of tobacco dependence. There is no such thing as a simple cure, however. Any treatment must be combined with lifestyle changes that prepare the person to live without tobacco. It is a lot of work, but the effort is more than justified by the payoff: a longer, better life that is free of nicotine addiction. SEE ALSO COSTS OF SUBSTANCE ABUSE AND DEPENDENCE, ECONOMIC; NICOTINE; TOBACCO: INDUSTRY; TOBACCO: SMOKELESS; TOBACCO TREATMENT: AN OVERVIEW; TOBACCO TREATMENT: BEHAVIORAL APPROACHES; TOBACCO TREATMENT: MEDICATIONS.

Tobacco: History of

Tobacco generally refers to the leaves and other parts of certain South American plants used by Native Americans because of the nicotine the plant contains. Tobacco plants are a species of the genus *Nicotiana*, belonging to the Solanaceae (nightshade) family. Other members of this family of plants include potatoes, tomatoes, eggplants, belladonna, and petunias.

Two species are most widely grown for use as tobacco. The major source of commercial tobacco is *Nicotiana tabacum*, a broadleaf plant that grows from 3 to 10 feet tall and produces ten to twenty leaves radiating from a central stalk. *Nicotiana rustica*, which in fact contains higher levels of nicotine than *N. tabacum*, is also known as Indian tobacco. Native Americans were the first to cultivate this plant, and it was probably the tobacco offered to Christopher Columbus. The word "tobacco" entered the English language around 1565. It derives from the Spanish word *tabaco*, which was probably taken from the Taino word for the roll of leaves containing *N. rustica* that the American natives of the Antilles smoked.

The History of Tobacco Use

Native Americans introduced tobacco to Europeans at the time of Columbus's exploration of the New World (1492–1506). The first written records of tobacco use date from this time, but there is **archaeological** evidence for tobacco's wide use in the Americas as early as 600–900 C.E. Native Americans considered tobacco a sacred plant because it was used in important rituals. For example, tobacco was used for seasonal ceremonies, sealing friendships, preparing for war, predicting good weather or good fishing, planting, courting, consulting spirits, and preparing magical cures. The desired effects of tobacco were a **trance** state, achieved by using the leaves in various ways, including smoking, chewing, snuffing (inhaling), drinking in the form of tobacco juice or tea, licking, and administering enemas by inserting into the anus.

Acute nicotine poisoning was a central aspect of the religious practice known as **shamanism** in many parts of South America. South American shamans, or high priests, would smoke or ingest tobacco to the point of producing a trance or coma. The shaman was able to calculate how much nicotine he could take to produce a coma state resembling death but from which he would recover. His followers, witnessing his recovery from apparent death, would believe more strongly in the shaman's magical powers.

In 1492 Columbus encountered natives in Hispaniola, an island of the West Indies, smoking tobacco in the form of large cigars. Enticed by the sacred and special regard in which they held tobacco, Columbus's crew experimented with tobacco smoking and soon became **enthusiasts**. Tobacco was brought back to Europe and, within a few decades, its use spread. People smoked it in the form of cigars or in pipes and used it as snuff or chewing tobacco. Within forty years of Columbus's arrival, Spaniards were growing tobacco in the West Indies. Tobacco use then became widespread in Europe and in the American colonies held by Spain and Portugal by the late 1500s.

archaeological relating to the scientific study of material remains from past human life and activities

trance state of partial consciousness

shamanism religion whose leaders perform rituals of magic, divination, and healing and act as intermediaries between reality and the spirit world

enthusiast supporter

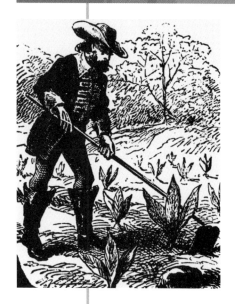

John Rolfe (1585–1622) tends a tobacco crop with a garden tool in Jamestown, Virginia, an English colony that made its first money by selling tobacco.

lucrative with the potential to make a lot of money

export merchandise shipped to another country as part of commercial business

In 1570 the tobacco plant was named "nicotiana" after Jean Nicot, the French ambassador to Portugal who introduced tobacco to France for medical purposes. Tobacco was said to be useful in the prevention of plague and as a cure for headache, asthma, gout, ulcers, scabies, labor pains, and even cancer. In the late 1500s Sir Walter Raleigh popularized the smoking of tobacco for pleasure in the court of Queen Elizabeth I (who reigned from 1558 to 1603); from there it spread to other parts of England.

James I of England (who reigned from 1603 to 1625), was strongly opposed to tobacco use and wrote the first major article opposing tobacco, titled "Counterblast to Tobacco," in 1604. King James described tobacco as "a custome loathsome to the eye, hateful to the nose, harmful to the brain, dangerous to the lungs, and in the black stinking fume thereof nearest resembling the horrible stygian [dark and gloomy] smoke of the pit that is bottomless." Despite James's opposition, however, tobacco use flourished. Eventually even James lessened his opposition to tobacco because of the **lucrative** income gained from taxing it.

During the 1600s tobacco use spread throughout Europe, Russia, China, Japan, and the west coast of Africa. Over the centuries, some rulers decreed harsh penalties for tobacco use. For example, Murad the Cruel of Turkey (who reigned from 1623 to 1640) ordered that tobacco users be beheaded, quartered, and/or hanged. Nevertheless, smoking persisted. In the American colonies, tobacco became the most important **export** crop and was of central importance in the economic survival of the colonies.

During the 1800s tobacco production was a central feature of American capitalism. Most tobacco was smoked as cigars or in pipes, or used as snuff. Cigarettes were hand-rolled. A skillful worker could roll four cigarettes per minute. Cigarette smokers were primarily boys or women of the lower class. The invention of the cigarette-rolling machine by James Bonsack in 1881 made tobacco use inexpensive and convenient. Bonsack went into business with W. B. Duke and Sons in Durham, North Carolina. Together they improved the machine, and by April 30, 1884, the device could roll 120,000 cigarettes per day.

Just as cigarettes were becoming widely available and affordable, tobacco manufacturers strongly promoted their use in massive advertising campaigns. Movie stars began to appear onscreen smoking cigarettes, which made the habit seem glamorous. The government issued cigarettes to soldiers during the world wars, and at home an increasing number of women began to smoke. All these factors increased the popularity of cigarette smoking in the United States and around the world in the mid-twentieth century. Smoking rates peaked in the United States for men in 1955, with 50 percent of men smoking, and in 1966 for women, with 32 percent of women smoking. As a result of clever marketing by the cigarette companies, smoking at that time was considered to be **sophisticated**, glamorous, individualistic, and even healthful.

sophisticated knowledgeable about the ways of the world; self-confident

While there had been occasional reports on the health hazards of cigarette smoking from the time of King James, the first large-scale studies showing the link between cigarette smoking and cancer appeared in the 1950s. Since then hundreds of studies have shown that cigarette smoking accounts for 30 percent of cancers—including some cancers of the lung, mouth, throat, esophagus, bladder, and kidney, as well as some leukemia, or blood cancer—and that it is the cause of some heart and **vascular** disease and stroke, emphysema and chronic obstructive lung disease, and other serious health problems. In 1962 the Royal College of Physicians in the United Kingdom and in 1964 the U.S. surgeon general issued reports on smoking and health, indicating that cigarette smoking most probably caused some lung cancers and other health problems. These reports marked the beginning of modern public-health efforts to control tobacco use.

vascular relating to the transport of fluids (such as blood or lymph fluid) through tubes in the body; frequently used to refer to the system of blood vessels

Landmarks in tobacco control in the United States include the following:

- 1965—Federal Cigarette Labeling and Advertising Act required health warnings on cigarette packages and an annual report to Congress on the health consequences of smoking.
- 1969—Public Health Cigarette Smoking Act strengthened health warnings on cigarette packs and prohibited cigarette advertising on television and radio.
- 1973—Little Cigar Act extended the broadcast ban on cigarette advertising to little cigars.
- 1984—Comprehensive Smoking Education Act required that four specific health warnings be printed on packaging on a rotating basis and stated that the cigarette industry must provide a list of substances added to cigarette.
- 1986—Comprehensive Smokeless Tobacco Health Education Act required three rotating health warnings on smokeless tobacco packages and in advertisements and a list of additives and nicotine content in smokeless tobacco products. It also prohibited smokeless tobacco advertising on television and radio and required reports to Congress on smokeless tobacco and a public information campaign on the health hazards of smokeless tobacco.

The four warnings currently rotated among cigarette packs are the following:

1. Surgeon General's Warning: Smoking Causes Lung Cancer, Heart Disease, Emphysema, and May Complicate Pregnancy

2. Surgeon General's Warning: Quitting Smoking Now Greatly Reduces Serious Risks to Your Health

3. Surgeon General's Warning: Smoking by Pregnant Women May Result in Fetal Injury, Premature Birth, and Low Birth-Weight

4. Surgeon General's Warning: Cigarette Smoking Contains Carbon Monoxide.

The three smokeless tobacco warnings that are rotated are the following:

1. Warning: This Product May Cause Mouth Cancer

2. Warning: This Product May Cause Gum Disease and Tooth Loss

3. Warning: This Product Is Not a Safe Alternative to Cigarettes

As a consequence of education and other public health activities, tobacco use has begun to decline in the United States. Currently, 25 percent of Americans, about 43 million people, smoke. About 45 million former smokers have quit. Unfortunately, the percentage of adults who smoke hit a plateau in the late 1990s. This is largely because the rate of adolescents who take up smoking is not declining. Many experts believe that adult smoking rates will not decline significantly until cigarette advertising that appeals to young people is regulated. These adolescents grow up to become addicted adult smokers. SEE ALSO ADVERTISING AND TOBACCO INDUSTRY; TOBACCO DEPENDENCE; TOBACCO INDUSTRY; TOBACCO: POLICIES, LAWS, AND REGULATIONS; TOBACCO, SMOKELESS.

Tobacco: Industry

The tobacco industry is composed of several different parts. At the core of the industry are primary suppliers, manufacturers, and distributors (both wholesale and retail). Advertising agencies and media outlets that promote the purchase and use of tobacco products also play an important role in the industry. Finally, law firms, public relations firms, and **lobbying** firms work from inside the tobacco industry to protect manufacturers and distributors of tobacco products from public-health regulation and control.

lobbying activities aimed at influencing public officials, especially members of the legislature

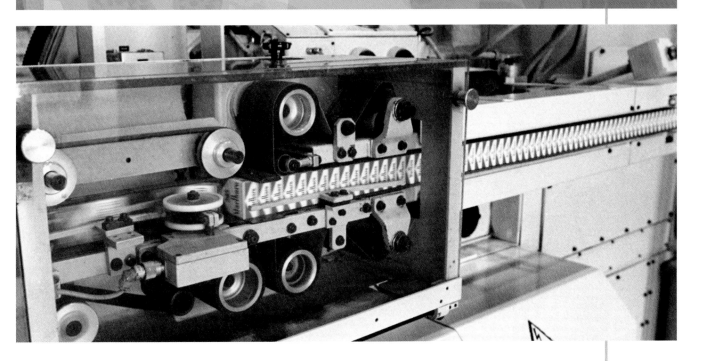

Although its overall popularity is declining in the United States, cigarette use is increasing worldwide at over 2 percent per year, especially in much of Asia, Eastern Europe, Russia, and the former Soviet republics. An integrated system of suppliers, manufacturers, marketers, and sales outlets is constantly evolving to supply this vast and growing market. In the past, efforts by lawyers and lobbyists for the tobacco industry managed to protect it from regulation advocated by a number of public health groups. However, since the 1990s, both the public and government have applied increasing pressure on the tobacco industry to admit tobacco's negative effects on health and to make changes in the way the industry operates.

The Philip Morris company, which owns this plant in Concord, North Carolina, is the largest cigarette manufacturer in the country, producing up to 165 billion cigarettes a year.

The Growth of the Industry

In the late nineteenth and early twentieth centuries, the tobacco industry comprised many small businesses that produced tobacco products for smoking, snuffing, and chewing. All of these products delivered **nicotine** to the user. A number of changes in the nineteenth century paved the way for the cigarette to become the major product of the tobacco industry. First, the industry developed types of tobacco that were easily processed into products for smoking. Second, the invention of cigarette-making machines (first used commercially in 1883 by the American Tobacco Company) made mass production possible. Safe matches were also introduced. Finally, the growth of railroads provided a network to transport cigarettes throughout the United States.

nicotine alkaloid derived from the tobacco plant that is responsible for tobacco's addictive effects

Duke of Durham, North Carolina. An important figure in the early success of the cigarette was Benjamin Newton (Buck) Duke, head of the American Tobacco Company. Duke realized that the mass production of cigarettes by machine made low prices possible. He believed that advertising could stimulate demand and a large market would develop to absorb the vastly expanded production. Duke engaged in price wars to weaken other manufacturers. Gradually, he bought out his competitors and turned the U.S. cigarette industry into a **monopoly**. By 1890 Duke controlled the cigarette market, and by 1910, just before his monopoly was broken, he controlled more than 80 percent of all tobacco products manufactured in the United States, except for cigars.

monopoly situation that exists when only one person or company sells a good or service in a given area

Antitrust Litigation. In 1907 the U.S. government filed an **antitrust** case against the American Tobacco Company. The result of this court case was the breakup of the trust four years later into a number of companies. Some of these companies, such as the R. J. Reynolds Tobacco Company (now RJR/Nabisco), still play major roles in the U.S. cigarette market.

antitrust relating to laws that prevent unfair business practices

In 1913 R. J. Reynolds developed and introduced a new brand of cigarette called Camel. Camel was the first brand to combine an ingredient of chewing-tobacco products with cigarette tobaccos. In addition to being cheaper than other brands, Camel relied on a national advertising campaign using magazines and billboards. Previously, cigarette advertising had relied on coupons and other promotions on cigarette packages. This new way to advertise tobacco products was extremely successful. Camel soon overwhelmed the competition and ushered in a dramatic expansion of the number of cigarette smokers in the United States. The other tobacco companies put out new products to compete with Camel, such as Lucky Strike and Chesterfield, and advertised in the mass media. Prices fell, and cigarette use increased sharply. This growth continued for about forty years, until the public became aware of the risk of lung cancer and other diseases related to smoking.

Two firms that were not part of the original tobacco trust have played major roles in the U.S. cigarette market. During the 1930s and 1940s, the Brown & Williamson Tobacco Company dominated the menthol category of the cigarette market with its Kool brand. Brown & Williamson continues to offer a full range of cigarettes for the U.S. and international markets. The other upstart company was Philip Morris, which began its U.S. operations as a specialty cigarette maker in New York in the first quarter of the twentieth century. In the mid-1950s Philip Morris hired an advertising agency to remake

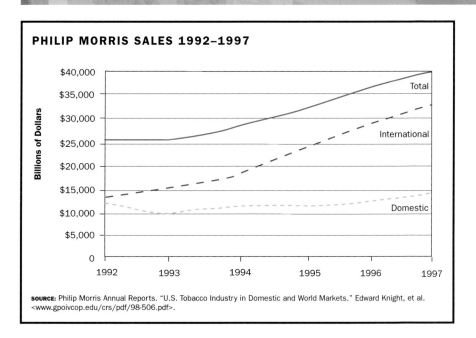

PHILIP MORRIS SALES 1992–1997

Billions of Dollars

Total

International

Domestic

1992　1993　1994　1995　1996　1997

SOURCE: Philip Morris Annual Reports. "U.S. Tobacco Industry in Domestic and World Markets." Edward Knight, et al. <www.gpoivcop.edu/crs/pdf/98-506.pdf>.

Philip Morris sales increased from 1992 to 1997, when they made nearly $40 billion in cigarette and tobacco sales.

the image of its Marlboro brand, originally targeted at ladies. The new campaign featured a rugged outdoorsman on horseback. By the mid-1970s Marlboro was the leading U.S. cigarette. By the 1990s, because of Marlboro's appeal to teens and young adults, Philip Morris overtook R. J. Reynolds to become the nation's largest tobacco-product manufacturer.

Innovation

The tobacco industry adapts to changing circumstances in many ways. Product innovation is a key strategy. Since the early 1950s, public-health concerns that cigarettes are a leading cause of illness and death have led to major changes in cigarette design. Two such changes are filters and so-called low-tar cigarettes. Multibillion-dollar advertising campaigns promoted these new, supposedly better products, yet years of study have produced evidence for only the smallest of benefits. Many accuse the tobacco industry of engaging in public relations gimmicks as a way to avoid any real response to public-health concerns.

Diversification

For more than two decades, the giant cigarette makers have invested their tobacco profits in other business enterprises. The practice of investing in a wide range of businesses is called diversification. Tobacco companies have invested in companies that produce soft drinks, cookies, and office products, as well as others that sell insurance and real estate. As a result, the tobacco companies own some of the most widely known consumer-product companies, such as Kraft and Nabisco.

These combined companies, such as RJR/Nabisco, are known as conglomerates.

None of the parent tobacco companies now have the word "tobacco" in their corporate names. The industry appears to want to hide behind harmless products as a way to deemphasize its production and promotion of tobacco products. Yet tobacco products remain by far the most profitable sector of each of these conglomerates, and tobacco products are always responsible for most of the company profits. In addition, not one of these companies has backed away from any available opportunity to sell tobacco products.

The tobacco companies make use of nontobacco subsidiaries (the companies they have bought) to support their tobacco businesses. For example, RJR/Nabisco fired the ad agency that did their Oreo Cookie advertising after that agency also produced ads promoting an airline offering smoke-free flights. Philip Morris has used one of its Kraft-General Foods warehouses for its coupon-redemption program for Marlboro cigarettes. Tobacco companies do not diversify to get out of the tobacco business. They diversify in order to make good investments and thus greater profits. The resulting product mix helps strengthen the core business in some way.

Price Wars

Price competition was a key tobacco industry strategy in the 1880s and in the early twentieth century. From the end of World War II (1945) until 1980, however, price competition was virtually absent from the U.S. cigarette market. In 1980 Liggett & Myers, a small firm that did not make big company profits, broke away from the other tobacco companies by introducing generic cigarettes, or cigarettes without a brand name or packaging. Brown & Williamson soon followed with its own generic products, and within a few years every cigarette manufacturer sold products at different price levels, from the heavily advertised, standard brands at the top to generic products at the bottom. Prices for the major brands continued to rise steeply through the early 1990s. Customers who might have stopped smoking because of high prices were kept in the market because of lower-priced products. By early 1993 lower-priced products accounted for more than 25 percent of all cigarette purchases.

This trend was a threat to profits. In addition, Philip Morris had become alarmed when sales of Marlboro sank to less than 25 percent of all cigarettes sold. The company decided to cut prices substantially while at the same time mounting the most elaborate advertising campaign ever seen in the industry. The competition was forced to cut prices as well. Sales of Marlboro once again surged, and the threat to profitability from lower-priced brands subsided.

Lobbying and Public Relations

In the 1950s proof that cigarettes caused lung cancer presented a serious challenge to the industry. In addition to putting filters on the product and making outrageous claims for their benefit, the industry began to follow a careful plan to improve its image. The industry hired the public relations firm Hill & Knowlton, which organized the Tobacco Institute to fulfill the industry's public relations and lobbying needs. The cigarette makers also formed the Tobacco Industry Research Committee (later reorganized and renamed the Council for Tobacco Research) to create the impression that the industry was involved in biomedical research on smoking and health.

The tobacco industry did in fact pursue studies of smoking, but the research conclusions were not released. Later, the public learned that the research clearly showed the addictiveness of nicotine and the link between smoking and various diseases. Many referred to the industry's unwillingness to release its findings as the "tobacco cover-up." Most companies continued to insist that tobacco is not addictive. However, in 1997 the Bennett S. LeBow company agreed to put warnings on cigarette packs stating that smoking is addictive. In addition, internal company documents showing the conclusions of industry research were leaked to the outside. These documents showed that the company was in fact aware of smoking's dangers long before these dangers came to the public's attention. Public criticism of the industry grew. People became angry when they realized that the industry understood the health dangers of smoking but refused to disclose their findings.

In addition, many states and individuals began to sue big tobacco companies for damages due to smoking. In several important individual cases, tobacco companies were ordered to pay large settlements. Four states also won very large settlements. Then, in 1998 the attorneys general of more than forty states and tobacco industry leaders agreed to a master settlement agreement instead of proceeding with separate lawsuits. The settlement requires the tobacco industry each year for ten years to pay $25 million to fund a charitable foundation that will support the study of programs to reduce teen smoking and substance abuse and the prevention of diseases associated with tobacco use. In exchange, the tobacco industry is protected against further lawsuits by states. Although this settlement will help fund many important antitobacco campaigns and health initiatives, it was not nearly as harsh toward the industry as other mea-

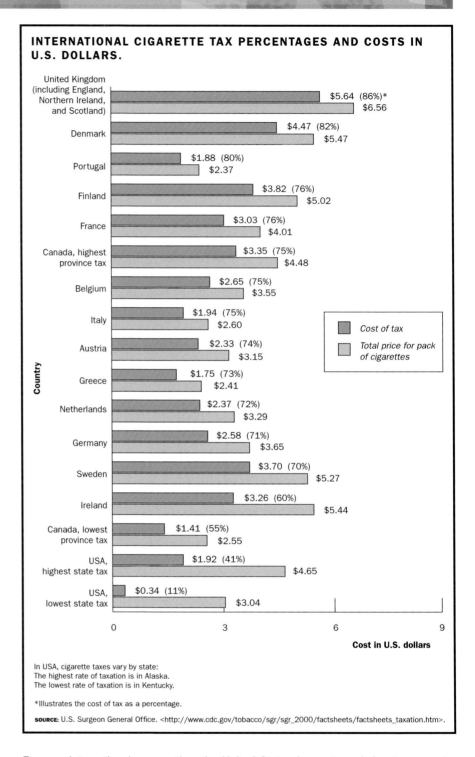

INTERNATIONAL CIGARETTE TAX PERCENTAGES AND COSTS IN U.S. DOLLARS.

Country

United Kingdom (including England, Northern Ireland, and Scotland) — $5.64 (86%)* / $6.56

Denmark — $4.47 (82%) / $5.47

Portugal — $1.88 (80%) / $2.37

Finland — $3.82 (76%) / $5.02

France — $3.03 (76%) / $4.01

Canada, highest province tax — $3.35 (75%) / $4.48

Belgium — $2.65 (75%) / $3.55

Italy — $1.94 (75%) / $2.60

Austria — $2.33 (74%) / $3.15

Greece — $1.75 (73%) / $2.41

Netherlands — $2.37 (72%) / $3.29

Germany — $2.58 (71%) / $3.65

Sweden — $3.70 (70%) / $5.27

Ireland — $3.26 (60%) / $5.44

Canada, lowest province tax — $1.41 (55%) / $2.55

USA, highest state tax — $1.92 (41%) / $4.65

USA, lowest state tax — $0.34 (11%) / $3.04

Cost in U.S. dollars: 0 | 3 | 6 | 9

Legend:
- Cost of tax
- Total price for pack of cigarettes

In USA, cigarette taxes vary by state:
The highest rate of taxation is in Alaska.
The lowest rate of taxation is in Kentucky.

*Illustrates the cost of tax as a percentage.

SOURCE: U.S. Surgeon General Office. <http://www.cdc.gov/tobacco/sgr/sgr_2000/factsheets/factsheets_taxation.htm>.

From an international perspective, the United States has extremely low taxes on tobacco products. These low American taxes are due in part to the successful lobbying efforts of the tobacco companies.

sures that were defeated (such as the McCain bill, defeated in the Senate in 1997). Some health advocates even believe that the tobacco settlement will benefit the tobacco industry in the long run. Also, in 1998, after years of being investigated on perjury charges, tobacco executives finally testified before Congress that nicotine is addictive under current definitions of the word and that smoking may cause cancer.

Smoking and the Young

Public campaigns to reduce youth smoking have grown in recent years. Between 1998 and 2000 smoking declined by 54 percent in middle schools and 25.2 percent in high schools. In 2001 youth smoking continued to decline, with significant declines in 8th- and 10th-grade students. Nevertheless, almost all long-term smokers begin smoking in the teen years, which is why so much public health attention is focused on preventing teen smoking. Laws have banned all cigarette advertising that aims to attract young smokers.

Efforts to make nicotine a drug regulated by the Food and Drug Administration (FDA) have been attempted for years. However, in 2000, the Supreme Court upheld a previous ruling that declares existing law does not provide the FDA authority over tobacco or tobacco marketing. Essentially, the Supreme Court ruling means that it is up to Congress to authorize the FDA to regulate nicotine, which it has not yet done. On the other hand, legislation to limit the influence of the tobacco industry on the public, especially young people, has led to many advertising restrictions. Tobacco companies are prohibited from sponsoring sports and other public events, and from advertising in public transit systems, shopping malls, and video arcades. More than 14,000 tobacco billboard advertisements nationwide have been torn down or replaced with antismoking messages. Cartoon characters such as Joe Camel used to advertise tobacco products are gone. Tobacco merchandise popular with young people, such as hats, shirts, and backpacks, were banned forever as of July 1, 1999. Payments for tobacco product placement in movies, videos, and other media were banned. Lobbying against a variety of tobacco control laws and ordinances was banned.

Conclusion

Cigarette smoking remains the leading cause of preventable death. Yet the tobacco industry continues to try to protect itself against regulation and increase their profits. Public interest groups must continue to fight for more government regulation in combination with efforts to reduce smoking, especially among the young. SEE ALSO AD-

DID YOU KNOW?

According to research by the economist Kenneth Warner, the tobacco industry needs to recruit 5,000 new young smokers *every day* to maintain the total number of smokers. These recruits replace the number of people who die from tobacco-related illness or quit smoking.

VERTISING AND THE TOBACCO INDUSTRY; NICOTINE; TOBACCO: DEPENDENCE; TOBACCO: MEDICAL COMPLICATIONS; TOBACCO: POLICIES, LAWS, AND REGULATIONS.

Tobacco: Medical Complications

The health dangers of smoking tobacco have been known for centuries. In 1604 King James I of England described tobacco as harmful to the brain and lungs, among other ill effects, and urged his subjects to avoid it. During the next 300 years, opinions varied as to whether tobacco is beneficial or harmful to the body. Some argued against tobacco as an immoral substance.

In 1926 a Cambridge University professor, Sir Humphrey Rolleston, gave a lecture to a medical society in which he listed some possible toxic effects of nicotine. These included irritation of the throat and upper air passages and heart disorders such as irregular heartbeat and angina, pain caused by insufficient blood reaching the heart. However, he did not believe that tobacco was a drug of addiction.

But even as Rolleston was lecturing, researchers were looking at evidence suggesting that smoking was responsible for the increasing number of lung cancer cases, a rare disease in the nineteenth century. By the 1960s most medical professionals and scientists agreed that tobacco smoking was the main cause of lung cancer, a contributing cause of other cancers, and a major cause of heart disease, diseased arteries, and lung diseases such as emphysema and chronic bronchitis. Yet from the 1920s to the 1960s, cigarette smoking became almost universally accepted as a social drug. In their advertisements, cigarette manufacturers presented cigarette smoking as a harmless enjoyment. By the 1960s the majority of adult males were smokers—in some age groups, more than 70 percent.

The turning point in the public's perception of the negative consequences of tobacco smoking was the publication of the *Report of the Royal College of Physicians* in England in 1962 and the *Report of the Surgeon General* in the United States in 1964. These two reports presented the evidence linking tobacco smoking to a variety of diseases. Many more reports on the health consequences of smoking followed.

As of 2002, cigarette smoking remained the most important cause of preventable disease and premature death in the developed countries of the world. Depending on the age at which a person starts to smoke, seven to thirteen years of life are lost to smoking-related

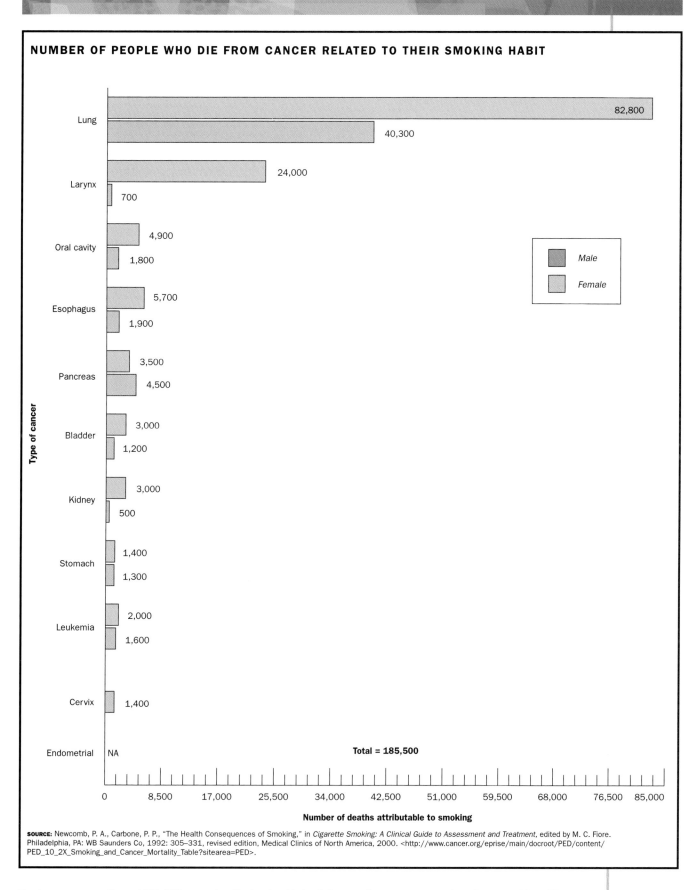

NUMBER OF PEOPLE WHO DIE FROM CANCER RELATED TO THEIR SMOKING HABIT

Legend:
- Male
- Female

Type of cancer	Male	Female
Lung	82,800	40,300
Larynx	24,000	700
Oral cavity	4,900	1,800
Esophagus	5,700	1,900
Pancreas	3,500	4,500
Bladder	3,000	1,200
Kidney	3,000	500
Stomach	1,400	1,300
Leukemia	2,000	1,600
Cervix		1,400
Endometrial		NA

Total = 185,500

X-axis: Number of deaths attributable to smoking — 0, 8,500, 17,000, 25,500, 34,000, 42,500, 51,000, 59,500, 68,000, 76,500, 85,000

Y-axis: Type of cancer

SOURCE: Newcomb, P. A., Carbone, P. P., "The Health Consequences of Smoking," in *Cigarette Smoking: A Clinical Guide to Assessment and Treatment*, edited by M. C. Fiore. Philadelphia, PA: WB Saunders Co, 1992: 305–331, revised edition, Medical Clinics of North America, 2000. <http://www.cancer.org/eprise/main/docroot/PED/content/PED_10_2X_Smoking_and_Cancer_Mortality_Table?sitearea=PED>.

Each year more than 185,000 people die in the United States from cancers related to smoking. The overwhelming majority of these people die from lung cancer.

diseases. Nonetheless, more than 63 million Americans continue to smoke or use smokeless tobacco.

Nicotine

Nicotine, the addictive component in tobacco, is a colorless liquid alkaloid that turns brown and begins to smell like tobacco when it is exposed to air. People who smoke become **physically dependent** on nicotine. They also become dependent on it in psychological and social ways. For example, people who are dependent on nicotine come to rely on smoking as a kind of comforting activity, often helping them keep their hands busy and active if they are feeling unsure or uncomfortable. So in addition to the chemical addictiveness of nicotine in tobacco, the rituals involved in holding, lighting, and puffing cigarettes can become nervous habits for some people.

Nicotine has both **stimulant** and **depressant** effects on the body. Nicotine is an interesting chemical because under some circumstances it can make the user feel more alert and aware (the stimulant effects), and under other circumstances it can make the user feel relaxed (the depressant effects). Nicotine also causes the brain to release endogenous opioids, chemicals that go to pleasure areas of the brain and give the smoker a feeling of enjoyment. Nicotine has positive reinforcement effects. This means that people who have experienced the pleasurable effects of nicotine are likely to want to experience them again. It also has negative reinforcement effects. This means that some smokers keep smoking not only to keep getting the pleasurable effects but also to avoid the discomfort of stopping nicotine use. The unpleasant symptoms caused by stopping are called **withdrawal**.

Nicotine is quickly absorbed through the skin, mucous membranes, and lungs. Absorption through the lungs produces measurable effects on the central nervous system in as little as seven seconds. This rapid rate of absorption means that each puff on a cigarette produces some reinforcement of the smoking habit.

Tobacco-Related Diseases

The scientific evidence that tobacco is a carcinogen, or cancer-causing substance, is overwhelming. It is also a leading cause of other diseases:

1. Smoking is the single major cause of cancers of the lung, larynx, pharynx (oral cavity), and esophagus; chronic obstructive pulmonary disease, including emphysema; and diseases of the blood vessels in the body.

physically dependent characteristic of someone who takes drugs for relief of uncomfortable physical symptoms, rather than for emotional or psychological relief

stimulant drug that increases activity temporarily; often used to describe drugs that excite the brain and central nervous system

depressant chemical that slows down or decreases functioning; often used to describe agents that slow the functioning of the central nervous system; such agents are sometimes used to relieve insomnia, anxiety, irritability, and tension

withdrawal physical and psychological symptoms that may occur when a person suddenly stops the use of a substance or reduces the dose of an addictive substance

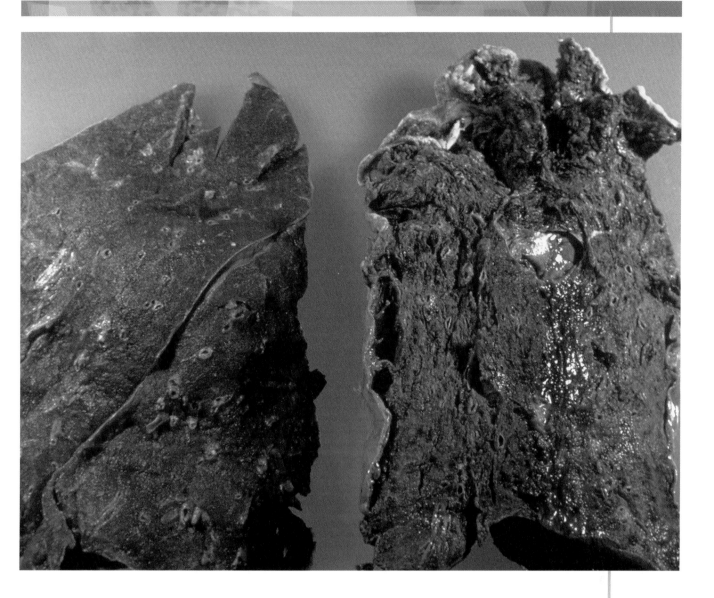

2. Smoking is one among several causes of stroke; coronary heart disease; cancers of the bladder and pancreas; aortic aneurysm; and mortality in infants.

3. Smoking is suspected of contributing to cancers of the cervix, uterus, stomach, and liver; gastric and duodenal ulcers; pneumonia; and sudden infant death syndrome.

When a normal lung (left) is compared to a smoker's lung (right), which is shredded and un-even, the detrimental effects of smoking become apparent.

Cancer. Tobacco smoking has been shown to be the major cause of lung cancer in both men and women. The increased risk for lung cancer is directly related to the amount smoked. The risk of death from lung cancer is about twenty times greater for men who smoke two packs a day than for those who have never smoked. It is about ten times higher for those who smoke one-half to one pack a day. How deep a smoker inhales also influences the risk of disease. Smoking in combination with drinking alcohol increases a person's chances of getting cancers of the oral cavity, larynx, pharynx, and esophagus.

Cardiovascular Disease. Smoking is one of three major causes of coronary heart disease. The risk of death from heart disease is 70 percent higher for men who smoke, with a similar effect for women. Smoking is more dangerous if the smoker also has conditions such as hypertension (high blood pressure) and elevated cholesterol levels. Smoking increases the risk for stroke. For example, women who smoke twenty-five cigarettes or more per day have a risk for stroke almost four times higher than nonsmokers. Smoking also increases the risk of atherosclerosis (formation of plaques or fat-like deposits), which block the flow of blood through arteries to the heart and other parts of the body. When this blockage occurs, the muscles may not receive sufficient oxygen. In the aorta, insufficient oxygen can lead to a rupture that is usually fatal.

Lung Disease. Tobacco smoking can cause chronic obstructive pulmonary disease, sometimes called emphysema or chronic bronchitis. This lung disease includes three related disorders: (1) too much mucous production in the airways, causing cough; (2) swelling of airways, making it difficult to completely blow out a breath; and (3) destruction of the walls of the alveoli, little air sacs in the lungs. Compared to nonsmokers, male smokers are three times as likely and female smokers are twice as likely to have a persistent cough.

Other Medical Complications. Other conditions caused by smoking include peptic ulcers; upper respiratory infections; osteoporosis, a disease that results in a decrease in bone mass; and cancers of the pancreas, bladder, and esophagus. In addition, tobacco use can change the way various medications are metabolized, or processed, in the body. This change in metabolism can prevent medications from having their full therapeutic effect on the body.

depression state in which an individual feels intensely sad and hopeless; may have trouble eating, sleeping, and concentrating, and is no longer able to feel pleasure from previously enjoyable activities; in extreme cases, may lead an individual to think about or attempt suicide

Psychiatric Disorders. Dependence on tobacco has been linked to **depression**. It is not yet known, however, whether depression prompts people to begin smoking or whether depression develops after a person has become dependent on tobacco. Mood disorders increase significantly during withdrawal from nicotine. People who try to quit smoking often relapse, or return to the habit, because of these negative changes in mood.

Secondhand Smoking. The smoke inhaled by the smoker is different from the smoke produced by tobacco burning between puffs. This

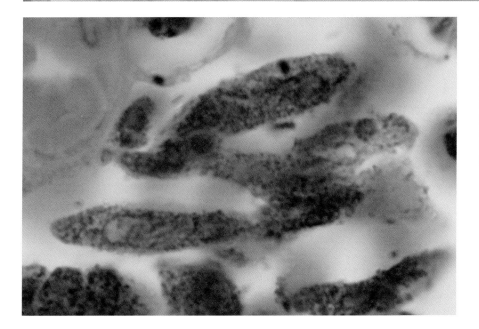

Cigarette smoking is correlated to numerous types of cancer, particularly cancers of the lung. Metastatic melanoma in the lung, magnified here at over 400 times its actual size, resembles fish swimming close together.

secondhand smoke, inhaled by a person who is merely in the same room as the person smoking the cigarette, has higher concentrations of carbon monoxide and substances believed to be carcinogenic. One of the main dangers of secondhand smoke affects the infants of mothers who smoke. These infants are far more likely to die before their first birthday, primarily as a result of respiratory complications and sudden infant death syndrome. Children of mothers who smoke seem in general more likely to suffer from colds, asthma, bronchitis, pneumonia, and other respiratory problems.

Smoking Rates and Disease

The overall increased mortality, or likelihood of death, from the tobacco-related diseases varies with the amount of tobacco smoked. For those who smoke two or more packs of cigarettes per day, it is about double that of nonsmokers; for those who smoke less, it is about 1.7 times higher than for nonsmokers. Quitting smoking can greatly reduce the risk for various diseases, but not all risks decline at the same rate. The risk for cardiovascular disease decreases sharply within a year of quitting smoking. The risks for cancer decline more slowly, with some heightened risk remaining ten years after quitting. By ten to fifteen years after quitting, the overall mortality of former smokers is not much higher than that of nonsmokers. Mortality rates do not increase as much for pipe and cigar smokers as for cigarette smokers, but pipe and cigar smokers still have much higher rates than nonsmokers do. For users of smokeless tobacco, the greatest mortality risk comes mainly from cancers of the oral cavity and throat.

Women and Smoking

Women who smoke tobacco have the same health risks as men. It is often said that women who smoke like men die like men. In 1986 deaths due to lung cancer among women exceeded deaths from breast cancer, becoming the leading cause of cancer death for women. Some women are at special risk. The combination of birth control pills and cigarette smoking greatly increases the risk of cardiovascular disease, including bleeding inside the skull. In addition, women who smoke have higher **infertility** rates than those who do not and are also more likely to have menstrual irregularities.

Smoking is particularly dangerous during pregnancy. Nicotine, which crosses from the mother's blood into the fetus's blood, constricts blood vessels. As a result, a decreased amount of oxygen is delivered to the fetus.

Women who smoke during pregnancy have higher rates of premature delivery. In the United States, smoking has been associated with a 20 percent increase in premature births among women who smoked a pack a day or more compared with those who did not smoke. Babies born to women who smoke during pregnancy weigh on average about seven ounces less than those born to nonsmokers. Low birth weight is related to numerous health problems in infants. Secondhand smoke also contributes to low birth weight. The greater the amount of tobacco smoked during the pregnancy, the higher the frequency of miscarriage and fetal death. Women who stop smoking early in pregnancy increase their likelihood of having normal deliveries and normal-birth-weight babies.

Education and smoking-prevention programs, particularly those directed at young people, have helped reduce the number of smokers in the United States. Smoking rates have decreased for white males in higher economic groups, but have decreased less for women and members of ethnic and racial minorities and lower economic groups. After increasing throughout much of the 1980s and 1990s, smoking rates are also decreasing in younger age groups in the United States. The rates of smoking among young adults ages 18 to 25 have decreased from 41.6 percent in 1998 to 38.3 percent in 2000. An estimated 13.4 percent of young people ages 12 to 17 were smokers in 2000, down from 18.2 percent in 1998.

In contrast to the general decline of smoking in the West, smoking rates may actually be increasing in developing and newly industrialized countries. In these countries, the cigarette remains a symbol of sophistication and affluence. SEE ALSO ADVERTISING AND THE TOBACCO INDUSTRY; NICOTINE; NICOTINE WITHDRAWAL; PREVEN-

---

infertility inability to have children

THE IMPACT OF SMOKING WHILE PREGNANT

Smoking during pregnancy has been proven harmful to both mother and child. When chemical-loaded smoke is inhaled, it travels through the placenta, the organ that passes nutrients and oxygen from the mother to the developing fetus.

The harmful chemicals in cigarette smoke restrict the fetus's development. It is deprived of oxygen and food, which increases its risk of stillbirth, premature delivery, and low birth weight, as well as brain damage, cerebral palsy, and being stricken by sudden infant death syndrome.

TION; PREVENTION PROGRAMS; TOBACCO: DEPENDENCE; TOBACCO TREATMENT: BEHAVIORAL APPROACHES; TOBACCO TREATMENT: MEDICATIONS.

Tobacco: Policies, Laws, and Regulations

Everyone has a big stake in tobacco. Smokers who become sick often wind up using tax money to help pay for their medical bills, while nonsmokers are put at risk when they breathe in the toxins from other people's cigarettes. Tobacco policies, laws, and regulations are intended to protect everyone—smokers and nonsmokers alike. Another main goal is to discourage young people from ever starting to smoke in the first place. Federal, state, and city governments have tried to achieve these goals by several means. Some of the most important are product labels, advertising restrictions, clean air rules, bans on sales to minors, special taxes, laws to prevent smuggling, and lawsuits against tobacco companies.

Labels and Advertising

In 1964 the U.S. surgeon general's first report on tobacco and health was issued. The next year, a federal law was passed requiring a warning label on cigarette packages: "Caution: Cigarette Smoking May Be Hazardous to Your Health." This warning has been strengthened and expanded over the years. Today, one of four different warning statements is required (on a revolving basis) on cigarette packages and advertisements. Somewhat different warning labels are required on smokeless tobacco and cigar packages and advertisements as well. Yet the labels are still smaller and the warnings weaker than those of many other countries. It is the job of the Federal Trade Commission (FTC) to make sure the U.S. warnings are displayed properly.

The FTC is also charged with monitoring tobacco advertising and marketing. In 1969 Congress passed a law that banned cigarette ads on television and radio. However, this law did not keep tobacco companies from heavily promoting their products. Tobacco ads and logos were seen everywhere, from newspaper and magazine ads, to billboards and signs on the sides of buses, to T-shirts and race cars. Then in 1998 the tobacco companies reached a massive settlement agreement with forty-six states. As part of this settlement, the companies agreed to remove all tobacco ads from billboards and public transportation.

Despite mandatory and visible warning labels about the health risks associated with smoking that appear on all packages of cigarettes, people continue to smoke.

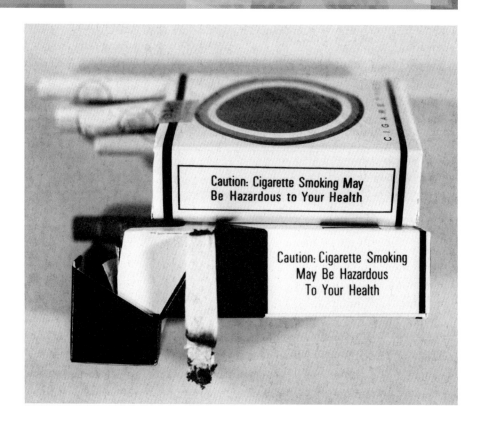

Caution: Cigarette Smoking May Be Hazardous to Your Health

Caution: Cigarette Smoking May Be Hazardous To Your Health

They also agreed to limits on sponsoring public events, handing out free samples, and giving away or selling clothes and other merchandise with their logos. In addition, they pledged to stop marketing to young people, even through methods that only indirectly appeal to teens.

The tobacco companies say they have lived up to this last promise, but critics disagree. A study published in the *New England Journal of Medicine* in 2001, for example, found that cigarette companies increased their advertising in magazines with young readers. The companies also increased their use of in-store marketing methods to attract young buyers, such as display racks, doormats with their logos, price discounts, and free gifts with the purchase of their products. So far, then, the limits on advertising have been less than a complete success. In fact, in the first year after the settlement, the FTC said the five biggest cigarette companies spent a staggering $8 billion on ads and promotion—up 22 percent more than the year before.

Another role of the FTC is to look into false or misleading sales practices. For years, the commission has investigated the claims that cigarette companies make about the amount of tar, nicotine, and carbon monoxide people get from their products. The concern is that a company may falsely imply its cigarettes are safer than they actually are. When a problem is found, the FTC can try to get the company to voluntarily stop making the claims in question. If that does not work, the commission can start a formal proceeding, much like a court trial, before an administrative law judge. If a violation of law is found, the judge can order the company to stop the practices. Some cases also are being decided in federal court.

Clean Air Laws

In 1972 another surgeon general's report first noted the health risks to nonsmokers from environmental tobacco smoke (ETS). Also known as secondhand smoke, this is a mixture of the smoke exhaled by others and the smoke that comes from the burning end of cigarettes. The following year, Arizona became the first state to restrict smoking in public places. Since then, many other states, cities, and large companies have taken similar action in an effort to keep indoor air cleaner and safer to breathe. As of 2001, forty-five states restricted smoking in state government buildings, and nearly half limited smoking in private work sites as well. In addition, thirty-one states had laws regulating smoking in restaurants.

Studies have shown that clean air laws are linked to less smoking and higher rates of quitting. One problem with such laws, however, is that they usually are not enforced unless someone calls to report a violation. Only then do officials investigate. If they find a problem, they typically can impose various warnings and penalties.

Work site smoking regulations not only protect nonsmokers; they also reduce the number of cigarettes that employees smoke during the day. This, in turn, can mean savings for employers, due to lower costs for lost work time, fire risk, damage to property, cleaning, health insurance, workers' compensation, disability, early retirement, and life insurance. The courts also have ruled that employers have a duty to provide a work site that is free of known hazards. As a result, many companies have taken steps to limit smoking, and 80 percent of workers are covered by some kind of workplace smoking policy. Yet fewer than half are protected by policies that ban smoking in both the work area and public or common areas.

The federal government has gotten involved as well. Smoking has been restricted in federal government buildings since 1979. In 1988 Congress banned smoking on many commercial airline flights within the United States. That ban later was extended to all such flights. In 1994 the Pro-Children Act was passed. It prohibited smoking in facilities where certain federally funded children's services are provided on a regular basis. The law applies to virtually all public schools and

> **IN THEIR OWN WORDS**
>
> "It is immoral for civilized societies to condone the promotion and advertising of products which when used as they are intended cause disability and death."
>
> —Louis W. Sullivan, former U.S. Secretary of Health and Human Services, 1991.

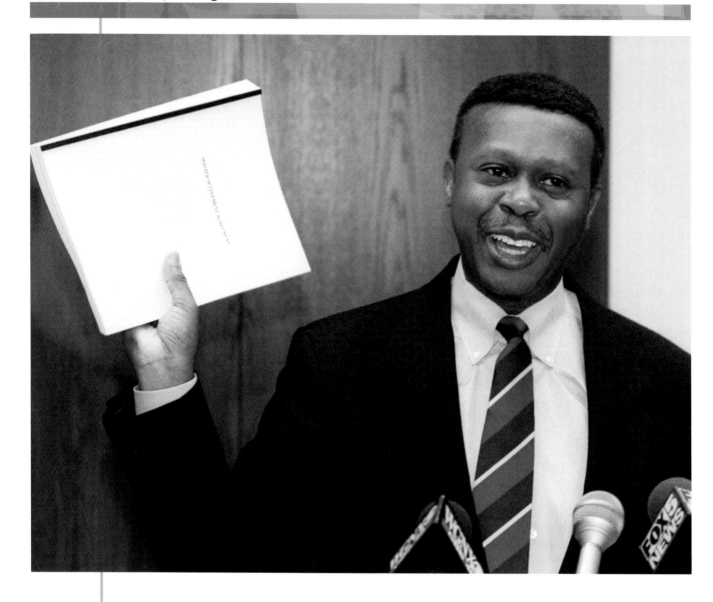

Georgia Attorney General Thurbert Baker, holds up a copy of a $206 billion tobacco company settlement, the largest civil settlement in U.S. history.

libraries. It also covers buildings that house Head Start programs and certain health and nutrition services for children. The U.S. Departments of Health and Human Services, Education, and Agriculture are jointly responsible for putting this law into action. Violators may be fined up to $1,000 per day. Nevertheless, many schools still lack a complete smoking ban on school property and at school-sponsored events.

Minors' Access Laws

Regulating the sale of tobacco to young people is mainly the job of the states. Every state now has a law that makes it illegal to sell cigarettes to anyone under age 18. Yet, illegal or not, many minors still are able to buy them. To address this problem, Congress passed the Synar Amendment in 1992. It says that state governments must send teen inspectors on yearly, unannounced visits to stores to see if merchants will sell tobacco to minors. If the sales rate is not less than 20 percent, the Substance Abuse and Mental Health Services Administration ☎ can withhold some federal funds for substance abuse services. By 2001, the national average sales rate to minors was 17 percent, down from about 40 percent in 1997.

☎ See *Organizations of Interest* at the back of Volume 3 for address, telephone, and URL.

That decrease in sales to minors is a big improvement, but it still is far from ideal. As a result, some states have taken further action. While all states ban giving away free samples to minors, a few prohibit such samples altogether, because it is so hard to control who gets them. For the same reason, more than two-thirds of states now restrict cigarette vending machines, although only two totally ban them. Several cities, including New York City, have their own vending machine laws as well. About two-thirds of states and many cities also require merchants to display signs stating the minimum age for buying tobacco products. In addition, some have laws that minors cannot sell cigarettes, since it can be hard for teens to refuse their friends.

Studies show these steps may be helping. For example, the Institute for Social Research ☎ oversees a large, long-term study of teen drug use and attitudes titled "Monitoring the Future." This study found that the percentage of 8th graders saying it would be "fairly easy" or "very easy" for them to get cigarettes if they wanted fell from 77 percent in 1996 to 68 percent in 2001. Of course, that means two-thirds of 8th graders still say they have ready access to cigarettes.

One problem is that many laws only penalize the salesperson when cigarettes are sold to minors. A 2000 report by the surgeon general noted that penalties need to be applied against store owners as well. To do this, it would be helpful if merchants had to be licensed to sell tobacco products. Then their licenses could be taken away temporarily or permanently if they failed to follow the law. Fines also could be imposed, and the fees collected could be used to pay for enforcement and education programs for merchants. At present, though, only thirty-four states require licenses for over-the-counter tobacco sales.

Taxes and Permits

Another approach is raising the cigarette excise tax, which is a tax levied on the manufacture, sale, or use of a particular product. This is widely regarded as one of the best ways to discourage smoking. Studies have shown that, for every 10 percent rise in the price of cigarettes, overall smoking decreases by 3 to 5 percent, and smoking by young people goes down by about 7 percent. State excise taxes vary widely, though. As of 2001, only three states had cigarette taxes of $1 or more per pack, and thirty-three had taxes of 50 cents or less. The average price and tax rate on cigarettes in the United States is well below that of most other developed countries, such as Canada or Switzerland. The tax rate on smokeless tobacco products is even lower.

In addition to state excise taxes, there are federal taxes and permits required as well. The federal Bureau of Alcohol, Tobacco, and Firearms ☎ (ATF) is the agency charged with making sure these requirements are met. Among other things, anyone who wants to manufacture tobacco products in the United States or import them for sale from other countries must get approval from the ATF first. Those who import tobacco products may be required to pay customs duties as well. The bureau also enforces laws dealing with contraband, the legal term for smuggled goods. To show that the proper taxes have been paid, the law requires that a stamp or mark be placed on all legally sold packages of cigarettes. The ATF defines contraband cigarettes as more than 60,000 cigarettes without such stamps or marks. Contraband cigarettes may be seized and destroyed, and those who smuggle them may be required to pay large fines.

Lawsuits Against Tobacco Companies

In recent years, many of the arguments about how tobacco products will be marketed and sold have occurred in the courts. Traditionally, the decision to smoke has been considered a personal choice. In the 1990s, though, people began to debate whether "choice" was the right word for such an addictive behavior. Smokers filed several class-action lawsuits, which means that large numbers of people sued the tobacco companies as a group, rather than individually. In 1996 the Liggett Group, the smallest of the nation's five big tobacco companies, offered to settle a class-action suit. It was the first time a tobacco company had taken financial responsibility for the health effects of its products.

In 1994 Mississippi became the first state to sue the tobacco industry. The state's main argument was that a vast sum of tax money was being spent to cover smoking-related health-care costs. Soon, the other states filed similar suits. In 1998, forty-six states and five U.S. territories signed an agreement with the tobacco industry, known as the Master Settlement Agreement (MSA). This agreement provided the states with funds to be used for tobacco prevention and control programs. It was the largest single legal settlement in history, totaling nearly $206 billion to be paid through the year 2025. As part of the MSA, the tobacco companies also agreed to limit their advertising and marketing practices. In addition, the companies were forced to open many of their private business documents to the public. Four

☎ See *Organizations of Interest* at the back of Volume 3 for address, telephone, and URL.

IN THEIR OWN WORDS

"The same people who tell us that smoking doesn't cause cancer are now telling us that advertising cigarettes doesn't cause smoking."

—Ellen Goodman, syndicated columnist, in an exposé on the power of the tobacco industry. From *The Boston Globe*, 1989.

other states—Mississippi, Florida, Texas, and Minnesota—settled their lawsuits separately for a total of $40 billion.

While the MSA was a giant step forward, it was not the final answer. For one thing, settlement funds go straight to the states, not to the federal government. Yet U.S. taxpayers also pay about $38 billion each year in federal taxes to treat tobacco-related illnesses. There are other costs, too. For example, the Social Security Administration pays nearly $2 billion per year in survivor's benefits to the children of parents who have died from smoking. In contrast, federal tobacco taxes bring in only about $5 billion per year. As a result, in 1999 the U.S. Department of Justice filed its own lawsuit against the tobacco industry.

Meanwhile, MSA funds began rolling into the states, and controversy brewed about how the money was used. As of early 2002, only five states were spending the minimum amount on tobacco prevention programs recommended by the Centers for Disease Control and Prevention (CDC)☎, even though this was typically only 20 to 25 percent of a state's settlement money. Yet there were many bright spots as well. Maine, one of the states meeting the CDC's standard, cut the smoking rate by high-school students by 36 percent. Massachusetts, another standout state, actually started its prevention program in 1993. In less than a decade, the state was already saving more than $2 for every dollar spent on prevention.

☎ See *Organizations of Interest* at the back of Volume 3 for address, telephone, and URL.

Clearly, tobacco policies, laws, and regulations make a difference. The surgeon general's 2000 report concluded that such approaches can play a key role in keeping many young people from becoming hooked on tobacco. They also can help increase the success rate of smokers trying to quit and decrease the health risks to nonsmokers. In the long run, they may help reduce tobacco's terrible toll of disease, disability, and death. SEE ALSO ADVERTISING AND THE TOBACCO INDUSTRY; LAW AND POLICY: DRUG LEGALIZATION DEBATE; NICOTINE; TOBACCO: INDUSTRY.

Tobacco: Smokeless

Tobacco is a plant native to the Americas, and Native Americans were the first to use it. In addition to smoking it, they used it in smokeless forms, mainly as a chewing material and in teas and other drinks. The ash was used in rituals throughout the Americas and the Caribbean. Tobacco was used along with many other plants for both ritual and medicinal purposes.

Christopher Columbus and other explorers brought tobacco to Europe, where it was taken up for recreation in both smoked form (cigars and pipes) and smokeless. Smokeless tobacco (ST) became popular in British society in the practice called sniffing. British colonists in the Americas preferred to chew tobacco or use snuff. In the 1800s chewing tobacco was widespread in the United States. This use decreased when the spitting that resulted (into spittoons or cuspidors or wherever the spit fell) was linked to the spread of tuberculosis, one of the most dreaded and fatal of diseases. In addition, the mass production of machine-rolled cigarettes further decreased use of smokeless tobacco. Around 1900, 52 percent of all tobacco used was smokeless. By 1952 that number had dropped to 6 percent. Sales of chewing tobacco declined until about 1970, and those who used it were mainly rural residents or baseball players.

The two most common types of ST used in the twentieth century were snuff and chewing tobacco. Snuff is a cured, ground tobacco that comes in three forms: fine-cut tobacco, moist snuff, and dry snuff. Snuff is used by placing a pinch between the cheek and gum or lower lip and gum. Chewing tobacco is also produced in three forms: loose-leaf tobacco, plug tobacco, and twist chewing tobacco. All three forms are used by placing a "chaw" in the cheek and periodically chewing.

In the 1970s the use of ST surged in the United States, with most smokers preferring moist snuff. Young people began using ST products much more than they did in the past. Use of ST among young people rose throughout the 1980s and peaked in 1995. Since then, a gradual decline in use by young people has been reported in national surveys. In 2001 an estimated 4 percent of 8th graders and 7.8 percent of 12th graders reported using ST within the past month. The renewed popularity of ST, which reached its peak in the 1990s, may have been the result of innovative advertising campaigns by tobacco companies. These campaigns used sports superstars, country-western entertainers, and rodeo celebrities to promote tobacco products. The advertising tried to replace the old image of the smokeless tobacco habit as unclean with a manly or macho image.

Smokeless tobacco, like cigarettes, contains nicotine, a drug that can lead to **physical dependence**. Cigarette smokers inhale smoke containing nicotine into their lungs, and the nicotine is then transported into the bloodstream. ST users absorb nicotine directly through the lining of their mouths. Each time smokers smoke a cigarette, they absorb approximately 1 milligram of nicotine into their system. By comparison, people who use chewing tobacco receive approximately 4.5 milligrams of nicotine per chaw, and people who use snuff receive approximately 3.6 milligrams of nicotine per pinch.

physical dependence condition that may occur after prolonged use of a particular drug or alcohol, in which the user's body cannot function normally without the presence of the substance; when the substance is not used or the dose is decreased, the user experiences uncomfortable physical symptoms

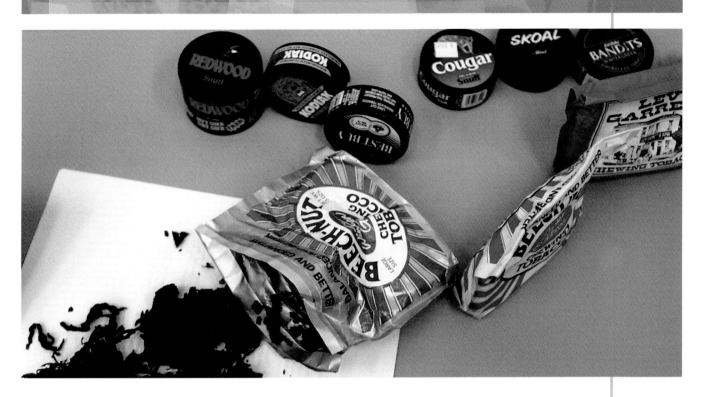

ST is sometimes viewed as a safe alternative to cigarettes, but this view is incorrect. In addition to dependence on nicotine, ST is directly related to a variety of health problems:

- bad breath
- abrasion (wearing down) of the teeth
- receding gums
- periodontal bone loss (affecting the structures that support the teeth)
- tooth loss
- leukoplakia (a condition in which thick white patches form on the mucous membranes of the mouth)
- various forms of oral (mouth) cancer

Smokeless tobacco may also play a role in cardiovascular changes and damage to the nervous and muscular systems.

Survey data as of 2001 indicate that users of smokeless tobacco are almost exclusively male. In a large national survey of smokeless tobacco use by young people, about 14.2 percent of male 12th graders used smokeless tobacco, while only 1.6 percent of female 12th graders used it. While ST users are mostly male, a 2000 study found that ST use is popular among some Native American women. Eastern Band Cherokee Indian women in North Carolina who used ST had an eight times greater risk of breast cancer than nonusers.

Chewing tobacco and snuff can cause bad breath as well as dental problems, and are related to cancers of the lips, tongue, and mouth.

As the use of smokeless tobacco has risen, education and programs to help people quit have become necessary. In 1994, Oral Health America created the National Spit Tobacco Education Program (NSTEP) as part of its Oral Health 2000 initiative. NSTEP is endorsed by Major League Baseball and encourages players and users to quit. But the main goal is to reduce ST use among kids. NSTEP's chairman is Hall of Fame broadcaster Joe Garagiola, and baseball stars Frank Thomas, Jeff Bagwell, and Hank Aaron endorse the program. Baseball star Lenny Dykstra, who had all his teeth pulled because of overuse of ST, did a public service announcement supporting the NSTEP cause, as did country music star Garth Brooks. During spring training in 1997, NSTEP counseled sixteen major league teams on ST education, providing intervention and programs aimed at helping people quit. Not only is it important to help the players quit, but it is equally important to reduce the number of ST-using players whom kids idolize. The national preventative health initiative, Healthy People 2010, is involved in several new programs to discourage all forms of tobacco use, including ST. Many quit-smoking programs and guides are now also addressing issues related to ST, from informing about the health risks to helping people quit ST use.

NSTEP offers users tips on quitting ST:

1. Be committed, and do not be discouraged by setbacks.

2. Quit with a friend or ask for support from friends who do not use ST.

3. Put three dollars in a jar every day to see the financial benefits of quitting.

4. Chew seeds or gum instead of tobacco while playing sports.

5. When the quit date is set, visit the dentist for a teeth cleaning, which should help ease the initial nicotine craving.

Users of ST who are dependent on nicotine may require therapy or use of a nicotine patch to kick this dangerous habit. SEE ALSO ADOLESCENTS, DRUG AND ALCOHOL USE; ADVERTISING AND THE TOBACCO INDUSTRY; NICOTINE; NICOTINE WITHDRAWAL.

Tobacco Treatment: An Overview

Because quitting tobacco is so difficult, many smokers seek some form of treatment to help them succeed. Nicotine is the addictive substance in tobacco, and nicotine addiction can be treated in several ways. The most effective methods are behavioral counseling and nicotine replacement therapy, particularly when they are combined.

Smoking Trends

Cigarette smoking is the most common form of tobacco use, and smoking is one of the nation's most serious public health problems. Tobacco use causes more than 430,000 deaths each year in the United States and is the leading preventable cause of death. Most adults in the United States have either smoked cigarettes or used some other tobacco product. In addition, an estimated 13.4 percent of young people ages 12 to 17 were smokers in 2000.

Although the number of Americans who smoked decreased in the late 1900s, the current number of smokers is still high. In the late 1990s, about one-quarter of adult Americans, or about 48 million people, smoked. Most of these people wanted to quit but were unable to do so because they found it too difficult. According to some figures from the late 1990s, only an estimated 2.5 percent of all smokers successfully quit each year.

> **IN THEIR OWN WORDS**
>
> "Nicotine is as addicting as heroin or cocaine."
>
> —C. Everett Koop, former Surgeon General, 1988.

A Note on Smokeless Tobacco

Like cigarettes, chewing tobacco and snuff present a similar risk of nicotine addiction. These products may prove more difficult to treat than cigarette use because they are sometimes viewed as less risky alternatives to cigarettes. One study quoted in a surgeon general's report on smoking reported that 77 percent of youth thought that cigarette smoking was very harmful, but only 40 percent rated smokeless tobacco as very harmful. Yet smokeless tobacco can cause cancer, bleeding gums and mouth sores that never heal, bad breath, stained teeth, and other related health problems. Once the negative publicity on smokeless tobacco use reaches a level close to the bad press on smoking, there should be a growing demand for using therapies to help smokeless tobacco users quit. Although a growing number of people use smokeless tobacco, most tobacco use is from cigarettes and most of the research on tobacco treatment has focused on helping smokers. Still, most of the tools that help smokers quit can also aid any nicotine addict.

The Effects of Quitting

When a person stops smoking or quits chewing smokeless tobacco, the body responds in a number of ways, some immediate and some over time. About twenty minutes after the last cigarette, blood pressure and pulse rate return to normal, and body temperature increases to normal. About eight hours later, the carbon monoxide level in the blood drops to normal, and after one day, an individual's chance of a heart attack decreases. After two days, nerve endings start to regenerate, and the ability to smell and taste improves. After two weeks, an individual's circulation improves and lung function increases by a maximum of 30 percent. After a year of smoking **abstinence**, the risk of coronary heart disease is reduced to half that of a smoker, and after five years of abstinence, the risk of death by lung cancer is cut in half. After fifteen years, the risk of coronary heart disease is equal to that of a nonsmoker.

Early Ideas About Quitting

Until the 1980s many people doubted that tobacco use was based on an addiction to or **dependence** on nicotine. In the 1950s and 1960s, a common view among experts was that smoking was just a bad habit. Experts at that time failed to realize that tobacco use was a form of drug use. Instead, they saw smoking and chewing tobacco as the kind of habit that could be broken by taking certain steps to change the behavior of the smoker. Behavioral approaches to stopping smoking or quit chewing have been in use ever since.

In the early twentieth century, self-help movements to treat alcohol or drug problems were very popular. The focus of these movements was to help people change the behaviors that contributed to their smoking habit. Such efforts at behavioral changes have a long history in society. Perhaps because minor behavioral problems are so commonplace, people tend not to seek professional help for dealing with them. As a result, over the years much of the "treatment" for cigarette smoking has amounted to individuals trying to quit on their own. However, researchers find that self-help treatments have not generally been effective for most people. In one study of 5,000 smokers, only 4.3 percent of individuals who had quit on their own remained abstinent for one year after they attempted to quit. Self-help treatments, combined with more formal treatment such as behavioral counseling, nicotine replacement, or a combination of the two, is likely to be more effective.

Group Therapy and Individual Therapy

A nicotine addict may see a therapist in one-on-one sessions in order to quit smoking. In these sessions, the smoker gets instruction and support from the therapist. Smokers and smokeless tobacco users can also seek such support in group therapy. Group programs have been used to provide hypnotism (a trance state in which smokers may be more suggestible), education, **behavioral therapy**, and combinations

abstinence complete avoidance of something, such as the use of drugs or alcoholic beverages

dependence psychological need to use a substance for emotional and/or physical reasons

behavioral therapy form of therapy whose main focus is to change certain behaviors instead of uncovering unconscious conflicts or problems

of therapies. There is no clear scientific evidence indicating which form of therapy is best, but group programs can be less expensive than individual programs. Some clients have strong personal preferences for one or the other form of treatment: Some enjoy the group support and like to share their experiences in a group; others find such involvement with groups unpleasant or embarrassing. For either type of therapy, the longer a person stays in treatment, and the greater the number of treatment sessions, the better the chances of success at quitting.

The Role of Doctors in Treatment

Physicians take an interest in preventing health problems in their patients. Thus, they often make special efforts to encourage patients to stop smoking or to quit chewing. In 1964 only about 15 percent of current smokers reported that a physician had advised them to quit smoking. By 1987 about 50 percent of current smokers had received such advice. Sometimes simple things like the advice of a doctor to quit and setting a date for quitting can lead to success. Doctors who take just a few minutes to give advice and provide a patient with pamphlets about smoking can make a difference. Physicians can also be helpful by referring patients to smoking treatment programs. Specialists who deal with patients already suffering from tobacco-related disease are in a good position to help those with a strong wish to quit. Yet cardiac or lung patients often fail to stop smoking. Being diagnosed with a smoking-related disease is no guarantee that the patient will quit smoking.

Efforts by Organizations

Several charitable organizations are devoted to reducing the rates of smoking and smoking-related diseases such as cancer, heart disease, and lung disease. The American Cancer Society, the Lung Association, and the Heart Foundation promote research and distribute public health information about smoking. Each has developed materials and programs to help people quit smoking. These materials, such as booklets and pamphlets, can reach many smokers at very low cost. U.S. government agencies concerned with smoking and smoking-related disease have also developed and promoted materials and procedures to encourage smokers to quit.

Charitable organizations also support efforts to ban or reduce smoking in the workplace. They provide smoking-treatment services to employees, such as employee assistance programs (EAPs). In addition to workplaces, restaurants and many other businesses now prohibit smoking on their premises. Just as social pressures encouraged many smokers to start the habit, social pressures might encourage them to stop. Once it was fashionable to be a cigarette smoker; now it is becoming fashionable to stop smoking.

Nicotine-Replacement Therapy

Nicotine-replacement therapy is considered an effective treatment for stopping smoking or ceasing to use smokeless tobacco. The most commonly used nicotine-replacement therapies are a gum that releases nicotine as it is chewed and a patch that slowly releases nicotine into the body through the skin. These therapies are available over the counter. Nicotine-replacement therapies can help reduce the nicotine **withdrawal** symptoms after a person stops smoking. As a result, the individual can focus on dealing with the behavioral challenges of stopping. For example, a smoker may be accustomed to having a cigarette while drinking a cup of coffee or while driving. He or she needs to learn how to separate those behaviors from the urge to smoke. People appear to prefer the nicotine skin patches over nicotine gum. They seem to have the fewest side effects and produce the greatest long-term abstinence rates.

Nicotine nasal sprays and nicotine vapor inhalers that deliver nicotine through the respiratory system are less common forms of nicotine-replacement therapy. They became available in the United States in the late 1990s. There have been reports of eye, nose, and throat irritation with the nasal sprays, but for some individuals these irritations decrease over time.

Other Drug Therapies

For someone who has tried repeatedly and yet failed to stop smoking for good, a medicine that could take away the desire to smoke would be welcome. A number of non-nicotine medications have been developed that reduce nicotine withdrawal symptoms, including irritability and anxiety. These medications mimic the effects achieved by smoking. As a result, they may help decrease an individual's desire for a cigarette. These medications include **antidepressants** (such as nortriptyline and bupropion or Wellbutrin), anxiolytics (medications usually prescribed to treat anxiety, such as buspirone, marketed as Zyban for use by people quitting smoking), and the blood pressure medication clonidine.

Hypnosis

Hypnosis is worth special mention because of its popularity as a smoking therapy. Hypnosis therapists make suggestions to the smoker

withdrawal physical and psychological symptoms that may occur when a person suddenly stops the use of a substance or reduces the dose of an addictive substance

antidepressant medication used for the treatment and prevention of depression

when he or she is in a **trance** and possibly more open to suggestions, such as "You will not want a cigarette" or "The thought of a cigarette will make you feel sick." Careful evaluations of hypnosis therapies show small or no treatment effects. These therapies are difficult to study, since there are no standard procedures. The methods and suggestions used vary from one therapist to the next. For those seeking hypnosis therapy, it is important to deal with therapists who have good reputations and who charge reasonable fees for their services.

trance state of partial consciousness

Combination Therapies

A wide range of behavioral therapies have been tested, and no single method stands out as particularly effective. Combination approaches are now widely used, in hopes that trying everything will lead to success at something. Currently, there is no reliable way to judge beforehand which smoker will be most helped by a particular technique. (The exception is that heavier, more dependent smokers are consistently more likely to benefit from nicotine replacement.) However, the something-for-everyone approach is reasonable.

One of the behavioral therapies involves the preparation of detailed contracts that spell out punishments if the smoker returns to smoking. For example, if the patient has a relapse, that is, returns to smoking, he or she must give $100 to someone he or she dislikes. Other procedures emphasize the extremely unpleasant effects of very heavy smoking, such as dizziness or nausea. In this type of therapy, the smoker eventually finds these effects so unpleasant that he or she will have a stronger desire to quit. Other behavioral techniques aim to prevent relapse, a common problem among smokers who have tried to quit.

Smokers have sometimes organized Smokers Anonymous programs. The program allows smokers to support each other and teach each other techniques that will help them to stop smoking and to keep from returning to smoking. However, unlike the great popularity of Alcoholics Anonymous (AA) ☎ groups, these programs have not generally become popular.

☎ See *Organizations of Interest* at the back of Volume 3 for address, telephone, and URL.

Conclusion

Tobacco addicts must understand that if one method does not help them, they should try another, and another, until they have stopped smoking. Any one attempt to stop smoking can be a failure, but this does not mean that all attempts will fail. Repeated attempts give the individual experience with assorted treatment techniques, so that the individual begins to learn what helps and what does not help.

Tobacco addiction often goes hand in hand with the abuse of alcohol or other drugs. Smokers who fail to stop smoking may have serious drug problems that require treatment before the smoking problem can be resolved. SEE ALSO ADDICTION: CONCEPTS AND DEFINITIONS; NICOTINE; TOBACCO TREATMENT: BEHAVIORAL APPROACHES; TOBACCO TREATMENT: MEDICATIONS.

Tobacco Treatment: Behavioral Approaches

physically dependent characteristic of someone who takes drugs for relief of uncomfortable physical symptoms, rather than for emotional or psychological relief

withdrawal physical and psychological symptoms that may occur when a person suddenly stops the use of a substance or reduces the dose of an addictive substance

The effects of nicotine on the body are one reason why it is so difficult to quit smoking. People become **physically dependent** on nicotine, and when they try to quit, they experience unpleasant **withdrawal** symptoms. One way they try to relieve these symptoms is to take up smoking again. However, the addictiveness of nicotine is not the only reason why quitting smoking is difficult. Cigarette smokers may smoke to regulate their moods or deal with stress. In this way they are psychologically dependent on tobacco. In addition, tobacco users tend to connect certain behaviors with smoking. To quit successfully, they need to change their behavior. While medications such as nicotine gum and skin patches can help smokers and nicotine addicts deal with their physical addiction to nicotine, behavioral approaches can help them to change certain behaviors that go along with smoking. The most effective treatment for tobacco combines medications with behavioral approaches.

Behavioral Treatments

abstinent describing someone who completely avoids something, such as a drug or alcohol

Since the 1960s, many behavioral techniques have been developed to help smokers and smokeless tobacco users quit, but only a few techniques have proved to be effective. One important part of any treatment is the support and encouragement that doctors and other health-care professionals can give. Doctors can improve a person's chances of becoming **abstinent** by recognizing the discomfort of quitting and expressing sympathy, by emphasizing that half of all smokers have quit for good, and by recommending therapies. Family members can also provide support by participating directly in treatment.

Problem Solving and Skills Training. In a behavioral treatment known as problem solving and skills training, people learn to recog-

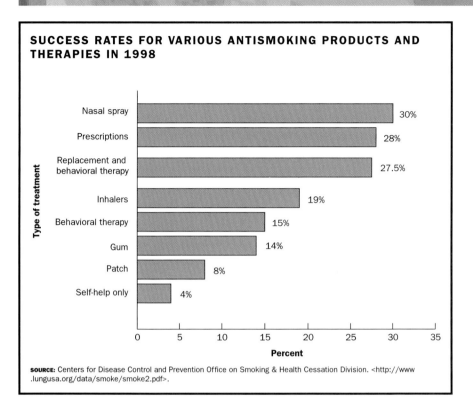

SUCCESS RATES FOR VARIOUS ANTISMOKING PRODUCTS AND THERAPIES IN 1998

Nasal spray — 30%
Prescriptions — 28%
Replacement and behavioral therapy — 27.5%
Inhalers — 19%
Behavioral therapy — 15%
Gum — 14%
Patch — 8%
Self-help only — 4%

Type of treatment (vertical axis)

Percent (horizontal axis, 0 to 35)

SOURCE: Centers for Disease Control and Prevention Office on Smoking & Health Cessation Division. <http://www.lungusa.org/data/smoke/smoke2.pdf>.

According to research by the Centers for Disease Control and Prevention, self-help was the least effective form of treatment for people trying to quit smoking in 1998, with only 4 percent reporting success.

nize their patterns of tobacco use and the situations in which they are most likely to smoke. For example, they may realize that their urge to smoke is strongest when they wake up in the morning, or that high-pressure situations lead them to light up a cigarette. By monitoring themselves, they learn how to deal with high-risk situations, or situations in which they are most likely to experience **craving** for tobacco.

craving powerful, often uncontrollable desire for drugs

A common problem for people trying to quit smoking is relapse, or a return to smoking after a time during which they do not smoke. Problem solving and coping skills are essential to preventing relapse. In skills training, the smoker learns to avoid situations that trigger the smoking urge, such as sitting in the smoking section of a restaurant. Instead, the smoker is encouraged to choose nonsmoking restaurants. Or the person can choose to take a night out in places where no smoking is allowed, such as movie theaters. Some situations that trigger the smoking urge are unavoidable, so for these times the person learns how to turn his or her attention away from smoking by using distractions, such as exercising. Craving to use tobacco products lasts only minutes, so using distractions can help the smoker wait out the time until the craving passes. Tobacco users are also taught to practice refusing tobacco or asking others not to use tobacco around them.

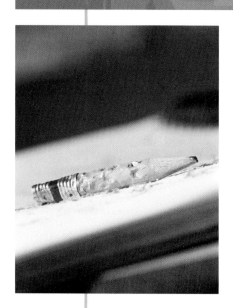

People trying to quit smoking commonly crave some type of oral activity like eating, drinking, or chewing. Nail biting, hand fidgeting, and pencil chewing are behaviors associated with nicotine withdrawal.

Rewards. Behavioral approaches also make use of rewards for not smoking. For example, the person trying to quit can use the money that is saved by not buying cigarettes to pay for a healthy and enjoyable activity like a vacation. Or the person could go to a movie as a reward for not smoking for seventy-two hours or some other short period.

Aversive Techniques. One behavioral approach to quitting smoking makes use of aversive techniques. An adverse, or aversive, reaction is a negative reaction against a particular thing or event. For example, in a technique known as rapid smoking, smokers are asked to smoke several consecutive cigarettes rapidly so that they will experience immediate adverse, unpleasant effects (such as nausea). The person then begins to connect the adverse reaction with the act of smoking, and feels less desire to smoke.

Relapse Prevention

Once a tobacco user has quit smoking, the challenge is to prevent relapse. "Relapse" means a return to the full program of smoking in which the individual had previously engaged. A slip, on the other hand, means smoking only one or a few cigarettes after a period of abstinence. Research has shown that slips, especially during the first few weeks after quitting, generally lead to relapse. As a result, smokers are advised not to take even one puff of a cigarette in order to prevent relapse. To remain abstinent, a person must change his or her behavior for good—not only during the period of treatment. Getting exercise, eating healthy foods, getting enough sleep and rest, and managing stress all contribute to remaining tobacco-free.

Conclusion

Combining medications and behavioral treatments for quitting smoking can increase success rates. These combinations can target different aspects of nicotine addiction. Nicotine gum or the prescription drugs can reduce the smoker's physical dependence on tobacco, which then allows the tobacco user to focus on the behavioral or psychological aspects of smoking.

Most cigarette smokers try to quit on their own, without medications or behavioral treatment. Their quit rates are the lowest of any approach. Society has changed in its attitudes to smoking, with more and more public places banning smoking on their premises. This trend, together with increased taxes on tobacco products, will put pressure on smokers to seek help in quitting the habit. SEE ALSO NICOTINE; NICOTINE WITHDRAWAL; TOBACCO: DEPENDENCE; TO-

BACCO: SMOKELESS; TOBACCO TREATMENT: AN OVERVIEW; TOBACCO TREATMENT: MEDICATIONS.

Tobacco Treatment: Medications

Although the nicotine in tobacco leads to a powerful addiction, people who want to stop smoking can be helped. Treatment to help people quit smoking is far less expensive than treatment of diseases caused by smoking, which will kill approximately one in two smokers who do not quit.

Examples of diseases that have been strongly linked to smoking include emphysema or chronic obstructive pulmonary disease, asthma, peptic ulcers, heart disease, and an increased risk of many types of cancer, including cancers of the mouth, pharynx, larynx, esophagus, stomach, pancreas, cervix, kidney, uterus, and bladder.

As early as the late 1890s, people were searching for medications that would help tobacco users quit. None of the products offered to the public between the early 1900s and the late 1970s were effective. As a result of important medical advances in the 1980s and 1990s, nicotine patches and nicotine gum came into use as effective treatments to help people quit smoking. Currently, the major accepted treatments for tobacco that use medications are nicotine replacement (products that provide nicotine through skin patches or gum) and symptomatic treatment (medications that do not provide nicotine, but that help decrease the craving for nicotine and the discomfort that occurs during withdrawal from the use of nicotine).

Nicotine Replacement

Of the 18 million smokers who try to quit each year, less than 7 percent do so successfully. In any given year, only about 1.7 million smokers quit for good. Most smokers who eventually quit successfully have between five and seven **relapses** before final success. Relapse is a common problem because of the unpleasant withdrawal symptoms smokers experience when they stop smoking. Smokers will often return to smoking to relieve those symptoms.

Nicotine replacement therapy substitutes a safer, more manageable, and less addictive form of nicotine to relieve the symptoms of nicotine withdrawal. The various forms of nicotine replacement include polacrilex (gum), transdermal delivery systems (patches), a vapor inhaler, and a nasal nicotine spray. These forms provide different doses and speeds of dosing.

relapse term used in substance abuse treatment and recovery that refers to an addict's return to substance use and abuse following a period of abstinence or sobriety

This man applies a NicoDerm® patch to his arm, which releases nicotine into his skin, and allows him to wean himself off cigarettes. NicoDerm® is one of three widely used U.S. nicotine patches that lasts for twenty-four hours.

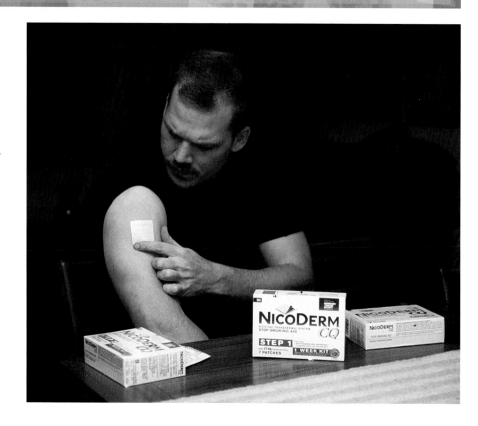

Nicotine replacement offers several advantages. (1) The nicotine in patches and gum does not contain all the toxins (poisons) present in tobacco or produced by burning tobacco. In fact, a burning cigarette produces an amazing number of chemical compounds—including tar, formaldehyde, carbon monoxide, ammonia, and hydrogen cyanide—many of which are known poisons to the human body. (2) Total daily nicotine intake is lower for most patients on nicotine-replacement systems. Much more nicotine is delivered to the body by inhaling from cigarettes. (3) Nicotine replacement allows doses to be controlled more effectively than with tobacco products. Someone trying to quit smoking can gradually cut back on the amount of nicotine he or she is getting by decreasing the patch dosage or the amount of nicotine gum chewed over time. (4) Nicotine replacement protects others in the smoker's household from the dangers of secondhand smoke.

Nicotine Gum. Nicotine polacrilex (Nicorette®) is a chewing gum containing nicotine that is available by prescription as well as over the counter. Nicotine from the gum may not be absorbed well if the client does not follow directions carefully. Patients may have less success with gum than with other forms of nicotine replacement because many dislike the taste and experience some discomfort, such as slightly sore mouths, throats, and jaws and stomach upset. Nevertheless, a study at the Addiction Research Center of the National Institute on

Drug Abuse (NIDA)☎ found nicotine gum to be effective in treating symptoms of tobacco withdrawal.

☎ See *Organizations of Interest* at the back of Volume 3 for address, telephone, and URL.

According to one manufacturer of nicotine gum, certain patients are more likely to benefit from this form of nicotine replacement. This treatment is most likely to benefit people who:

- have a high physical dependence on nicotine, preferring cigarette brands with nicotine levels over 0.9 milligrams
- find the first cigarette in the morning the hardest to give up
- smoke at least fifteen cigarettes per day
- smoke their first cigarette within fifteen minutes of awakening
- do most of their smoking in the morning

Patients who use nicotine gum should be warned that chewing many pieces of the gum at the same time or one after the other may cause a severe nicotine overdose.

Skin Patches. Four brands of nicotine patch are widely available in the United States. All deliver a given dose of nicotine through the skin over either a twenty-four hour (Habitrol, Prostep, and Nico-Derm®) or a sixteen-hour (Nicotrol) period. While Habitrol and Prostep are prescription items in the United States, Nicotrol is sold over the counter. The four brands deliver nicotine at different rates and have different skin-contact effects (causing rashes or irritation in some users), but there is no evidence that any one brand is more effective than the others. There is as yet no way to tell which patch will work better for an individual patient.

The nicotine patch is highly effective: It doubles the rate of successful attempts to quit smoking. Different studies have reported that from 22 to 42 percent of patients quit after six months of using the patch. The success rate is higher when combined with counseling.

The University of Wisconsin's Center for Tobacco Research and Intervention suggests that patients may benefit from use of a skin patch if they have a strong desire to quit and fit into at least one of the following categories:

- smoke at least 20 cigarettes per day
- smoke their first cigarette within thirty minutes of waking up
- have experienced a strong **craving** for cigarettes during the first week of previous attempts at quitting

craving powerful, often uncontrollable desire for drugs

The nicotine patch should be applied as soon as the patient wakes up, and the user should stop all smoking during patch use. The patch should be applied to a hairless part of the body, with a different site every day. The same site should not be used again for one week. The recommended length of treatment for the four patches varies from six to sixteen weeks. Some researchers have concluded that, in general, the chances of success are better from longer-term use. Side effects include a skin reaction at the patch application site in 30 percent of patients. The patch may also cause some sleep problems, but these problems may actually be a symptom of the withdrawal rather than a side effect of the treatment.

Nasal Spray. A nicotine nasal spray (Nicotrol NS) is available only with a prescription. The spray is packaged in a pump bottle that smokers can inhale (up to eighty sprays per day) when they feel a craving to smoke. The spray can cause a person to become dependent on it (more so than with the patch or gum). For this reason, the manufacturer recommends that the spray be used for a maximum of three months. People with sinus conditions, allergies, or asthma should not use the spray, and it is not recommended for treatment of young smokers. Very heavy smokers may benefit from using the nasal spray in combination with the gum and skin patch.

Nicotine Inhaler. A nicotine inhaler (Nicotrol Inhaler) is also available only with a prescription. It contains nicotine mixed with menthol that is delivered to the mouth as a vapor. Most of the nicotine is absorbed through the mucous membranes of the mouth and throat, and does not get as far as the lungs. The most common side effects of the inhaler include a sore throat, irritation of the mouth, and coughing.

Non-Nicotine Medications

antidepressant medication used for the treatment and prevention of depression

Medications that do not deliver nicotine are also sometimes used to treat nicotine addiction. Bupropion (Wellbutrin) is an **antidepressant** that reduces withdrawal symptoms and cravings to smoke. The most common side effects of bupropion are agitation and insomnia (inability to sleep), dry mouth, headache, nausea, and a skin rash. In studies, bupropion used together with a nicotine replacement helped 50 percent of a group of smokers to quit after one year of treatment. Buspirone (BuSpar) is an anti-anxiety medication that is used to help patients with tobacco withdrawal symptoms. It has a very low potential for abuse and does not interact with alcohol.

The Treatment of Nicotine Withdrawal

Clonidine (Catapres) is a medication that has been tried in the treatment of nicotine withdrawal discomfort. In studies, heavy smokers who took clonidine on days when they did not smoke found that it reduced anxiety, irritability, restlessness, tension, and craving for cigarettes. Researchers also gave clonidine to smokers trying to quit. After six months, 27 percent of those given clonidine reported that they did not smoke. Surprisingly, clonidine seemed to be effective only for women. Clonidine does have side effects, such as drowsiness, so doctors should recommend it with great caution.

Benzodiazepines. Nicotine strongly influences the smoker's mood. Smokers smoke more than usual during stressful situations. Therefore, those trying to quit often relapse (begin smoking again) during stressful situations. Treating the mood changes that result from abstinence may improve the chances of quitting smoking. In some extremely unusual circumstances, **benzodiazepines** (a type of tranquilizer) have been prescribed for this purpose. Because these drugs are extremely addictive, doctors only rarely resort to this treatment. More studies are needed to determine its effectiveness for treatment of smokers trying to quit.

Conclusions

Treatments that combine medications with behavioral approaches appear to have the best results. People smoke for different reasons (to prevent withdrawal, to ease anxiety, to relax, to achieve pleasant effects), so a treatment program that targets several reasons for smoking may be successful in most cases. Despite gaps in our knowledge, programs to quit smoking are improving constantly, and smokers do not have to be alone in their attempts to quit. The National Cancer Institute maintains a web site with constantly updated information about programs sponsored by a variety of organizations, including the American Cancer Society, the American Lung Association, and the Office on Smoking and Health ☎ of the Centers for Disease Control. SEE ALSO ADDICTION: CONCEPTS AND DEFINITIONS; NICOTINE; TOBACCO: DEPENDENCE; TOBACCO: MEDICAL COMPLICATIONS; TOBACCO TREATMENT: AN OVERVIEW; TOBACCO TREATMENT: BEHAVIORAL APPROACHES; TOLERANCE AND PHYSICAL DEPENDENCE.

Tolerance and Physical Dependence

People who begin taking drugs often do so to achieve a certain effect that they find enjoyable or positive in some way. Prescription medications may be taken initially to treat pain, **depression**, or anxiety.

benzodiazepine drug developed in the 1960s as a safer alternative to barbiturates; most frequently used as a sleeping pill or an anti-anxiety medication

☎ See *Organizations of Interest* at the back of Volume 3 for address, telephone, and URL.

depression state in which an individual feels intensely sad and hopeless; may have trouble eating, sleeping, and concentrating, and is no longer able to feel pleasure from previously enjoyable activities

Improper use of prescription and other drugs (including alcohol) may make a person feel alert, powerful, confident, relaxed, friendly, sexy, or talkative. These rewarding consequences increase the likelihood that a person will continue using a drug. Furthermore, two other important consequences that influence continued drug use are tolerance and physical dependence.

Physical dependence occurs when a person's body becomes accustomed to and dependent on the presence of a particular drug. When the dose is lowered or the drug is stopped, the person will begin to notice withdrawal symptoms. Resuming use of the drug eliminates the withdrawal symptoms. Some withdrawal symptoms feel like a flu bug. The individual may feel hot and sweaty, chilly and shaky. They may develop a runny nose and eyes, and itchy skin. Diarrhea and anxiety may also occur.

Physical dependence is not the same as addiction. Physical dependence is a totally biological response of the body; addiction includes psychological or behavioral factors. A person can be physically dependent on a drug but not addicted to it. For example, a patient who has been in the hospital after major surgery may be put on regular doses of narcotic painkillers. When these are stopped, he or she may notice symptoms of withdrawal. This person has become physically dependent on (but not addicted to) painkillers.

When drug users become tolerant to a drug's effects, they must increase the dose to feel the same effects of the original dose. An individual being treated for severe pain may develop tolerance to a pre-

IN THEIR OWN WORDS

"If addicts can be punished for their addiction, then the insane can also be punished for their insanity. Each has a disease and each must be treated as a sick person."

—William O. Douglas (1898–1980), U.S. Supreme Court Justice in *Robinson v. California,* 1962.

After a person has become used to a certain dosage of a drug, they may experience a range of withdrawal systems when use of the drug is decreased or stopped.

WITHDRAWAL SYMPTOMS ASSOCIATED WITH DIFFERENT SUBSTANCES

	Alcohol	Amphetamine	Caffeine	Cocaine	Opioids	Nicotine
Craving					X	X
Tremor	X					
Sweating, fever	X				X	
Nausea or vomiting	X				X	
Malaise, fatigue	X	X		X		
Hyperactivity, restlessness	X	X	X	X		X
Headache	X					
Insomnia	X	X	X		X	
Hallucinations	X					
Convulsions	X					
Delirium	X					
Irritability	X	X		X		X
Anxiety	X		X	X		X
Depression	X			X		
Difficulty concentrating						X
Gastrointestinal disturbance			X			
Increased appetite						X
Diarrhea					X	

scription painkiller. The health-care provider may need to increase the dose in order to appropriately treat the patient's pain.

A person who has several alcoholic drinks a night may find that he or she has to drink increasing quantities to achieve the effects obtained from the original amount. An alcoholic can appear normal at **blood alcohol concentrations (BACs)** that would make a social drinker pass out. That person's body has developed tolerance to alcohol's effects.

blood alcohol concentration (BAC) amount of alcohol in the bloodstream, expressed as the grams of alcohol per deciliter of blood; as BAC goes up, the drinker experiences more psychological and physical effects

Tolerance can cause a person to take more of a certain drug regardless of the initial reasons for drug use. For example, a person may regularly drink alcohol to feel comfortable in social situations. If that person becomes able to drink large amounts of alcohol without getting sleepy or dizzy, his capacity to drink increases regardless of the reasons for his drinking.

A drug abuser who has become tolerant to a drug's effects may increase the dose of drug. But high doses often produce unwanted effects, such as dysphoria (a feeling of uneasiness) or physical illness. Once the user experiences these negative effects, he or she may stop using the drug. However, the drug abuser may also become tolerant to the drug's negative effects, and so continue drug use. In general, tolerance and physical dependence make stopping a drug very difficult.

Addiction is a condition that occurs due to both physical and psychological factors. The individual's body becomes physically dependent, and he or she develops tolerance to the drug's effects. However, a person who is addicted to drugs also develops psychological dependence on the drug. Drug use may cause multiple problems for an individual: in school, on the job, in personal relationships, in finances, and in health. Yet a person who is addicted to drugs overrides these negative consequences of drug use, and continues to seek out and use drugs. This person is truly addicted. Researchers would like to better understand how issues of physical dependence, tolerance, and addiction interact to make drug use such a hideous snare. SEE ALSO ADDICTION: CONCEPTS AND DEFINITIONS; ALCOHOL: WITHDRAWAL; BENZODIAZEPINE WITHDRAWAL; COCAINE: WITHDRAWAL; NICOTINE WITHDRAWAL; NONABUSED DRUGS WITHDRAWAL.

Toughlove

The term "toughlove" (or tough love) describes a style of caring in which a person or a group reasserts power over another person for whom he or she is responsible. In its most common use today, the term describes the means by which parents of abusive, delinquent, or drug-abusing children can regain parental control. Toughlove is also the name of a self-help program for these parents and their children.

Toughlove, the self-help program, was developed by Phyllis and David York in 1980. They found that rescuing their daughter, who engaged in highly destructive behavior, did more harm than good. Instead, they permitted natural and logical consequences to correct their daughter's behavior while they sought emotional support from their friends. They wrote and published *Toughlove* (1980) and founded an organization called the Toughlove Support Network (which is described in their later book, published in 1984). The network's mission is to promote what they view as a mode of **intervention** for individuals, families, and communities.

The Toughlove Philosophy

According to the Toughlove philosophy, parents are the ones with the dominant power in a family. Children misbehave when parents fail to assert themselves or to take responsibility for their role as parents, but when parents' expectations are stated clearly, a child will no longer control the family. Parents are urged to describe the behavior they expect from their children. Wondering about the causes of child misbehavior is discouraged. Parents do not need to understand why their child misbehaves. Instead, they must act in coalition with other parents to assert control of themselves and their home environment.

Toughlove parents are taught not to feel guilty about their child's misbehavior, because children are responsible for their own actions. A Toughlove parent of a destructive child might say: "We have had enough. We are not rescuing you from the trouble you have caused. We love you enough to say no." Proponents of Toughlove believe that drug and alcohol abuse is the most important factor causing the disruptive behavior among teens. Once parents suspect drug and alcohol abuse, it is important that they investigate by questioning their child's friends, school officials, other family members, and anyone else their child meets frequently. When parents find drug and alcohol abuse, they must require **abstinence**. Strict discipline and setting limits are seen as the only means of enabling children to behave and to have a chance of regaining control of their lives.

Parents must confront their child about the drug and alcohol abuse and state the behavior they expect. Toughlove recommends that they require the child to stop using drugs and seek treatment if needed. If a child refuses to comply, he or she is to be ejected from

intervention when referring to substance abuse, it means an attempt to help an addict admit to his or her addiction, recognize the ill effects the addiction has had on the addict and on his or her relationships, and get help to conquer the addiction

abstinence complete avoidance of something, such as the use of drugs or alcoholic beverages

the home. Many uncooperative children are sent to live with another Toughlove family until they are serious about meeting their own parents' requirements. Children who refuse to live with another Toughlove family are out on their own until they agree to their parents' rules.

To gain help in maintaining firmness and setting appropriate rules, parents attend a support group consisting of other parents who endorse the Toughlove principles. Toughlove support groups are organized by the parents without any professional leadership. Besides providing support for parents, Toughlove groups evaluate the effectiveness of treatment programs and the effectiveness of professionals who treat children for alcohol and drug abuse.

Toughlove parent groups emphasize that old-fashioned values for raising children are superior to those commonly used in today's world. Members believe that child-development professionals are **advocates** for modern child-raising methods that blame parents for child misbehavior. They describe the Toughlove group as their island of support within a pro-child social environment made up of the police, educators, social workers, and the courts. The groups offer a persuasive and comforting rationale for the use of strict discipline that addresses the needs of parents who were experiencing great stress and feelings of failure.

advocate supporter or defender of a cause or a proposal

Critics of Toughlove

Toughlove has been criticized as being simplistic and heavy-handed. Researchers have noted that parents in Toughlove groups who did not believe their child was abusing drugs or alcohol were nevertheless instructed in how to document such abuse. Other possible causes of their child's misbehavior were ignored, because the Toughlove solution is supposed to apply in all situations. The practice of throwing an unruly child out of the house is especially controversial. Although most children go to live with other Toughlove families, some are forced to leave with nowhere to go and can become homeless, a predator or a victim, or a threat to themselves and others. For example, John Hinckley, who attempted to kill President Ronald W. Reagan in 1982, had been cast out of his home by parents who endorsed Toughlove and who later warned other parents to be cautious in disciplining their children.

Neither the Toughlove program nor the style of caring identified with it has been evaluated. On the one hand, there is anecdotal evidence from parents to vouch for it. On the other, as illustrated by the Hinckley family, Toughlove solutions can make matters worse. At present, it is not known whether the positive or the negative is the more common outcome, or whether positive outcomes result from factors having nothing to do with Toughlove. SEE ALSO ADOLESCENTS, DRUG AND ALCOHOL USE; FAMILIES AND DRUG USE; PREVENTION; PREVENTION PROGRAMS.

Treatment: History of, in the United States

The history of the treatment of alcohol and other drug problems in the United States has not followed a simple path. Various views on what causes addiction have often come into conflict. For example, one widely held belief about addicts is that people exercise free will in choosing to use drugs. A different but very common view is that drug addiction is a disease that overwhelms a person's free will. Since treatment efforts began, experts have been searching for insights into the best methods of intervention. This article provides an overview of the treatment methods used from the nineteenth century to the twenty-first century.

The History of the Treatment of Alcoholism

Mutual Aid. In the nineteenth century, people who drank heavily were called "habitual drunkards." (The term "alcoholic" came into use in the twentieth century.) The effort to help habitual drunkards began with the Washington Total Abstinence Movement, or the Washingtonian Movement, in 1842. This movement began a tradition of mutual aid, the banding together of people in similar circumstances to help one another. Mutual aid developed throughout the 1800s in connection to American Protestantism. The Salvation Army, which arose in the United States in the mid-1870s, is also a mutual aid society, as is Alcoholics Anonymous (AA) ☎ and the many other groups inspired by AA. Mutual aid is now more often referred to as "self-help," but this term misses the meaning of people helping each other.

☎ See *Organizations of Interest* at the back of Volume 3 for address, telephone, and URL.

Washingtonian societies were dedicated to sobering up hard drinkers, usually (but not always) men. Although some famous teetotalers (people who drink no alcoholic beverages at all) like Abraham Lincoln were members, the societies were open to anyone, including the poor, (sometimes) nonwhites, and women. The societies stressed Christian charity, economic self-improvement, and democratic principles.

The Asylum Movement. Samuel Woodward, a Massachusetts superintendent of an asylum, or a home for the mentally ill, was the father of institutional treatment of habitual drinkers. Woodward argued that drunkards could not be treated successfully on a voluntary basis. What they needed, he said, was to be committed (involuntarily) to a "well-conducted institution," or asylum.

The first such asylum, funded by the State of New York, opened in Binghamton in 1864. Other asylums opened in Kings County, New York (1869), Massachusetts (1893), Iowa (1904), and Minnesota (1908). The asylum movement led to dozens of private institutions that treated well-to-do drunkards and, by the 1890s, drug addicts. But overall, the movement for public treatment was a failure. State legislatures did not support them, partly because of their cost, and partly because physicians never could produce a strictly medical "cure" for addiction. Instead, doctors believed recovery could be achieved through bed rest, a healthy diet, and therapeutic baths (hydrotherapy), and the discipline of useful labor.

By the time of Prohibition in 1920, all public asylums for drunkards had been closed or converted to other use. However, the asylum movement did leave a legacy for the treatment for addictions: It stressed an understanding of addiction as a **compulsion**, and the belief that doctors and medicine were necessary for successful treatment.

compulsion irresistible drive to perform a particular action; some compulsions are performed in order to reduce stress and anxiety brought on by obsessive thoughts

The Mental Hygiene Movement. The mental hygiene movement, which began in 1908, took the approach that addiction was strongly influenced by a person's environment—the addict's family and social influences. The movement also believed that addiction could be the result of a biological defect and could be incurable, although if the condition was addressed early on it could be stopped from progressing. Mental hygienists stressed the importance of family, friends, and occupation in creating a healthy environment for an addict's continuing sobriety. Mental hygiene developed into what is called community mental health.

The emphasis on the addict's environment challenged the strictly biological view of the asylum movement. Mental hygienists believed that only voluntary access to free or inexpensive care would attract patients in the early stages of drinking or drug-taking careers. The Massachusetts Hospital for Dipsomaniacs and Inebriates (1893–1920) is an example of how views were changing at that time. It began as a hospital run on the asylum model but in 1908 was completely reorganized to follow a mental hygiene course. Most of its admissions were legally voluntary; the hospital established a statewide network of **outpatient** clinics; it worked closely with local charities, probation

outpatient person who receives treatment at a doctor's office or hospital but does not stay overnight

offices, employers, and the families of patients. Known finally as Norfolk State Hospital, it was a preview of what treatment was to become, beginning in the 1940s.

The mental hygiene movement changed the emphasis of the asylum tradition but did not entirely abandon its practices. For example, Norfolk created on its campus a "farm" for the long-term detention of "incurables." From 1910 to 1925, many local governments across the United States established farms to hold repeated public drunkenness offenders and drug addicts. Some of these persisted until the 1960s, and some have been reopened in recent years to accommodate homeless people with alcohol and drug problems.

Modern Alcoholism Treatment

Alcoholics Anonymous (AA), which grew out of the mental hygiene movement of the 1920s and 1930s, has had an enormous influence on the treatment of alcoholism. AA looks at alcoholism as a disease, and this view has affected public and political attitudes toward heavy drinking and treatment methods. Although experts disagree about its effectiveness, AA has spread throughout the United States and around the world, and many groups such as Narcotics Anonymous ☎ follow AA's **Twelve Steps**.

During the early 1960s, some state hospitals, particularly in Minnesota, incorporated recovering alcoholics and the principles of AA into their treatment programs. A treatment was developed called the Minnesota model of short-term inpatient care (usually twenty-eight days). This inpatient treatment was to be followed by AA fellowship. Across the country, local councils on alcoholism began to press states and localities for outpatient clinics, keeping alcoholics out of jail, and treatment resources. However, progress was slow. By 1967 only 130 outpatient clinics and only 100 halfway houses (transitional housing) and recovery homes existed to treat alcoholics. Alcoholics continued to be barred from most hospital emergency rooms.

Several important court decisions in the 1960s supported the view that alcoholism is a disease. In 1970, Congress passed the Comprehensive Alcohol Abuse and Alcoholism Prevention, Treatment and Rehabilitation Act (called the Hughes Act, after Senator Harold Hughes of Iowa, a recovering alcoholic). The goal of this act was to encourage a more humane and decent response to people with alcohol-related problems. President Richard M. Nixon signed the legislation establishing the National Institute on Alcohol Abuse and Alcoholism ☎ (NIAAA). This legislation made federal funds available for the first time specifically for alcoholism treatment programs. By

☎ See *Organizations of Interest* at the back of Volume 3 for address, telephone, and URL.

Twelve Steps program for remaining sober developed by Alcoholics Anonymous; adopted by many other groups, such as Narcotics Anonymous

1980, thirty states had passed laws to ensure that public drunkenness would not be treated as a crime. A system of community-based alcoholism treatment services began to emerge.

History of the Treatment of Drug Addiction

During the late 1800s, many people were addicted to morphine as a result of poor medical treatment or attempts at self-treatment. But morphine addiction declined after the turn of the century as physicians and pharmacists changed their practices and new laws began to be applied to the dispensing of medicines. At the same time, a growing number of urban young people began to experiment with drugs, especially smoking opium, morphine, and cocaine. By 1910 the public saw drug addiction as the problem of petty thieves, loose-living actors, gamblers, prostitutes, and other suspicious types, along with racial minorities and undisciplined youths. While habitual drunkards were often portrayed as occasionally bothersome fools, drug addicts were portrayed as dangerous and exotic.

Because of the link between drug addiction and crime, many believed that drug addicts should be confined under strict conditions for long periods. The mental hygienists at Norfolk State Hospital believed addicts could not remain sober and favored imprisoning them. State hospitals saw addicts as threats to hospital routine and order.

As the number of state laws against the sale or possession of **opiates** and cocaine increased in the 1890s, and as enforcement tightened after 1910, county jails and state prisons faced a major problem. Jailers proposed solving this crisis through two treatment strategies. First was the creation of special institutions for drug addicts, such as the narcotic hospitals that opened at Lexington, Kentucky (1935), and Fort Worth, Texas (1938). These hospitals were more like jails, although they were authorized to admit voluntary patients of "good character" whose applications were approved by the U.S. surgeon general. Before they were closed in the 1970s, the two facilities had admitted more than 60,000 individuals.

The second form of treatment proposed by jailers was to set up clinics to provide drugs to registered addicts. Addicts were to receive a certain dose of morphine (occasionally heroin, and very rarely, smoking opium), which would then be reduced over a short time to whatever dose prevented **withdrawal**. At this point, it was believed, the drug addict would stop taking drugs.

However, few of the clinics worked this way. Many clinic operators believed that their primary aim was to stop illegal drug selling by supplying addicts with drugs through medical channels. Most clinic

opiate derived directly from opium and used in its natural state, without chemical modification (e.g., morphine, codeine, and thebaine)

withdrawal group of physical and psychological symptoms that may occur when a person suddenly stops the use of a substance or reduces the dose of an addictive substance

operators believed that reducing doses to the point of withdrawal was useless if the addict did not then get institutional treatment. As a result, clinic doctors rarely bothered to reduce doses. Following World War II, the clinics closed. The period from 1923 through 1965 was a time of strict enforcement of increasingly severe laws against drug possession and sales. Drug addiction was a problem assigned to the criminal justice system, with many drug addiction hospitals being run by state prison systems.

Modern Drug Treatment

In 1961 the American Bar Association and the American Medical Association published a joint report favoring outpatient treatment for drug addicts and limited maintenance treatment programs for heroin addicts as alternatives to prison sentences. In 1962 the U.S. Supreme Court struck down a California law that made drug addiction a crime. The emerging view was that drug addicts required medical treatment, not imprisonment.

methadone potent synthetic narcotic, used in heroin recovery programs as a non-intoxicating opiate that blunts symptoms of withdrawal

Methadone. An important reason for this change in attitude was the success of experiments in treating heroin addicts through **methadone** maintenance. Methadone maintenance treatment centers have become widespread, although the treatment continues to be a source of controversy. Critics argue that it encourages users simply to replace one drug with another. Supporters argue that methadone maintenance allows former heroin addicts to live productive and healthy lives.

Heroin addiction is more common in areas where there is a great deal of poverty. Many experts argue that no form of treatment is effective without job and community development to support recovering addicts and to prevent relapse, or a return to drug use following treatment. They recommend that individual treatment using medications must be combined with strategies to improve general living conditions. Many workers in antipoverty programs supported methadone as a useful treatment, but many others did not. In 1966, when New York City launched a major expansion of treatment for drug addiction, it chose to make drug-free therapeutic communities the centerpieces of its effort.

detoxification process of removing a poisonous, intoxicating, or addictive substance from the body

Throughout the middle to late 1960s, publicly supported programs for drug addiction expanded, offering a variety of treatments: therapeutic communities; methadone maintenance programs; compulsory (court-ordered) treatment involving residential rehabilitation; twelve-step programs; religious programs; and a number of traditional mental-health approaches offering **detoxification** followed by **psychotherapy**. Yet the total number of treatment programs in the United States remained small.

Community-Based Treatment. A 1966 federal law encouraged the establishment of community-based treatment programs. This expansion of treatment capacity was important also for its attention to problems related to a variety of drugs. It came at a time of sharp increase in marijuana use among middle-class youth, an epidemic of amphetamine use, growing experimentation with LSD, and media focus on the counterculture, or the youth revolt.

President Nixon took office in 1969, and on June 17, 1971, he declared a "War on Drugs." Nixon created, by executive order, the Special Action Office for Drug Abuse Prevention (SAODAP). The creation of SAODAP marked the federal government's first commitment to make treatment widely available. In fact, SAODAP's goal was to make treatment so available that addicts could not say they committed crimes to get drugs because they could not obtain treatment.

Over the next several years, a variety of community-based programs were initiated and/or expanded, including drug-free outpatient programs, methadone maintenance, and therapeutic communities. SAODAP put less emphasis on hospital-based programs. SAODAP also stressed treatment within the military as an alternative to court martial.

During the first two years after SAODAP was created, treatment greatly expanded. In early 1971 there were thirty-six federally funded treatment programs in the United States. Two years later, there were almost 400. Between 1976 and 1982, however, the level of federal support for treatment was cut almost in half, as presidential administrations turned their attention toward prevention campaigns and pursuing policies designed to limit the importation and trafficking of drugs.

Despite a reduction in federal funds since the 1970s, there has been a selective increase in private funding of drug treatment facilities. Beginning in the 1970s, a few insurance industry leaders began to provide coverage for the treatment of alcohol and drug dependence. In response, private hospitals (both nonprofit and for-profit) expanded their treatment capacities dramatically. Commonly, programs consisted of a brief period of inpatient detoxification followed by several weeks of inpatient rehabilitation. After release from the hospital, treatment continued through participation in AA, Narcotics Anonymous, or Cocaine Anonymous. ☎ However, people without in-

psychotherapy treatment of a mental or emotional condition during which a person talks to a qualified therapist in order to understand his or her problems and change his or her problem behaviors

☎ See *Organizations of Interest* at the back of Volume 3 for address, telephone, and URL.

surance either had no access to treatment or had to turn to publicly supported programs.

Tobacco Treatment

Today, tobacco use is widely considered to be a problem of drug dependence (the drug being nicotine). For most of the twentieth century, however, it was not treated as such by either the medical or criminal-justice establishment.

Tobacco use was frowned on in the nineteenth century by the same groups who disapproved of drunkenness. As far back as the 1890s, advertisements for medicines claimed to help people break the tobacco habit. In the early twentieth century, a wave of temperance groups that advocated sobriety swept across the country, and more than twenty states passed tobacco prohibition laws, though most were quickly repealed. Public concern with tobacco use declined dramatically from the 1920s through the 1950s. Cigarette smoking became an accepted practice among men and grew steadily among women. This situation changed abruptly with the publication of the 1964 *Report of the U.S. Surgeon General* that linked cigarette smoking to cancer. Since then, increasing attention has been paid to treatment of the tobacco habit. The treatment approach considered most effective is a combination of medications, such as nicotine chewing gum and skin patches, and some kind of behavioral therapy. SEE ALSO ALCOHOL: HISTORY OF DRINKING; ALCOHOLICS ANONYMOUS (AA); LAW AND POLICY: CONTROLS ON DRUG TRAFFICKING; METHADONE MAINTENANCE PROGRAMS; PREVENTION; PREVENTION PROGRAMS; TOBACCO: HISTORY OF; TEMPERANCE MOVEMENT; TREATMENT TYPES: AN OVERVIEW; U.S. GOVERNMENT AGENCIES.

Treatment Programs, Centers, and Organizations: A Historical Perspective

Drug and alcohol abuse are age-old problems, but the development of treatment programs occurred fairly recently. Most formal treatment programs were founded in the second half of the twentieth century. Many came about because of an increased focus on social programs during the mid-1960s. In that period, President Lyndon B. Johnson created a policy called the Great Society, which stressed that communities should take responsibility for social problems and learn how to solve them. As a result of Great Society policies, new terms such as "community-based" and "storefront" (referring to programs

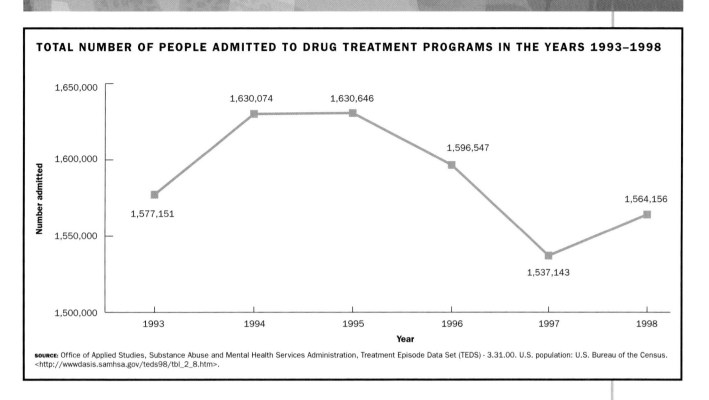

TOTAL NUMBER OF PEOPLE ADMITTED TO DRUG TREATMENT PROGRAMS IN THE YEARS 1993–1998

SOURCE: Office of Applied Studies, Substance Abuse and Mental Health Services Administration, Treatment Episode Data Set (TEDS) - 3.31.00. U.S. population: U.S. Bureau of the Census. <http://wwwdasis.samhsa.gov/teds98/tbl_2_8.htm>.

that operated out of storefronts in various communities) emerged. The programs that developed from this time forward took varying approaches to treatment for substance abuse. This article presents an overview of some significant drug and alcohol abuse treatment programs, centers, and organizations.

> The number of people admitted to drug treatment programs rose in 1998, after declining over the previous two years.

Hazelden Foundation

Hazelden (PO Box 11, CO3, Center City, MN 55012–0011; 800–257–7810), established in 1949, was one of the pioneering programs that developed the approach to treatment that is now widely known as the Minnesota Model. Today, the private, nonprofit Hazelden Foundation operates residential (live-in) **rehabilitation** programs. The main headquarters is located in Center City, Minnesota, with additional facilities in Illinois, Minnesota, New York, and Florida. The programs offer Minnesota Model treatment for thousands of alcoholics and drug-**dependent** men and women each year. In 2000 Hazelden granted its first master of arts degrees in the field of addiction counseling.

The stay at a residential treatment center lasts an average of twenty-eight days, but there is no time limit. Rehabilitation is done by a staff of trained counselors who are also working on their own programs of recovery. The staff identifies each person's needs and designs an individual treatment plan, with the individual helping to determine the best

rehabilitation process of restoring a person to a condition of health or useful activity

dependent psychologically compelled to use a substance for emotional and/or physical reasons

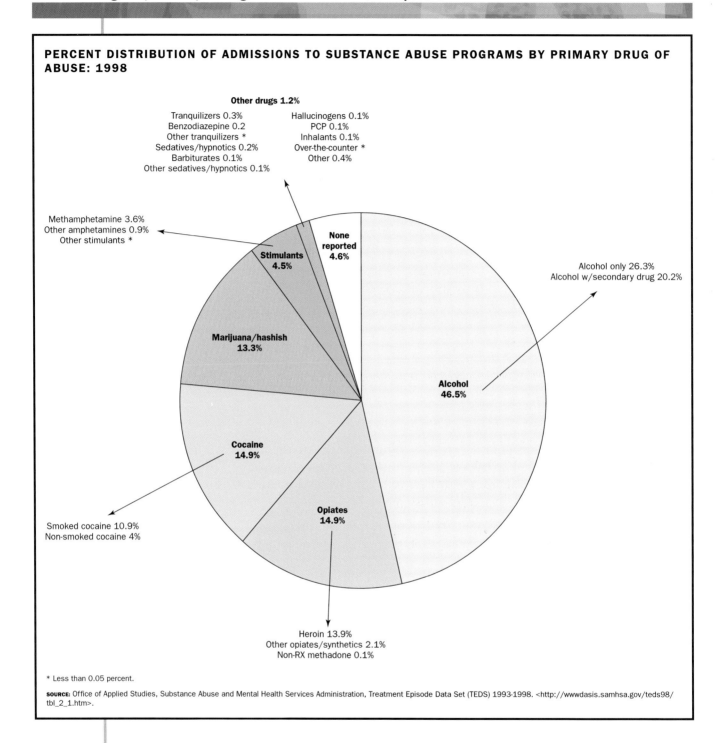

PERCENT DISTRIBUTION OF ADMISSIONS TO SUBSTANCE ABUSE PROGRAMS BY PRIMARY DRUG OF ABUSE: 1998

Other drugs 1.2%

Tranquilizers 0.3%
Benzodiazepine 0.2
Other tranquilizers *
Sedatives/hypnotics 0.2%
Barbiturates 0.1%
Other sedatives/hypnotics 0.1%

Hallucinogens 0.1%
PCP 0.1%
Inhalants 0.1%
Over-the-counter *
Other 0.4%

Methamphetamine 3.6%
Other amphetamines 0.9%
Other stimulants *

None reported 4.6%

Stimulants 4.5%

Alcohol only 26.3%
Alcohol w/secondary drug 20.2%

Marijuana/hashish 13.3%

Alcohol 46.5%

Cocaine 14.9%

Opiates 14.9%

Smoked cocaine 10.9%
Non-smoked cocaine 4%

Heroin 13.9%
Other opiates/synthetics 2.1%
Non-RX methadone 0.1%

* Less than 0.05 percent.

SOURCE: Office of Applied Studies, Substance Abuse and Mental Health Services Administration, Treatment Episode Data Set (TEDS) 1993-1998. <http://wwwdasis.samhsa.gov/teds98/tbl_2_1.htm>.

Alcohol was cited as the primary drug of abuse in nearly half of all admissions to substance abuse programs in 1998.

course of treatment. Treatment at Hazelden makes use of the beliefs and strategies of Alcoholics Anonymous. ☎

Daytop Village

Daytop Village, Inc. (54 West 40th Street, New York, NY 10018; 212–354–6000), which began in 1964, was developed to treat convicted felons who were addicted to drugs. This new approach offered an alternative to imprisonment, in the form of a residential treatment center, based on an approach called the therapeutic community, developed by a group known as Synanon. This approach has proven highly effective for both adolescents and adults, regardless of the types of drug they use. It involves four basic types of treatment: (1) behavior management and behavior shaping, (2) emotional and psychological life, (3) ethical and intellectual development, and (4) work and vocational life. By the mid-1970s, Daytop was also offering separate, nonresidential programs to adults and adolescents.

The Daytop treatment system views drug dependence as the result of a mix of factors: a person's education, medical history, emotional and spiritual life, and social influences. Treatment, according to the Daytop model, must attend to all of these factors. Many successful treatment programs have been built on a foundation of Daytop ideas.

Marathon House

In 1966 social workers for Progress for Providence (Rhode Island) became concerned about a growing community presence of heroin, heroin dealers, and addicts. After training at Daytop Village, representatives from Progress for Providence established Marathon House, the first New England-based therapeutic community, in Coventry, Rhode Island, in October 1967. Later, additional treatment facilities, including one for male adolescents, were opened throughout New England. In 1999 Marathon became an affiliate of Phoenix House.

Phoenix House

Founded in 1967, Phoenix House (164 W. 74th Street, New York, NY 10023; 212–595–5810) is a therapeutic community program that developed out of the treatment approach begun at Synanon. Phoenix House provides drug-free residential and **outpatient** treatment for adults and adolescents, plus **intervention** and prevention services. Phoenix House operates programs in prisons and homeless shelters. It is one of the largest nongovernmental, nonprofit drug-abuse service agencies and has a 1–800–COCAINE substance-abuse information and referral service.

Haight-Ashbury Free Clinic

The Haight-Ashbury Free Clinic (558 Clayton Street, San Francisco, CA 94117; 415–487–5632) was founded in June 1967 by doctors and community volunteers to provide medical services for the waves of young people, known as hippies, who came to San Francisco during

☎ See *Organizations of Interest* at the back of Volume 3 for address, telephone, and URL.

outpatient person who receives treatment at a doctor's office or hospital but does not stay overnight

intervention when referring to substance abuse, it means an attempt to help an addict admit to his or her addiction, recognize the ill effects the addiction has had on the addict and on his or her relationships, and get help to conquer the addiction

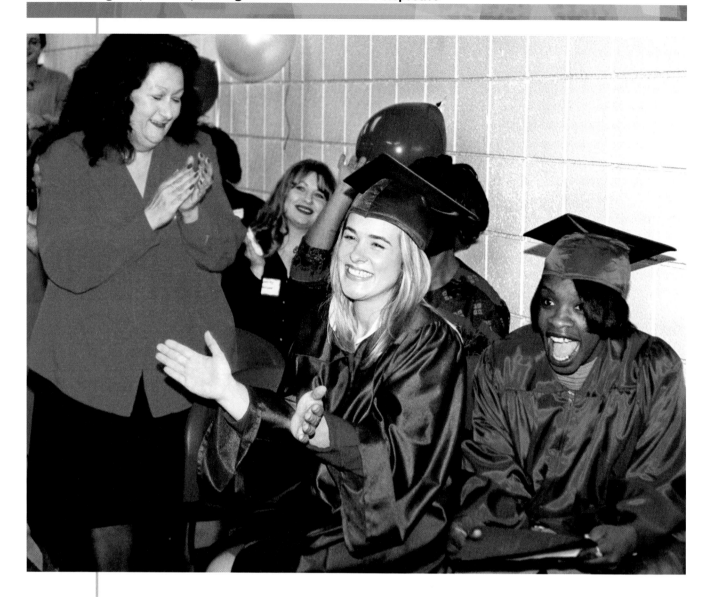

Graduates celebrate commencement at the Phoenix House in California. The organization serves over 5,000 adults and teens in eight states by providing treatment for and prevention of substance abuse.

sedative-hypnotic
drug that has a calming and relaxing effect; "hypnotics" induce sleep

the "summer of love." These young people often lived in crowded, unclean conditions, and many contracted respiratory, skin, and sexually transmitted diseases. The Free Clinic offered an alternative to the established medical care system. Counselors at the Free Clinic viewed health care as a right, not a privilege, and provided services without charge and without criticism of the patients' lifestyle. The Free Clinic developed ways to treat addiction to heroin, **sedative-hypnotics**, **stimulants**, and **psychoactive** drugs. Haight-Ashbury Free Clinics, Inc. provides community medical services to the working poor, the unemployed, and the homeless.

Gateway Foundation

In 1968 the not-for-profit Gateway Houses Foundation became the first therapeutic community in Illinois. Modeled on Daytop Village, it was established as a residential setting in which former drug addicts could help other drug abusers find a way to live drug-free, useful lives in the community. Outpatient programs were also developed for individuals who did not need long-term residential treatment. The agency changed its name to Gateway Foundation in 1983 to better describe the services offered. Gateway also offers community-based education and prevention programs.

The therapeutic community remains the core of Gateway's programs. Individuals participate in support groups that use the **Twelve Steps** during and after treatment. Gateway Foundation's successful treatment center within the Correctional Center of Cook County (the largest U.S. county jail) resulted in treatment programs for inmates in other Illinois and Texas prison programs. Treatment for all Gateway clients includes work and social-skills development, continuing education, and employment counseling.

Oxford House

Oxford House, Inc., is a movement of halfway houses, or transitional homes that help recovering individuals make the transition from inpatient treatments to a less-structured life. Oxford Houses do not receive financial support from the government. The first Oxford House was established in Silver Spring, Maryland, in 1975, in response to a decision by the state of Maryland to save money by closing a publicly supported halfway house. The men living in it decided to rent and operate the facility themselves. Operated democratically, residents of the house determined how much each would have to pay to cover expenses, developed a manual of operations, and agreed to evict anyone who returned to substance use. The concept spread, and by 2000 there were approximately 350 houses in North America.

Each Oxford House makes use of AA and Narcotics Anonymous (NA)☎ strategies, though the houses are not connected to those two organizations. Individuals can remain in residence as long as needed to become sober. The average length of stay is thirteen months.

Second Genesis, Inc.

Second Genesis, Inc. (7910 Woodmont Avenue, Suite 500, Bethesda, MD 20814; 301–656–1545), is a long-term, residential and outpatient rehabilitation program for adults and teenagers with substance abuse problems. Founded in Virginia in 1969, Second Genesis operates residential therapeutic communities and outpatient services in Maryland, Virginia, and Washington, D.C. Second Genesis admits adults, women and their young children, and teenagers.

stimulant drug that increases activity temporarily; often used to describe drugs that excite the brain and central nervous system

psychoactive term applied to drugs that affect the mind or mental processes by altering consciousness, perception, or mood

Twelve Steps program for remaining sober developed by Alcoholics Anonymous; adopted by many other groups, such as Narcotics Anonymous

☎ See *Organizations of Interest* at the back of Volume 3 for address, telephone, and URL.

The Second Genesis residential program has been described as a school that educates people who have never learned how to feel worthy without hurting themselves and others. Through highly structured treatment, Second Genesis combines the basic values of love, honesty, and responsibility with work, education, and intense group pressure to help correct the problems that prevent people from living by these values. Discovering self-respect in a family-like setting, residents are taught to replace behavioral problems and substance abuse with positive alternatives.

Walden House

Walden House (520 Townsend Street, San Francisco, CA 94103; 415–554–1100) is a therapeutic community that began in San Francisco. It offers residential facilities for adults and adolescents, a day treatment program, outpatient services, and a nonpublic school and training institute. Walden House is a highly structured program designed to treat the behavioral, emotional, and family issues of substance abusers. The heart of Walden House is a long-term residential treatment program in several phases. All of the household tasks, groups, and seminars promote responsibility and emotional growth. Walden House emphasizes self-help and peer support.

Founded in 1969 as a response to the drug epidemic of the 1960s, Walden House has grown into one of the largest substance-abuse programs in California. The program pioneered the use of alternative treatments with substance abusers, for example, herbs, diet, and physical exercise. Walden House has designed many special programs to treat particular populations, including clients with AIDS, homeless people, minorities, pregnant women, mothers, and clients referred from the criminal-justice system as an alternative to imprisonment.

Operation PAR

Operation PAR, Inc. (Parental Awareness & Responsibility) is a therapeutic community founded in 1970 by Florida state and county officials and a concerned parent. In the years since its founding, PAR has developed one of the largest nonprofit systems of substance-abuse education, prevention, treatment, and research in the United States. At present, PAR operates more than twenty-five substance-abuse programs in nineteen locations in Florida. The program targets individuals who behave in **aggressive** and antisocial ways as a result of substance abuse. The facility is an important alternative to imprisonment for criminal courts throughout central Florida. Approximately 70 percent of clients have histories of significant involvement with the criminal-justice system. PAR offers individual and group coun-

aggressive describing hostile and destructive behavior

seling, AA and NA support groups, educational services, job training and a job placement program, work experience, recreational therapy, and parenting therapy and classes.

Project Return Foundation, Inc.

Project Return Foundation, Inc. (10 Astor Place, 7th Floor, New York, NY 10003; 212–979–8800) is a nonprofit human-services agency that operates several New York City programs following the therapeutic community approach. The agency was founded by two recovering addicts in 1970 as a self-help and community center for substance abusers.

Project Return also operates an anti-AIDS education/prevention program; a medically supervised, drug-free **outpatient** program; and a facility for substance abusers who are HIV-positive. In total, nearly 1,000 men and women receive daily treatment and rehabilitation services through programs run by Project Return Foundation, Inc.

outpatient person who receives treatment at a doctor's office or hospital but does not stay overnight

Abraxas

The Abraxas Foundation was founded in Pennsylvania in 1973 to offer drug treatment to individuals in the state's juvenile and adult justice system. The state required that the program use a then-abandoned U.S. forest-service camp, Camp Blue Jay, within the Allegheny National Forest. By 1988 all Abraxas facilities served male or female adolescents. For example, Abraxas V in Pittsburgh was developed as an all-female residential facility. In 1990 a project was developed to provide community-based services to youths returning to Philadelphia from state institutions. The success of this project led to its expansion to Pittsburgh.

From its beginnings, Abraxas has made education an essential part of its therapeutic community treatment. The Abraxas School, a private high school on the Abraxas I treatment campus, offers a full curriculum of courses and special educational services for the resident population. Alternative schools have been developed in Erie and Pittsburgh because of the tremendous difficulty troubled adolescents have returning to public high schools.

Institute on Black Chemical Abuse (IBCA)

Founded in 1975, the Institute on Black Chemical Abuse (2616 Nicollet Avenue South, Minneapolis, MN 55408; 612–871–7878) is an organization that provides programs and services for the African-American community. IBCA seeks to encourage and support the exploration, recognition, and acceptance of African-American identity and experience, including the unique history of African Americans in the United States and the role that racial identity plays in drug dependence. Programs are designed to address the devastating effects of the drug-abuse problem on this community. IBCA offers outpatient treatment and home-based support.

IBCA's efforts in the community include education and prevention for people who face the problems of substance abuse. IBCA also educates and trains clergy members working with these issues in the community. The IBCA prevention programs have involved school and business leaders in programs aimed at establishing community awareness of substance-abuse issues. The Drug Free Zones program, in particular, has received national recognition.

Jewish Alcoholics, Chemically Dependent Persons and Significant Others Foundation, Inc. (JACS)

JACS is a nonprofit volunteer membership organization (850 Seventh Avenue, New York, NY 10019; 212–397–4197). JACS provides support programs and conducts retreats for recovering Jewish substance abusers and their families. These programs aim to strengthen family communication and reconnect individuals with Jewish traditions and spirituality. The programs are designed to help participants find ways in which Judaism can assist their continuing recovery. Participants and rabbis explore the relationship between Jewish spiritual concepts and Twelve-Step programs. JACS also provides community outreach programs offering information on alcoholism and substance abuse to Jewish spiritual leaders, health professionals, and the Jewish community.

Society of Americans for Recovery (SOAR)

Society of Americans for Recovery (600 E. 14th Street, Des Moines, IA 50316; 515–265–7413) is a national organization of concerned people whose aim is to prevent and treat dependence on alcohol and other drugs, and to educate the public about substance abuse and about its successful treatment. The organization sponsors regional conferences throughout the country and publishes a newsletter. The organization tries to fight the negative stereotype that society forms of alcoholics and addicts, and it supports **lobbying** for more funding of treatment. It also encourages people to learn more about addictions and recovery and to meet others who are active in communities on behalf of substance-abuse issues.

lobbying activities aimed at influencing public officials, especially members of the legislature

Betty Ford Center

This eighty-bed hospital for recovery from dependence on drugs or alcohol was named in honor of President Gerald Ford's wife, who was treated successfully and who promotes such therapy. The center is located southeast of Palm Springs, California, on the campus of the Eisenhower Medical Center. The staff at the center views alcoholism and other types of dependence as long-term, progressive diseases that will be fatal if they are not treated. The program at Betty Ford is designed so that patients learn to become responsible for their own actions and recovery. Because substance abuse affects the family, the center has created the family-treatment program, a five-day intensive process that includes education and individual and group therapy. SEE ALSO APPENDIX OF ORGANIZATIONS; ETHNIC, CULTURAL, AND RELIGIOUS ISSUES IN DRUG USE AND TREATMENT; HALFWAY HOUSES; LAW AND POLICY: COURT-ORDERED TREATMENT; PREVENTION; PREVENTION PROGRAMS; TREATMENT: HISTORY OF, IN THE UNITED STATES.

Treatment Types: An Overview

Perhaps there is no other illness to which the saying "an ounce of prevention is worth a pound of cure" is more applicable than it is to substance abuse and dependence. The reason for this is that once a person becomes **dependent** on, or addicted to, alcohol or some other drug, certain **physiological** changes occur inside the body, which make it extremely difficult to give up using that particular substance. For example, alcohol affects a variety of neurotransmitters (chemicals that help transmit messages between brain cells), and the overall effect is the inhibition or reduction of brain cell activity. When alcohol is removed, the affected nerve cells are overstimulated, and this results in **craving**. Similar changes also take place when a person abuses other drugs, such as heroin or cocaine, and some of the brain cells may become permanently damaged in the process.

It is therefore very difficult to cure dependence on substances; however, there are a number of ways in which it can be successfully treated. These include **psychological** approaches as well as treatments that involve the use of medications.

Psychological Approaches

Alcoholics Anonymous (AA) ☎ is the oldest and most popular self-help organization that has been established for (and by) alcoholics. Its aim is to help alcoholics recover from their addiction by using a psychological/spiritual approach. The organization has grown tremendously over the past few decades, and it is now estimated to have approximately 100,000 groups worldwide.

dependent psychologically compelled to use a substance for emotional and/or physical reasons

physiological relating to the functions and activities of life on a biological level

craving powerful, often uncontrollable desire for drugs

psychological relating to the scientific study of mental processes and behaviors

☎ See *Organizations of Interest* at the back of Volume 3 for address, telephone, and URL.

Over 40 percent of those admitted to substance abuse programs in 2000 reported abusing more than one type of drug.

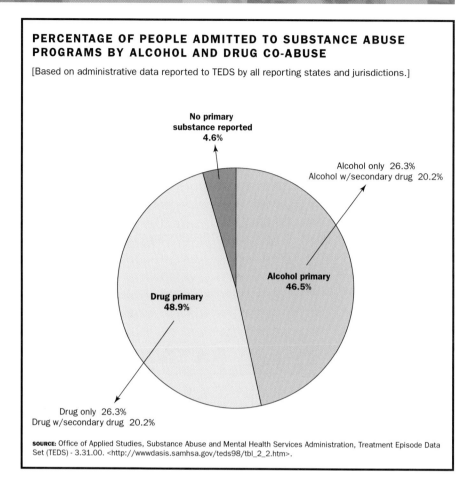

PERCENTAGE OF PEOPLE ADMITTED TO SUBSTANCE ABUSE PROGRAMS BY ALCOHOL AND DRUG CO-ABUSE

[Based on administrative data reported to TEDS by all reporting states and jurisdictions.]

No primary substance reported 4.6%

Alcohol only 26.3%
Alcohol w/secondary drug 20.2%

Alcohol primary 46.5%

Drug primary 48.9%

Drug only 26.3%
Drug w/secondary drug 20.2%

SOURCE: Office of Applied Studies, Substance Abuse and Mental Health Services Administration, Treatment Episode Data Set (TEDS) - 3.31.00. <http://wwwdasis.samhsa.gov/teds98/tbl_2_2.htm>.

☎ See *Organizations of Interest* at the back of Volume 3 for address, telephone, and URL.

narcotic addictive substance that relieves pain and induces sleep or causes sedation; prescription narcotics includes morphine and codeine; general and imprecise term referring to a drug of abuse, such as heroin, cocaine, or marijuana

The concepts of AA have also been applied to other substance use disorders. For example, there is an organization called Narcotics Anonymous ☎ for those addicted to **narcotics**.

The program of Alcoholics Anonymous is based on a twelve-step process:

1. Admitting powerlessness over alcohol.

2. Believing that a power greater than yourself could restore sanity and normalcy in your life.

3. Making a decision to turn your life over to the care of God.

4. Making a moral inventory of yourself.

5. Admitting to God, yourself, and to others the exact nature of your weaknesses.

6. Being ready to have God remove these weaknesses.

7. Asking God to remove the weaknesses or shortcomings.

8. Making a list of all persons you have harmed, and being ready to make amends to them all.

9. Making direct amends to such people wherever possible, except when to do so would injure them or others.

10. Continuing to take personal inventory, and promptly admitting it when you are wrong.

11. Seeking to improve your conscious contact with God through prayer and meditation.

12. Having had a spiritual awakening as the result of these steps, you try to carry this message to others, and to practice these principles in all parts of life.

The twelve-step model of treatment is usually applied on an **outpatient** basis, but there are **inpatient** rehabilitation clinics that are based on the AA twelve-step process. Therapy at such rehabilitation units usually consists of education as well as individual and group therapy sessions.

Behavior Modification. Behavior modification techniques involve rewarding desirable behavior and providing negative consequences for inappropriate behavior. For example, one counselor developed a voucher system in which negative urine tests (which indicate no drug use) were rewarded with gift certificates that could be used to purchase a variety of items. This behavioral group remained in treatment longer and had longer periods of abstinence, compared to a control group that had received standard drug counseling.

"Contingency contracting" is another effective behavior modification technique that is occasionally used for treating substance abuse. With contingency contracting, negative consequences follow undesirable behavior. For example, patients who are concealing their drug use from their bosses, family members, or anyone else may be asked to sign a "contract" that allows their therapist to inform one or more specific individuals if their drug use resumes.

Cognitive Therapy. The aim of cognitive therapy is to change the negative, inappropriate thoughts that lead to substance abuse and dependence. Cognitive psychotherapy for addiction recovery is usually a long process consisting of several phases or stages. Each of the stages has a primary goal, and different types of psychological interventions become appropriate, depending on the goal. During the first two phases, called pretreatment and stabilization, the focus is placed on challenging the denial of patients regarding the consequences of their disease and addressing the symptoms of **withdrawal**.

outpatient person who receives treatment at a doctor's office or hospital but does not stay overnight

inpatient person who stays overnight in a facility to get treatment

withdrawal physical and psychological symptoms that may occur when a person suddenly stops the use of a substance or reduces the dose of an addictive substance

Newspapers are one place where clinics and counselors may advertise services available to help those with drug- or alcohol-related problems.

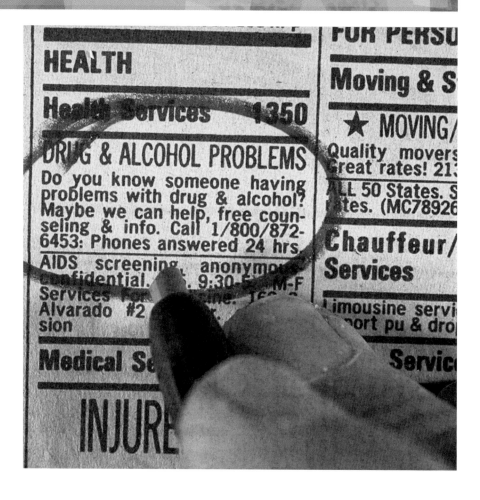

relapse term used in substance abuse treatment and recovery that refers to an addict's return to substance use and abuse following a period of abstinence or sobriety

During the third and fourth stages of early and middle recovery, the patients' major goals are to learn to function without drugs and alcohol, and to develop a healthy lifestyle. During these stages, the focus of cognitive therapy is on **relapse** prevention. Relapse is often due to ineffective coping skills in so-called high-risk situations (for instance, a high-risk situation might develop if the addict attends a party where he or she is strongly tempted to use drugs). Therefore, the therapeutic work of this approach is to develop effective coping responses, as well as to learn to handle a lapse (taking a single drink or drug) so that it does not turn into relapse. The final stages, late recovery and maintenance, emphasize personal growth in areas such as self-esteem, spirituality, intimacy, and work, while individuals are maintaining a drug-free lifestyle.

Treatments Using Medications

Although medications should not be relied upon as the only means of treating substance use disorders, they can be useful and effective components or parts of a comprehensive treatment program that addresses the psychological, social, and spiritual needs of the patient.

The drug disulfiram (Antabuse) has been used to treat alcoholics for over fifty years. Disulfiram acts on the liver to inhibit the metabolism of alcohol, and it results in the production of large amounts of a toxic substance called acetaldehyde. Therefore, if a person who had taken disulfiram drinks some alcohol—even in very small amounts—he or she will experience very unpleasant symptoms, such as nausea and vomiting, as a result. The symptoms vary with each individual, but they are generally proportional to the amounts of disulfiram and alcohol ingested. Severe reactions from unsupervised ingestion of alcohol may cause respiratory depression, unconsciousness, and even death. Because of the possibility of severe reactions, the use of disulfiram has been declining in the United States. Instead, newer drugs are being used to combat alcohol dependence, most of which can be described either as an **agonist** or as an **antagonist**.

Agonists. Agonists usually activate the same brain cells that are activated by the original drug that an individual is addicted to. However, the effects of agonist medications are less intense and tend to last longer than those of the addictive drugs they replace. For example, **methadone** is often given to heroin addicts, because it is metabolized (or broken down) by the body more slowly than heroin, and it does not have such an intense physical effect on a person's body. Because methadone reduces the craving and the withdrawal symptoms that occur when a heroin addict stops using the drug, methadone treatment makes it easier for the addict to quit. Eventually, some patients are able to stop using methadone itself as well. Even when addicts are kept on methadone maintenance treatment for a long time, they may be able to turn their lives around, they can work, and they can be acceptable members of their families and of society in general, which was not the case while they were addicted to heroin.

Antagonists. Antagonists work by preventing the abused drug from producing its usual (intense, pleasurable) effect. Antagonists have no potential for abuse and they produce no withdrawal syndrome. Naltrexone is an antagonist medication that has been used with some success for the treatment of alcohol dependence. It is usually used after **detoxification** to maintain abstinence. Unfortunately, however, relatively few patients take an antagonist as prescribed because of its lack of pleasant effects, its lack of effect on withdrawal (if the patient stops taking the medication), and its inability to stop the craving. Nevertheless, a review of a large number of studies found that naltrexone, when taken as prescribed, is moderately effective in reducing the number of drinks consumed by alcoholics.

agonist chemical that can bind to a particular cell and cause a specific reaction

antagonist agent that counteracts or blocks the effects of another drug

methadone potent synthetic narcotic, used in heroin recovery programs as a non-intoxicating opiate that blunts symptoms of withdrawal

detoxification process of removing a poisonous, intoxicating, or addictive substance from the body

Treatment of Adolescents

Adolescent drug and alcohol use often stems from different causes than it does for adults. For example, several studies have found that the influence of peers (friends, classmates) is very important, and having friends who are substance abusers is one of the biggest risk factors for the development of teen drug abuse and dependence.

In treatment, adolescents must be approached differently from adults. This is true for several reasons: adolescents are still developing or growing; they have different values and belief systems; they are influenced by environmental considerations, such as strong peer influences, that most adults are not influenced by; and they are still in school. Treatment approaches should also account for age, gender, ethnic group, cultural background, family structure, intellectual and social development, and readiness for change. Furthermore, younger adolescents have different developmental needs than older adolescents, and treatment approaches should be developed appropriately for different age groups.

Treatment should involve family members, because family history may play a role in the origins of the problem, and successful treatment cannot take place in isolation. Treatment providers should have specific training in the principles of adolescent development, and treatment programs should avoid mixing adult clients with adolescent clients. Treatment options can vary. Brief interventions, which involve screening, guidance, and educational interventions, are primarily appropriate for adolescents who have mild or moderate substance use disorders. Brief interventions may also occur in primary care settings as part of a routine medical exam.

Treatment may also include various intensities of outpatient treatment, as well as twenty-four-hour intensive inpatient care for adolescents requiring a high level of supervision. Inpatient care generally includes detoxification—a three- to five-day program with intensive medical monitoring and management of withdrawal symptoms. Residential treatment is a long-term model that includes **psychosocial** rehabilitation among its goals. The duration of residential treatment can range from thirty days to one year, and it is especially beneficial for adolescents with coexisting personality and substance abuse disorders.

Therapeutic communities are intensive and comprehensive (addressing many areas of the patients life) treatment centers. Although originally developed for adults, they have been modified successfully to treat adolescents with the most severe alcohol or substance use disorders for whom long-term care is considered the best choice. The

psychosocial describing something that relates to both life experiences as well as mental processes

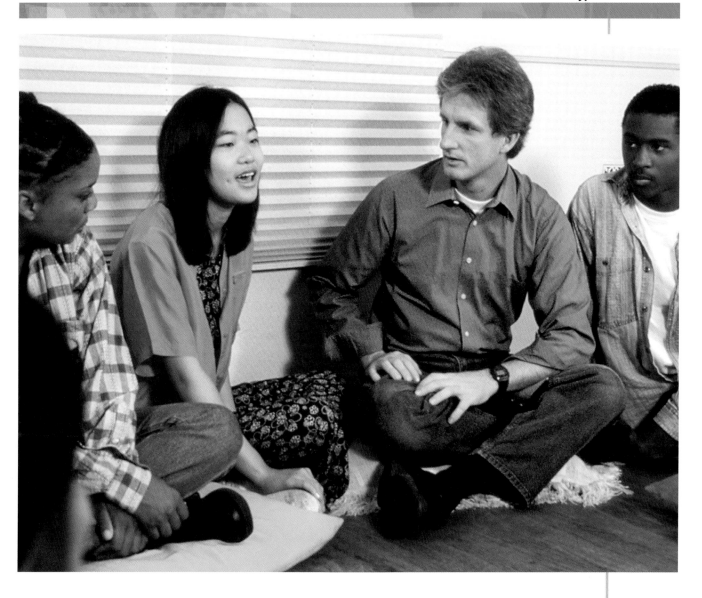

community itself is both therapist and teacher in the treatment process. The core goal is to promote a safe, healthy lifestyle and identify behaviors that can lead to alcohol and substance abuse that need to be changed. The community provides a safe and nurturing environment within which adolescents can begin to experience healthy living. Adolescents typically spend twelve to eighteen months living in a therapeutic community.

Self-help groups, such as AA, can be helpful when used in addition to other outpatient services and residential programs for teenagers. Self-help groups offer positive role models, new friends who are learning to enjoy life free from substance use, people celebrating sober living, and a place to learn how to cope with stress. Many adolescents involved with these twelve-step programs have a fellow member serve as a sponsor to provide guidance and help in

Group therapy aims to help individuals overcome the feeling that they are suffering alone with their drug problem and to encourage hope for a successful recovery.

times of crisis or when the urge to return to drinking or using drugs becomes overwhelming.

Treatment programs can also include family therapy to bring about positive changes in the way family members relate to—and communicate with—each other. This type of therapy may help decrease family conflict and improve effectiveness of communication. Family members, both parents and youth, can learn how to listen to one another and solve problems through negotiation and compromise.

It is extremely important that adolescents are assessed for coexisting mental disorders. Such disorders (if any) should be addressed and treated before substance abuse treatment takes place. Since substance use problems often occur along with other behavior disorders, many providers offer skills training in impulse control, anger management, problem solving, assertiveness, time management, and stress management.

During the final phase of treatment, providers work with adolescents to develop an aftercare plan to make sure they do not start using alcohol or other drugs again. Continuing (long-term) care programs are often needed to help adolescents reduce their risk for relapse. Self-help groups and group homes that offer transitional living arrangements can also be helpful for adolescents trying to recover from substance use disorders. SEE ALSO SPECIFIC DRUGS FOR TREATMENT ENTRIES; ADDICTION: CONCEPTS AND DEFINITIONS; AL-ANON; ALATEEN; ALCOHOLICS ANONYMOUS (AA); BRAIN CHEMISTRY; BRAIN STRUCTURES; NARCOTICS ANONYMOUS (NA); TREATMENT PROGRAMS, CENTERS, AND ORGANIZATIONS: A HISTORICAL PERSPECTIVE.

U.S. Government Agencies

The U.S. Department of Health and Human Services (DHHS) is a government department that includes individual agencies devoted to public health. Some of these agencies have the specific purpose of reducing drug abuse through prevention programs as well as treatment programs for substance abusers. These agencies include the following:

☎ See *Organizations of Interest* at the back of Volume 3 for address, telephone, and URL.

- The National Institute on Drug Abuse (NIDA) ☎ conducts and funds research on drugs of abuse and their effects on individuals. NIDA is part of the National Institutes of Health.

- The National Institute on Alcohol Abuse and Alcoholism (NI-AAA) ☎ conducts and funds research on alcohol abuse and al-

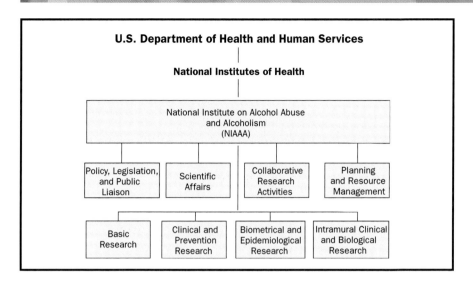

U.S. Department of Health and Human Services

|

National Institutes of Health

|

National Institute on Alcohol Abuse and Alcoholism (NIAAA)

- Policy, Legislation, and Public Liaison
- Scientific Affairs
- Collaborative Research Activities
- Planning and Resource Management
- Basic Research
- Clinical and Prevention Research
- Biometrical and Epidemiological Research
- Intramural Clinical and Biological Research

The U.S. Department of Health and Human Services includes various agencies, such as the National Institute on Alcohol Abuse and Alcoholism (NIAAA), that work to reduce substance abuse through research, prevention, treatment, and legislative methods.

coholism. NIAAA is also a component of the National Institutes of Health.

- The Substance Abuse and Mental Health Services Administration (SAMHSA) promotes prevention programs for substance abuse and mental disorders and treatment programs for these disorders. SAMHSA includes the Center for Substance Abuse Prevention (CSAP) ☎ and the Center for Substance Abuse Treatment ☎. CSAP leads the nation's efforts to prevent alcohol and other drug use, with a special emphasis on youth and families at particularly high risk for drug abuse. CSAT works to improve treatment services and ensures that services are available to people most in need.

☎ See *Organizations of Interest* at the back of Volume 3 for address, telephone, and URL.

Drug and alcohol abuse are complex behaviors that often result in a number of negative consequences. Understanding the various aspects of substance abuse requires drawing connections between areas of research. Since many people with substance abuse disorders abuse both drugs and alcohol, the research programs of NIDA and NIAAA are interrelated. In addition, many individuals who suffer from alcohol or drug abuse also suffer from mental illness. As a result, both NIDA and NIAAA promote studies of individuals who have more than one diagnosed disorder. But in general, these organizations work to expand awareness and information in the following areas:

AIDS. A current focus of concern in government health agencies is acquired immunodeficiency syndrome (AIDS). This disease has become a growing health problem among injecting drug users. Drug users who share needles have an increased risk of infection with human immunodeficiency virus (HIV), the virus that causes AIDS. Thus, NIDA works together with the Centers for Disease Control and Prevention on AIDS prevention programs and with the National

Institute of Allergy and Infectious Diseases to provide HIV therapy to injecting drug users with HIV.

Substance Abuse and Pregnancy. The effects of drug and alcohol abuse by pregnant women on fetuses and infants is another high-priority focus within the DHHS. Among other agencies, NIDA conducts research and demonstration programs, which are programs designed to serve as models for other agencies wishing to run similar programs in this area.

Combining Services. Recent research has shown that the most effective treatment for drug abusers is a combination of services that address not only their drug-abuse problems but also other health problems. Drug abusers can also benefit from education and job training. Accordingly, NIDA and the centers within SAMHSA are exploring the best ways to provide many different and necessary services to substance abusers.

In addition to the specific groups mentioned above, many other agencies are involved in prevention and treatment efforts. For example, the Food and Drug Administration decides when new medications for addiction can be put on the market. Both the Department of Education and the Department of Justice have significant programs aimed at prevention. The Department of Veterans Affairs and the Department of Defense have also made major commitments to treatment.

The following five sections discuss a few of the specific agencies that work directly in the areas of prevention and treatment of drug and alcohol abuse.

The National Institute on Drug Abuse (NIDA)

NIDA is the world's largest institute supporting research on the health aspects of drug abuse and addiction. NIDA supports almost 85 percent of all drug-abuse research, through financial grants to scientists at major research facilities in the United States and in other countries. NIDA's own staff also conducts research. NIDA was formally established in 1974 as one of three research institutes within the Alcohol, Drug Abuse, and Mental Health Administration, but in 1992, NIDA (along with NIAAA), was transferred to the National Institutes of Health.

ecstasy designer drug and amphetamine derivative that is a commonly abused street drug

NIDA research focuses on all drugs of abuse, from heroin and cocaine to newer drugs such as methamphetamine and **ecstasy**. In addition to illegal drugs, NIDA supports research to combat what may be the nation's most serious and costly public-health problem—tobacco use. NIDA's nicotine research continues to increase our understanding of nicotine addiction and the reasons why people start smoking. This research often leads to effective prevention and treatment approaches. Because drug abuse is the main way in which the HIV virus spread, NIDA researches prevention and treatment strategies to combat HIV/AIDS and other infectious diseases. NIDA is also responsible for the development of medications to treat drug addiction.

Through scientific research, NIDA has built a base of information on how drugs affect us—what they do to our bodies; to our behavior, thoughts, and emotions; to our relationships; and to our society. Understanding what factors place individuals at risk for turning to drug abuse is of great importance to prevention and treatment providers, educators, and policy makers.

Research has shown that treatment can be an effective tool in helping some people to recover from addiction. NIDA is researching ways to improve the effectiveness of treatment and to find ways to keep patients in treatment for longer periods in order to improve their chances of success. To support the great number of research programs, the research community needs an adequate supply of scientists with up-to-date skills and knowledge. NIDA contributes by sponsoring drug-abuse research programs in the biomedical and behavioral sciences. These programs include support of research training in medical schools and universities.

A final important function of NIDA is to make research findings available to the widest audience possible. NIDA has an extensive outreach and public education program to rapidly provide research-based information to scientists, health-care professionals, policy makers, and the general public. For example, NIDA staff works with community-based networks to hold town meetings at locations across the country. NIDA also has a Science Education Program, which develops materials for students from kindergarten to grade twelve and teachers.

The National Institute on Alcohol Abuse and Alcoholism (NIAAA)

NIAAA is the main federal agency for research on the causes, consequences, treatment, and prevention of alcohol-related problems. NIAAA supports both biological and behavioral research; the training of scientists to conduct research; programs that develop professional positions in the health field; and research on alcohol-related public policies. NIAAA is one of eighteen research institutes of the prestigious National Institutes of Health, a component of the DHHS.

NIAAA supports research by providing financial grants to scientists at leading U.S. research institutions. NIAAA's own staff scientists also conduct research. Findings from these research areas are made available to health professionals, scientists, and the public. Publications, reports, and database services are accessible online.

Research funded by the NIAAA or conducted by NIAAA staff specializes in six areas:

predispose to be prone or vulnerable to something

1. *Genetics.* NIAAA supports research aimed at discovering the genes that **predispose** individuals to alcoholism and the environmental factors (influences such as family, peers, and community) that influence its development.

2. *Alcohol and the Brain.* Many of the behaviors related to alcohol use problems are the result of alcohol's effects in the brain. NIAAA research is designed to learn how these effects influence the development of alcohol abuse and alcoholism. Brain imaging techniques are an important tool used in animal and human studies.

craving powerful, often uncontrollable desire for drugs

relapse term used in substance abuse treatment and recovery that refers to an addict's return to substance use and abuse following a period of abstinence or sobriety

detoxification process of removing a poisonous, intoxicating, or addictive substance from the body

3. *Development of Medications.* NIAAA is strongly committed to developing medications to lessen the **craving** for alcohol, reduce risk of **relapse**, and ensure safe **detoxification** of individuals undergoing treatment. Naltrexone, the first medication approved as a safe and effective treatment for alcoholism since 1949, was developed from neuroscience (brain) research. NIAAA expects that findings from neuroscience and genetics research in coming years will result in the approval of more medications.

4. *Prevention.* NIAAA prevention research is aimed at developing effective measures to reduce alcohol-related problems. These studies target such areas as injuries and violence related to alcohol use, alcohol in the workplace, and drinking and driving. Many prevention researchers conduct their work in high-risk neighborhoods of large cities.

5. *Treatment.* NIAAA emphasizes research to improve treatment of alcohol abuse and alcoholism.

6. *Identifying and Understanding Populations and Drinking Behavior.* Research enables the NIAAA to monitor the health of the population, to develop prevention and treatment services for alcohol problems, and to establish social policies that deal with alcohol-related problems. NIAAA-supported research examines the specific drinking patterns that lead to alcohol-related problems. It also considers the role of several factors—age, gender, race/ethnicity, genes, environment—that affect the rates of alcohol-related injury or disease.

Substance Abuse and Mental Health Services Administration (SAMHSA)

This agency of the DHHS was established in 1992. SAMHSA's main responsibilities are to promote prevention programs for substance abuse and mental disorders and treatment programs for these disorders. The agency works with states, communities, and organizations to make sure that people who have mental or substance abuse disorders or who are at risk of developing them get the services they need. SAMHSA provides grants (funds) to states to help them maintain and improve their substance abuse and mental health services. Some agency grants provide resources to communities in order to identify and address the needs of their members at the earliest stages of a disorder.

SAMHSA houses four centers: the Center for Substance Abuse Prevention ☎, the Center for Substance Abuse Treatment ☎, the Center for Mental Health Services, and the Office of Applied Statistics.

Center for Substance Abuse Prevention (CSAP). This agency was originally established as the Office for Substance Abuse Prevention. It was created in 1986 for the prevention of alcohol and other drug problems among U.S. citizens, with special emphasis on youth and families living in high-risk environments. Since 1992 the agency was renamed and is now part of the SAMHSA.

CSAP has two major goals: First, the group tries to encourage a standard of no use of any illegal drug and, second, to encourage a standard of no illegal or high-risk use of alcohol or other legal drugs. (High-risk alcohol use includes drinking and driving; drinking while pregnant; drinking while recovering from alcoholism and/or when using certain medications; having more than two drinks a day for men and more than one for women.)

☎ See *Organizations of Interest* at the back of Volume 3 for address, telephone, and URL.

The prevention work of CSAP is based on five principles:

1. The earlier prevention begins in a person's life, the more likely it is to succeed.

2. Prevention programs should make use of the latest findings of scientific research, including knowledge on which practices are most effective.

3. Prevention programs should be aimed at people of different ages and backgrounds, and should address a wide variety of risk factors.

4. Programs must be evaluated both as they proceed and at their conclusion.

5. The most successful programs are likely to be those begun and conducted at the community level.

CSAP performs many kinds of prevention work, including the following demonstrations for specific high-risk groups and individuals in high-risk environments: assisting communities in developing alcohol- and drug-use prevention programs and early intervention programs; maintaining a national clearinghouse for publications on prevention and treatment; and supporting the National Training System, which develops new drug-use prevention materials and delivers training.

CSAP's staff meets regularly with various federal organizations, including the departments of defense, justice, education, transportation, labor, housing and urban development, the Bureau of Indian Affairs, and others, to sponsor joint prevention efforts. CSAP also develops partnerships with the research community, parent groups, foundations, policy makers, health-care practitioners, state and community leaders, educators, law-enforcement officials, and others to increase opportunities for prevention and early intervention.

Center for Substance Abuse Treatment (CSAT). CSAT was established in January 1990 as the Office for Treatment Improvement. In 1992, the agency was renamed and is now part of the SAMHSA.

The purpose of CSAT is to make effective treatment and recovery services more available for people with drug and alcohol problems. CSAT works to ensure that the system of state and local government agencies and public and private treatment programs providing addiction-treatment services make use of advances in treatment technology. To carry out this responsibility, CSAT works with states, communities, and treatment providers to improve the quality and effectiveness of treatment. CSAT provides grants (funds) and technical assistance to organizations that provide treatment and encourages co-operation among agencies—drug-treatment providers, human services organizations, educational and vocational services, the criminal justice system. CSAT works to make sure that specific patient populations, especially minority racial and ethnic groups, adolescents, the homeless, women of childbearing age, and people in rural areas, get the services they need.

Research has revealed much knowledge about addiction and treatment. Two basic facts drawn from this research guide the work of CSAT:

1. Addiction is a complex problem. Addiction cannot be treated without also addressing other problems a person may face, such as poor health, mental health disorders, or being poor and disadvantaged.

2. Addiction is often a long-term problem with many relapses (when a person returns to drug use after a period of being drug-free). The gains made during treatment often are lost following a person's return to the community.

Based on these facts, CSAT encourages programs that provide care in many areas of a person's life and that do not simply stop when drug treatment is completed. People at high risk for drug use—those who have been affected by problems such as crime, abuse, poverty, and homelessness—need the most attention. At the core of CSAT's overall approach is, quite simply, the belief that treatment works. Treatment has proved effective in reducing the use of illegal drugs and alcohol, improving rates of employment, reducing rates of HIV, reducing criminal activity, and reducing death rates among patients.

Recently, CSAT's emphasis shifted from improvement of services to the development of knowledge about the effectiveness of different treatments.

Center for Mental Health Services (CMHS). SAMHSA's Center for Mental Health Services works to make high-quality care available to people who have mental illnesses or are at risk for developing them. CMHS also helps the families of these individuals by creating a nationwide network of community-based mental health services. Its education programs are helping to change the public's negative image of these illnesses. CMHS provides grants (funds) to organizations that develop and apply knowledge about community-based services for adults with serious mental illnesses and children with serious emotional disturbances. The center also collects and analyzes national mental health services data to help inform future decision making

☎ See *Organizations of Interest* at the back of Volume 3 for address, telephone, and URL.

about services. CMHS's information clearinghouse is called the Knowledge Exchange Network ☎ (KEN).

Office of Applied Studies (OAS). SAMHSA's Office of Applied Studies gathers available data on substance abuse practices in the United States. It then analyzes the data and publishes its conclusions. OAS directs the annual National Household Survey on Drug Abuse, the Drug Abuse Warning Network, and the Drug and Alcohol Services Information System, among other studies. Through these studies, SAMHSA is able to identify trends in substance abuse and, soon, also in mental health care. SAMHSA programs bring the latest knowledge from scientific research to community-based programs in prevention and treatment. The results are being measured in the improved quality of people's lives. SEE ALSO PREVENTION; PREVENTION PROGRAMS; RESEARCH; SUBSTANCE ABUSE AND AIDS.

Users

Do you ever get a song stuck in your head? The tune comes back to you, over and over again. Even when you do not want to think about that song, it keeps coming back. It nags you. Living with alcohol, tobacco, and other drugs can be like that. You start smoking tobacco, and then one day when you wake up, the first thought that comes to mind is, "I need a smoke." You cannot make the thought go away. Even when you do not want to think about cigarettes, the idea keeps coming back. It nags you and nags you. For most tobacco smokers, that nagging feeling is followed by getting up and finding a cigarette, lighting it up, and smoking it. Ask a smoker: "If you were to stop smoking, which cigarette of the day would be the hardest to give up?" Most of the time, regular smokers say that the hardest cigarette to give up is the first cigarette in the morning.

Once people begin to use alcohol, tobacco, or other drugs, the drug becomes a nagging part of their daily lives. They end up spending a lot of time talking about drugs, going out and trying to get drugs, and taking the drugs. For drugs like alcohol and cocaine, it is easy to take too much and get sick. Then, even after sleeping, the user often has a hangover, and getting rid of the hangover takes time.

This is part of the natural history of using alcohol, tobacco, and other drugs. Natural history of drug use is the story of using drugs as it unfolds in the lives of drug users. The first part of the story of using drugs may be the excitement of doing something new. But for many drug users, the later chapters of the story include this nagging feeling about the drug. The nagging feeling often does not go away until the drug is used again. The rest of this natural history often includes spending more and more time talking with people about the drug, getting the drug, using the drug, and recovering from hangovers or other effects of using the drug. These activities begin to fill the life of a drug user so that more and more of each day is filled with drugs and drug stuff. This includes the pain and suffering you can sometimes see in the lives of people who take drugs.

Who Uses Drugs and When Do They Start?

Studies of young people and drug use show that the use of tobacco and other drugs often starts earlier for boys, later for girls. Girls may be a little more sheltered and protected by their parents or other family members. Or, boys may tend to break rules more than girls do. Using drugs is a type of rule breaking.

The age when most people start to use drugs is different for different drugs. Many people start smoking tobacco at age 18, with some people starting when they are older, and others starting when they are a little younger. About two-thirds of high-school seniors have smoked tobacco at least once, and almost one-quarter of high-school seniors smoke tobacco every day. Across the entire United States, about one-quarter of the whole population smokes tobacco regularly. But if you have not started smoking tobacco cigarettes by the time you are 30, you probably will not become a regular smoker.

For alcohol, the age of starting to drink is a little older than the age of starting to smoke tobacco. About 4 out of 5 high-school seniors have tried drinking alcohol, but only 1 out of 20 of the seniors drink every day. This probably is a consequence of the legal age of drinking, which is 21 throughout the United States. About one-eighth of the entire U.S. population drinks alcohol often. However, most people start drinking alcohol before they turn 30. If you have not started drinking alcohol by age 30, you probably will not become a regular drinker.

For illegal drugs like marijuana and amphetamines, the fraction of people using them is even lower than the fraction of people who drink alcohol. For example, about 1 in every 9 young people in the United States has used an illegal drug recently. For most of them, the most recently used illegal drug is marijuana . Not counting marijuana, about 1 in 20 young people in the United States has used an illegal drug in the past month. Most drug users start using illegal drugs like marijuana and cocaine in their late teens or early twenties, after they start smoking tobacco or drinking alcohol. As with tobacco and alcohol, most people do not start smoking marijuana, or taking cocaine or other illegal drugs, after age 30. If people are going to start using illegal drugs, they typically begin before age 30.

Drug Use and Mental Health

depressed feelings of intense sadness and hopelessness

Once drug use starts, a person in good mental health can become **depressed** and worried. Some of these feelings are effects of the drug that go along with hangovers and the sense of being nagged all the time. Some of these unpleasant feelings are the results of drug use taking over the drug user's daily life so that more and more time is spent with the drug, and less time is spent doing other activities the person used to enjoy, like sports or music. Drug users can also become depressed because they are not living up to their own expectations for themselves, or the expectations of parents, teachers, friends, and other people who care about them. Falling short of expectations over and over again can be a distressing way of life, especially when drugs are nagging you and you cannot stop thinking about drugs long enough to do everything else you would like to do.

Marijuana is the most frequently used drug by teenagers aged 12 to 17 according to a U.S. study conducted in 1999 and 2000.

Risk and Protective Factors

Many factors can contribute to a person's becoming a drug user. Other factors protect against drug use.

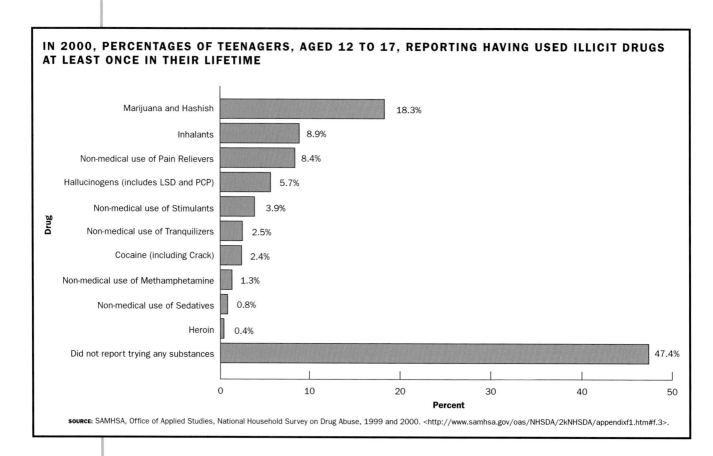

IN 2000, PERCENTAGES OF TEENAGERS, AGED 12 TO 17, REPORTING HAVING USED ILLICIT DRUGS AT LEAST ONCE IN THEIR LIFETIME

Marijuana and Hashish — 18.3%
Inhalants — 8.9%
Non-medical use of Pain Relievers — 8.4%
Hallucinogens (includes LSD and PCP) — 5.7%
Non-medical use of Stimulants — 3.9%
Non-medical use of Tranquilizers — 2.5%
Cocaine (including Crack) — 2.4%
Non-medical use of Methamphetamine — 1.3%
Non-medical use of Sedatives — 0.8%
Heroin — 0.4%
Did not report trying any substances — 47.4%

Drug (y-axis) / Percent (x-axis: 0, 10, 20, 30, 40, 50)

SOURCE: SAMHSA, Office of Applied Studies, National Household Survey on Drug Abuse, 1999 and 2000. <http://www.samhsa.gov/oas/NHSDA/2kNHSDA/appendixf1.htm#f.3>.

Dependence. Some drug users become **dependent** on drugs. Their bodies cannot function without drugs. Sometimes these users get into trouble at school or are arrested by the police. The accompanying figure uses a clock face to show the fraction of people who have become dependent on each drug. For instance, about one out of every three people who use tobacco become dependent on it, so tobacco is placed at the three o'clock position on the clock. One out of every six people who use cocaine has become dependent on it, so cocaine is shown at the six o'clock position. For alcohol dependence, the fraction is one in every seven or eight alcohol drinkers. About one in every nine to eleven marijuana users has become dependent on marijuana.

dependent psychologically compelled to use a substance for emotional and/or physical reasons

Personality. Young people who break the rules against using drugs often have a history of breaking other rules and getting into trouble even before drug use starts. Of course, some young people who use drugs are not troublemakers. They may just be curious and want to see what drug use is all about, even when they know it might get them into serious trouble. Or, they might not know about drug dependence and other serious problems caused by drug use.

Social Factors. Drug use can affect all types of people. No one really is immune. It sometimes is said that people of color are more likely to become drug users, but studies show that this statement is not generally true. It sometimes is said that drug use is more common in cities than in rural areas. This statement may be true for drugs like cocaine and heroin, but it is not true for drugs like tobacco and alcohol. In the United States, tobacco smoking by teenagers is most common in states with large rural populations, such as North and South Carolina, Kentucky, West Virginia, and Montana.

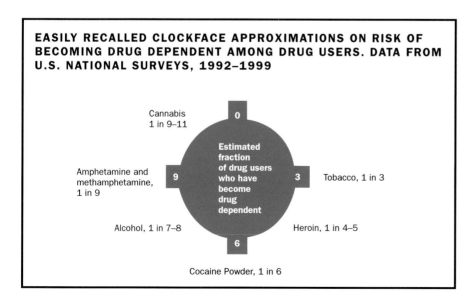

EASILY RECALLED CLOCKFACE APPROXIMATIONS ON RISK OF BECOMING DRUG DEPENDENT AMONG DRUG USERS. DATA FROM U.S. NATIONAL SURVEYS, 1992–1999

Cannabis 1 in 9–11

0

Estimated fraction of drug users who have become drug dependent

Amphetamine and methamphetamine, 1 in 9

9

3

Tobacco, 1 in 3

Alcohol, 1 in 7–8

Heroin, 1 in 4–5

6

Cocaine Powder, 1 in 6

This clockface shows the increasing risk of becoming addicted to various drugs. Of these drugs, tobacco users have the highest risk, with one out of every three people who use tobacco becoming addicted.

epidemic rapid spreading of a disease to many people in a given area or community at the same time

The science of epidemiology includes the study of drug **epidemics**. Epidemiologists chart the rise and fall of drug use from year to year. These epidemics are shaped by how many people are active drug users, how many started using drugs within the last year, and how many people in each category fall into different social groups. Epidemiologists examine whether people are poor or wealthy, whether they are well behaved or troublemakers, and what ethnic group they belong to. The accompanying figure shows the rise and fall of a recent epidemic of cocaine use in the United States.

Some epidemiological studies indicate that in the early years of an epidemic the drug users tend to be wealthier and come from the upper social classes. However, in the later years, this changes and the drug users tend to be poorer and come from the lower social classes. In the twenty-first century, it generally is the poorer people of the world who are more likely to start smoking cigarettes. Some people of upper and middle social classes still smoke cigarettes, but the risk of starting to smoke tobacco tends to be greater for poor people.

Parents. Parents may also have a great effect on whether or not their children use drugs, drink alcohol, or smoke tobacco. Some studies show that the children of parents who smoke are more likely to become smokers, and that the children of parents who drink alcohol frequently are more likely to become drinkers. In some recent studies, teenagers were asked about their own marijuana use. They were

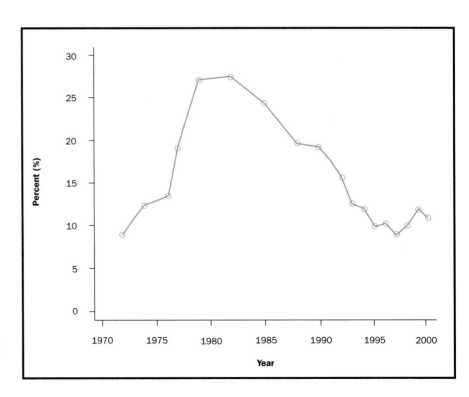

Cocaine use in the United States has steadily declined after reaching a peak in the early 1980s.

also asked about their parents' approval and disapproval of regular to-bacco smoking. When their parents strongly disapproved, about 1 in 16 to 20 teenagers were recent marijuana smokers. When their parents neither approved nor disapproved, about 1 in 5 teenagers had smoked marijuana recently.

In addition to showing approval or disapproval, parents can affect their children's drug judgment in several ways. Parents provide social models for young people, who may imitate what they see. Inheritance and genetic factors also are involved, with drug dependence tending to run in families. Drug dependence also is more common among monozygotic, or identical, twins (who share all of their genes) than among dizygotic, or fraternal, twins (who share 50% of the same genes, on average). Parents also can have an effect by supervising and monitoring their children. For example, when parents help children choose their friends, the children seem to be less likely to start using drugs in the early teen years.

Religion. Religion and church-related activities may help to prevent drug use. Many religions prohibit the use of certain drugs. Islam prohibits alcohol, and the Church of Latter-day Saints restricts many drugs, including tobacco and alcohol. The community formed by a place of worship also can help to prevent drug use. People who belong to that community may tend to come into contact with more people who do not use drugs. In many communities of faith, drug use is less common.

The Effects of Drug Use on School and Work

Schoolwork and academics can be greatly influenced by drug use. Teenagers who use drugs, including alcohol and tobacco, are sometimes more likely to do poorly in school. They may skip classes. Their grades can drop as their drug use rises. Drug users also tend to have a greater risk of dropping out of school before they get their high-school diploma. Drug use becomes more important than their grades and class work.

Drug use can cause harm on the job as well. Drugs can distort a person's senses and reasoning abilities. Drug users sometimes misjudge distances and directions. These effects might lead to situations in which a person cannot do his or her job properly. Drug users can endanger their coworkers or customers who count on them for service. Users who are going through **withdrawal** symptoms can also have trouble performing on the job.

Many employers now give a drug test to anybody who applies for a job, and will not hire a person who has taken drugs recently. Also,

withdrawal physical and psychological symptoms that may occur when a person suddenly stops the use of a substance or reduces the dose of an addictive substance

some employers give this test to employees, to make sure that workers are not starting to use drugs. An employee who has taken drugs recently may be fired from his or her job because of drug use.

Epidemiological studies have shown some interesting relationships between drug use and occupations. For example, alcohol problems seem to be more common in jobs involving daily activities that expose the workers to a high risk of injury. Alcohol problems also seem to be more common among bartenders and others who work in places where alcohol is sold.

Conclusion

There is no average drug user. The use of alcohol, tobacco, and other drugs occurs among males and females and across many personality types, conditions of urban or rural living and points in between, social classes, occupations, and age groups. Some groups may be more likely to start using drugs or to become drug dependent once drug use starts, but everyone is at some risk for drug use. SEE ALSO ADDICTION: CONCEPTS AND DEFINITIONS; ADOLESCENTS, DRUG AND ALCOHOL USE; DRUGS OF ABUSE.

Violence and Drug and Alcohol Use

Violence connected to drug and alcohol use has had a significant impact on society. Substance abuse can cause people to act violently as a direct result of drugs' effects on the brain. Drugs can also lead to violence in indirect ways. For example, drug users are more likely to commit crimes, some of which may be violent, in order to obtain drugs or the money to buy drugs. Evidence suggests that the sale and distribution of illegal drugs causes violence in both sellers and buyers.

Researching Drugs and Behavior

aggression hostile and destructive behavior, especially caused by frustration; may include violence or physical threat or injury directed toward another

The link between drugs and **aggression** and violent behavior depends on the type of drug and the person who uses the drug. Some drugs directly activate brain mechanisms that control aggression, mostly in individuals who have already shown aggression in the past. Research using animals has allowed scientists to study the direct effects of drugs on aggression and violent behavior.

One type of animal research is known as the experimental-psychological approach. In this type of experiment, scientists set up and control the environment of research animals. In the 1960s researchers developed models of aggression by observing animals who were housed in crowded conditions over long periods of time, exposed to painful electrical shocks, denied scheduled rewards, or restricted in their food intake. By comparing animals' behavior in these conditions to their behavior in normal living conditions, scientists gain insight into the causes of violence and aggression.

With humans, researchers have created similar conditions by setting up and controlling the environment in laboratory settings. The aim of such research is to cause aggressive behavior similar to the behaviors people show in the world outside of the laboratory. The ethical dilemma of such research is to reduce risk to the research subjects while at the same time trying to realistically capture the essential elements of violent behavior and its causes.

In another type of research, scientists study the brain directly in order to understand how changes in this organ may lead to aggression. After studying the brain tissue of violent patients, researchers developed techniques to destroy specific areas of the brain in laboratory animals. This stimulated the animals to become enraged and bite. Obviously this type of research is very limited in its scope and difficult to translate to humans.

Nonetheless, research on aggression has helped scientists understand the link between drugs and alcohol and violence. Statistics link alcohol to aggressive and violent behavior in humans on a very large scale that is consistent over the years and encompasses many types of violent acts. Experimental studies have shown that after drinking alcohol, individuals are prone to aggressive and competitive behavior. While it may be true that alcohol consumption is often associated with socially acceptable behavior, individuals react to it differently depending on their genes, their life experiences, and their environment. Alcohol impairs judgment and disrupts patterns of social interaction, and these effects can lead to violence. In the brain, research has shown that alcohol affects the two **neurotransmitters** that play a role in aggressive behavior.

Drinking and Family Violence

Research shows that alcohol is a contributing factor to violence in American households. Alcohol is most often a factor in husband-against-wife violence. The husband has been drinking in approximately one-quarter to one-half of cases of wife beating. The most common pattern is that either the husband or both the husband and the wife drink, but not usually the wife alone. Studies show that

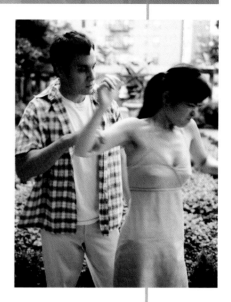

Alcohol impairs judgment and increases aggressive behavior, and is often a factor in husband-against-wife violence.

neurotransmitter
chemical messenger used by nerve cells to communicate with other nerve cells

ESTIMATED NUMBER OF CHILDREN IN HOUSEHOLDS WHERE ONE OR MORE PARENT IS DEPENDENT ON ALCOHOL, BY CHILDREN'S AGES: 1996

Ages of children (years)	Estimated number of children
Under 2	678,923
2 years to 5 years	1,551,952
6 years to 9 years	1,616,156
10 years to 13 years	1,225,437
14 years to 17 years	1,115,056
Total	6,187,524

SOURCE: Office of Applied Studies, Substance Abuse and Mental Health Services Administration, National Household Survey on Drug Abuse, 1996. <http://www.samhsa.gov/oas/nhsda/Treatan/treana08.htm#E10E4>.

In 1996 over six million children in the United States lived in homes where one or more parent was dependent on alcohol.

paranoid psychosis symptom of mental illness characterized by changes in personality, a distorted sense of reality, and feelings of excessive and irrational suspicion; may include hallucinations (i.e., seeing, hearing, feeling, smelling, or tasting something that is not truly there)

predisposition condition in which one is vulnerable or prone to something

hallucinogenic of a substance that can cause hallucinations, or seeing, hearing, or feeling things that are not there

stimulant drug that increases activity temporarily; often used to describe drugs that excite the brain and central nervous system

husbands or partners with alcohol problems are more likely to commit violence against their wives or partners.

According to a 2000 study by the Bureau of Justice Statistics, two-thirds of victims who suffered violence by a current or former spouse, boyfriend, or girlfriend reported that alcohol had been a factor. Among spouse victims, three out of four incidents involved someone who had been drinking. By contrast, only 31 percent of the crimes committed by strangers were thought to be related to alcohol.

Research also shows that violence against women may lead to their own use of alcohol and drugs. Women may use drinking as a way to deal with physical and emotional pain and fear that result from living in a violent relationship. Women in alcohol treatment programs had higher rates of father-to-daughter violence than women in a comparison group. These findings show that the relationship of alcohol and family violence must be carefully interpreted. While alcohol may not necessarily cause violence in family relationships, its use may be a response to violent victimization.

How Different Drugs Affect Behavior

Drug users who inject amphetamine may develop **paranoid psychosis**, a state in which they commit violent acts. Individuals who have a **predisposition** to violence are more likely to suffer from this effect. While low amphetamine doses can increase certain negative social behaviors, higher doses often lead to severe social withdrawal.

Although there are few studies on cocaine's effect on aggression and violence, evidence shows aggressive individuals may tend to engage in violent acts after using the drug. However, as discussed below, with crack cocaine the real problem is the violence associated with the supplying, dealing, and buying of the drug. Phencyclidine (PCP), another drug that does not directly cause violence, may cause violent behavior in an individual with a violent history.

Marijuana and hashish, whose active ingredient is tetrahydrocannabinol (THC), tend to decrease aggressive and violent behavior. Because marijuana and related drugs are easily available at a relatively low cost, there is less violence associated with dealing and buying it than is the case with cocaine. LSD, popular in the 1960s but less so today, has rarely been associated with violent behavior.

Ecstasy (MDMA), is a drug that has both **hallucinogenic** and **stimulant** effects. It is associated with reduced aggression and an increase in empathy among users while they are taking it. However, several days after using the drug, individuals may suffer feelings of

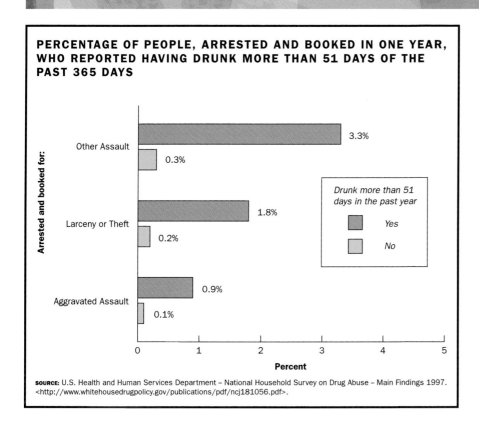

PERCENTAGE OF PEOPLE, ARRESTED AND BOOKED IN ONE YEAR, WHO REPORTED HAVING DRUNK MORE THAN 51 DAYS OF THE PAST 365 DAYS

Arrested and booked for:

Other Assault — 3.3% / 0.3%
Larceny or Theft — 1.8% / 0.2%
Aggravated Assault — 0.9% / 0.1%

Drunk more than 51 days in the past year
Yes
No

Percent

SOURCE: U.S. Health and Human Services Department – National Household Survey on Drug Abuse – Main Findings 1997. <http://www.whitehousedrugpolicy.gov/publications/pdf/ncj181056.pdf>.

A National Household Survey on Drug Abuse in 1997 found that people who had drank more than fifty-one days out of the past year were much more likely to be arrested for crimes (including assault and larceny) than people who drank less often.

depression, hostility, and social fears. These symptoms are more likely to appear in long-term heavy users. Ecstasy can also bring about a reduced concern for personal safety, leading to reckless behavior that may have a violent outcome. Ecstasy affects the neurotransmitter serotonin by destroying the neurons that produce it. Evidence suggests that low levels of serotonin play a role in violent and aggressive criminal behavior. Long-term use of ecstasy could therefore contribute to an increased tendency for violent behavior.

Drug Addiction, Crime, and Violence

Violence connected with drug use is largely connected to getting money to maintain the drug habit, and to establishing and conducting the business of drug dealing. Competition for drug markets and customers, and disputes among individuals involved in selling drugs, play a role in drug-related violence. In addition, locales where drugs are sold on the streets tend to be disadvantaged economically and socially. As a result, legal and social controls against violence are not as effective as in more affluent areas.

Although the number of drug-related **homicides** has been declining in recent years, drugs are still one of the main factors leading to homicides. According to the Federal Bureau of Investigation's *Crime in the United States: Uniform Crime Reports*, in 1998 murders

homicide murder

narcotic addictive substance that relieves pain and induces sleep or causes sedation; prescription narcotics includes morphine and codeine; general and imprecise term referring to a drug of abuse, such as heroin, cocaine, or marijuana

related to **narcotics** were the fourth-most documented circumstance out of twenty-four possible categories. Over half of adult males arrested in thirty-four American cities in 1999 tested positive for drug use, according to the Department of Justice's report, *Arrestee Drug Abuse Monitoring (ADAM) Program: 1999 Annual Report on Drug Use Among Adult and Juvenile Arrestees.* In more than half of the cities reporting data, 65 percent or more of the arrestees had recently used marijuana, cocaine, methamphetamine, opiates (such as heroin), and/or PCP, according to preliminary findings of the 2000 ADAM report. Use of at least one of these drugs ranged from 51 percent in Des Moines to 79 percent in New York City.

The link between crime and drugs goes beyond those who are under the influence at the time of the arrest. In 1998 an estimated 61,000 convicted jail inmates said they had committed their offense to get money for drugs, according to the Bureau of Justice Statistics. More than 11 percent of inmates who committed a crime to get money for drugs were convicted of a violent offense in 1999.

According to the National Crime Victimization Survey, approximately 7.4 million individuals age 12 or older in 1999 were victims of violent crimes. Victims were asked if they could tell whether the offender had been drinking or using drugs. About 28 percent of the victims of violence reported that the offender was using drugs and/or alcohol. Based on this information, approximately 1.2 million violent crimes occurred in which the victims were sure that the offender had been drinking, and for about one in four of these, victims believed the offender was also using drugs.

Among young people, studies show that violence has increased since the mid-1980s. According to the 1999 National Household Survey on Drug Abuse, more than 5 million of the estimated 23 million youths aged 12 to 17 reported participating in a violent act, such as fighting at school or work. Youths who participated in violent behaviors were more likely to have used alcohol and illicit drugs than those who did not participate in violent behaviors. For example, 26 percent of youths who had participated in a serious fight at school or work reported past month use of alcohol, and 18 percent reported drug use.

Drug Trafficking and Violence

For many years, the trafficking of drugs in the United States was controlled by traditional organized crime groups operating inside and outside the country. From the 1950s to the 1970s, La Cosa Nostra, better known as the Mafia, controlled an estimated 95 percent of all heroin entering New York City, as well as most of the heroin distributed throughout the United States. This monopoly was effectively ended in 1972 by French and U.S. drug agents. Today, the traffic in illegal drugs is controlled by international organized crime syndicates (organizations) from Colombia, Mexico, and other countries.

These groups often model their operations after international terrorist groups. They maintain tight control of their workers through compartmentalized structures that separate production, shipment, distribution, **money laundering**, communications, security, and recruitment, so that workers are unaware of their colleagues' activities. Like terrorists, they make use of technologically advanced airplanes, boats, radar, communications, and weapons to distribute and protect their investment. They also use vast counterintelligence networks to keep one step ahead of competitors and law-enforcement officials. Drug traffickers and terrorists often use similar methods to achieve their goals. Many drug trafficking organizations engage in acts that could be considered terrorist in nature, such as killing innocent people in public, large-scale bombings, kidnapping, and torture.

In addition, drugs form an important part of the financial infrastructure of terrorist groups. The sale of drugs is the primary source of income for many of the more powerful terrorist organizations. Twelve of the twenty-eight terrorist organizations identified by the U.S. Department of State traffic in drugs. For example, the Taliban regime in Afghanistan, which protected Osama bin Laden and his Al Qaeda network, used money from the sale of opium and heroin to finance its operations.

money laundering
activity in which a person or group hides the source of money that has been illegally obtained

Conclusion

Violence and crime can be connected to drug and alcohol abuse in a variety of ways. These include an individual's response to a particular drug or alcohol, a person's coping mechanism to try and escape someone else's abuse, violent crimes associated with drug trafficking, or violent crimes committed while under the influence of drugs or alcohol. Violence would exist in our society even if substance abuse did not. Yet there is no doubt that many violent behaviors are directly related to drug and alcohol abuse. SEE ALSO CHILD ABUSE AND DRUGS; CRIME AND DRUGS; DRUG TRAFFICKERS; TERRORISM AND DRUGS.

Wood Alcohol (Methanol)

Wood alcohol, or methanol, is a form of alcohol that is used as an industrial solvent, in antifreeze, and in the manufacture of chemicals. When swallowed, wood alcohol is metabolized or adapted by body enzymes to create formaldehyde and formic acid. Both of these substances are poisonous. Formic acid can cause blindness. Only desperate alcoholics drink wood alcohol, but it is sometimes drunk by accident by people experimenting with various alcohol substitutes. Any consumption of wood alcohol should be treated as a medical emergency, and the 911 emergency line should be called for immediate help. SEE ALSO ALCOHOL: CHEMISTRY.

Workplace, Drug Use in the

Drug use by employees and workers has become an important issue for American business. Employers of all types (large and small businesses, nonprofit organizations, government, and so on) are concerned about illegal drug use because it has serious effects on job performance, **productivity**, safety, and health. Most of the illegal drug users in the United States are employed. According to the 2000 National Household Survey on Drug Abuse, of the estimated 11.8 million illegal drug users over age 18, 9.1 million (77 percent) were employed either full or part time.

Because of increasing concerns about drug abuse by workers, most business organizations have established written policies on drug use and require drug testing of workers. Most also offer employee education and employee assistance programs for workers with a drug problem. Programs in the workplace reach out to workers and their

productivity quality of yielding results or benefits

Illicit drug use and heavy alcohol use is most frequently reported by people working in the food industry, including waiters, waitresses, and bartenders, according to National Household Surveys on Drug Abuse conducted in the 1990s.

PERCENTAGE OF FULL-TIME WORKERS, AGE 18–49, REPORTING CURRENT ILLICIT DRUG AND HEAVY ALCOHOL USE, BY OCCUPATION CATEGORIES

Occupational Category	Current Illicit Drug Use	Current Heavy Alcohol Use
Overall	7.7	7.5
Executive, Administrative & Managerial	8.9	7.1
Professional Specialty	5.1	4.4
Technicians & Related Support	7.0	5.1
Sales	9.1	4.1
Administrative Support	3.2	5.1
Protective Service	3.0	7.8
Food Preparation, Waiters, Waitresses & Bartenders	18.7	15.0
Other Service	12.5	11.4
Precision Production & Repair	4.4	11.6
Construction	14.1	12.4
Extractive & Precision Production	4.4	5.5
Machine Operators & Inspectors	8.9	9.0
Transportation & Material Moving	10.0	10.8
Handlers, Helpers & Laborers	6.5	13.5

SOURCE: Office of Applied Studies, Substance Abuse and Mental Health Services Administration, National Household Survey on Drug Abuse, 1994 and 1997.
<http://www.samhsa.gov/oas/nhsda/A-11/WrkplcPlcy2-20.htm#TopOfPage>.

families. As a result, the workplace has become an effective place for drug prevention, treatment, and rehabilitation efforts.

The Development of Workplace Drug Policies

When drug-free workplace programs began in the 1960s, they had many critics. Drug testing of employees was controversial because early drug testing methods were poor and workers were concerned about individual rights and privacy. The U.S. military began to conduct drug testing in 1971, and was the first workplace to offer treatment, rather than punishment, to those who tested positive for drug use. In 1980 new technology became available that provided reliable, inexpensive testing methods for marijuana and other commonly abused drugs. This development, along with the military's commitment to addressing the drug problem among its personnel, was pivotal in the decision to begin widespread drug testing and to begin strict policies forbidding the illegal use of drugs on or off the job.

In the 1980s the National Transportation Safety Board discovered that drugs were involved in railroad and airline accidents. The transportation and utility industries then adopted drug-free workplace policies for employees in positions that affected public safety. Early drug-free policies required that drug-using employees be fired. Many businesses were uncomfortable with this approach, especially when the employees' drug use did not pose a threat to anyone except the users themselves. Today's drug-free workplace policies take a more positive, helping-hand approach. These policies have two basic purposes: (1) to minimize the risk of hiring drug users by testing job applicants for illegal drugs, and (2) to get the substance-abusing employee into treatment and back on the job.

Drug Testing

The federal government encourages and in some instances requires both public and private businesses to develop drug-free workplace programs. For example, the Federal Railroad Administration began hearings on drug rules for the railroad industry in 1984 and issued regulations requiring the testing of employees as well as other policies. These federal regulations went into effect in 1986. In September 1986, President Ronald W. Reagan issued an executive order that required all federal government agencies to develop drug-free workplace programs to ensure that the more than 2 million federal employees were not illegally using drugs on or off the job. In the same decade, the Department of Transportation (DOT) issued regulations for the transportation industries, such as the airlines, trucking, railroad, and mass transit companies. These regulations required:

(1) written policies prohibiting the illegal use of drugs on or off the job, and (2) drug testing of employees before being hired, if their boss had reasons to suspect drug use, and after any accident, and random drug testing for workers in specified safety-sensitive occupations. Congress passed the Drug-Free Workplace Act of 1988, which requires all federal grant recipients and most federal contractors to certify that they will provide a drug-free workplace. In general, the law required employers to:

1. Develop and publish a written policy and ensure that employees read and consent to the policy as a condition of employment.

2. Initiate an awareness program to educate employees about the dangers of drug abuse, the company's drug-free workplace policy, any available drug counseling, employee assistance programs, and the penalties that may be imposed on employees for drug-abuse violations.

3. Require that all employees notify the employer or contractor of any conviction for a drug offense in the workplace.

4. Make an ongoing effort to maintain a drug-free workplace. Nothing in the law required companies to test their employees for drugs. However, as a side effect of fulfilling the act, most companies did create drug-testing policies.

By the end of the twentieth century, these drug-testing regulations affected nearly 10 percent of the entire U.S. workforce.

After a major subway accident in New York City in 1994, the DOT regulations expanded to include alcohol. The engineer involved in the accident was found to be using both alcohol and drugs. The Nuclear Regulatory Commission also issued regulations requiring written policies and extensive testing of personnel at nuclear sites. Other government agencies, for example, the Department of Energy, also expanded their policies on drug and alcohol use.

The Prevalence of Drug-Free Workplace Programs

In 1988 the Bureau of Labor Statistics (BLS) surveyed businesses throughout the United States about their policies on drug abuse. The survey found that half the nation's nonagricultural workforce was employed by organizations with a formal policy on drugs, and that 20 percent of paid workers were employed in establishments with some type of drug-testing program. In the years since the BLS survey, the number of corporate and other employers and the employees covered by these policies has continued to increase sharply. A 2001 survey by

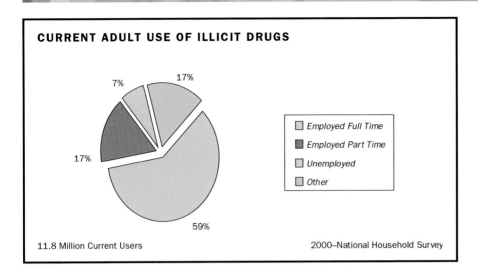

CURRENT ADULT USE OF ILLICIT DRUGS

7%

17%

17%

59%

- Employed Full Time
- Employed Part Time
- Unemployed
- Other

11.8 Million Current Users

2000–National Household Survey

A 2000 survey found that people who are employed part time make up more than half of the total number of adults currently using illicit drugs.

the American Management Association indicates that more than two-thirds of major businesses surveyed employees for illegal drug use. Nearly 20 percent select employees for random testing as part of the drug-free workplace effort. For most American companies, the drug-free workplace concept has become a standard business practice. A person seeking employment in the United States will most likely have to pass a drug test to get the job.

The drug test itself is a crucial but often controversial part of a standard drug-free workplace policy. The question of whether to use drug-testing technology raises many difficult issues—moral, social, ethical, medical, scientific, and legal. Many citizens are very concerned that drug testing is an invasion of a person's civil rights and freedoms. They view the drug-testing process, generally collection of urine, as degrading and dehumanizing. Some people question whether the goal of a drug-free workplace justifies requiring workers to provide urine samples on random demand. Unions and **civil libertarians** often ask, Where will it stop? Where do you draw the line? Some fear that demands for employee AIDS testing and pregnancy testing will be the next workplace battlegrounds.

civil libertarian person who believes in the right to unrestricted freedom of thought and action

Government employees, unions, and civil libertarians argue strongly that drug testing is an invasion of privacy and constitutes an illegal search and seizure (of body fluids). Therefore, they argue, such actions violate individual rights guaranteed by the Constitution. In general, constitutional protections apply only to testing conducted and required by government agencies (federal, state, and local). Therefore, employee drug testing conducted by private employers is not covered by the constitutional safeguards. However, government-mandated drug testing of employees in the private sector (for example, transportation and nuclear power workers) must be in accordance with the Constitution. Several of these constitutional questions have been brought before the Supreme Court. In general, the Court has upheld drug testing when safety or security is a concern.

Management and workers continue to struggle with a number of drug-testing issues. Some question the accuracy and reliability of drug testing. One repeated concern relates to the quality of the laboratories offering drug-testing services. To combat this complaint, Congress required strict technical and scientific procedures for federal workplace drug-testing programs, as well as standards for all laboratories in 1987. A national laboratory certification program was also begun to ensure the quality of drug testing done in laboratories. The use of a government-certified lab has become the standard by which drug-testing programs are measured. These tough federal standards have nearly eliminated concerns about drug-testing accuracy and reliability. In addition, better testing technology will continue to be developed, making it much more difficult for the casual drug user to escape detection. Urine testing may be replaced by tests of saliva and sweat, making the test procedure less objectionable.

Employee Assistance Programs

A vital part of workplace drug policies is employee assistance programs (EAPs). EAPs were developed in the 1970s to focus on alcohol abuse and to assist employees in dealing with the stresses of employment and personal life. Typically, EAPs provide short-term counseling and make referrals for employees who need treatment or long-term counseling. These programs also conduct management training and health workshops and seminars on topics such as quitting smoking and losing weight.

As managers began to develop drug policies, they struggled with the question of what to do if they discovered that an employee was using drugs. Generally, corporate lawyers and security officers would suggest dismissing the employee, while corporate medical and EAP staff would recommend treatment. The issue proved difficult to resolve for many corporations. The cost of treatment and the uncertainty of success weighed heavily on the minds of financial officers responsible for making a profit in a bad economy. Most corporations have set aside resources for EAPs to implement the helping-hand approach.

EAPs also faced problems when asked to take part in an antidrug effort. Some EAP providers had difficulty expanding their programs to deal with illegal drug users. People who abuse illegal drugs have different needs and present different issues from, for example, people who have a drinking problem. EAP counselors promise to keep their clients' substance-abuse problems confidential, but they may feel troubled about not reporting illegal drug use. Also, EAP providers may feel pressure to "cure" an employee's drug problem—before that employee is fired. Despite these problems, EAPs not only help employees but are also a good investment because they help companies maintain experienced, healthy workers. New training programs in substance abuse for EAP professionals have made the EAP provider more skilled in dealing with the drug-using employee.

A Difficult Balance

Employers face a difficult balancing act when upholding their drug-abuse policies. On the one hand, many employers feel a moral obligation to do all they can to achieve a drug-free workplace. They have corporate responsibilities to provide a healthy and safe workplace for all employees and to protect investors in their companies from financial losses resulting from drug abuse. On the other hand, employers have obligations to their workers—to respect the individual rights and civil liberties of loyal and trustworthy employees (who for the most part are not involved with drugs). Striking a balance between these two obligations is a continuing challenge for employers. For the most part, members of the U.S. business community agree that the workplace is an appropriate site for confronting drug abuse. They have sent a clear message to the workforce and to the community that drug use will not be tolerated.

Conclusion

Although drug abuse in the workplace is still a significant concern of American employers, substantial progress has been made since the early 1980s. Accidents, absenteeism (not showing up for work), and positive drug tests have all declined. In the future, workplaces are likely to continue expanding drug-testing and employee assistance programs. As the country has gained confidence in the accuracy and reliability of drug testing, lower thresholds will be permitted that will make it much more difficult for the casual user to escape detection. There is new technology becoming available to test saliva and sweat for drugs that will minimize the intrusiveness of the testing process. Educating high-school and college students that they must be drug-free to get and hold a job will contribute to the reduction of drug abuse among young people. Workplace efforts are the most organized drug education, prevention, and treatment programs in the country today, and will most likely grow and expand. They may be one of the best ways to solve the drug problem in America. SEE ALSO COSTS OF

> **IN THEIR OWN WORDS**
>
> "The real victim of the war on drugs might be the constitutional rights of the American people."
>
> —Richard Matsch, U.S. District Court Judge, 1989.

Substance Abuse and Dependence, Economic; Drug Testing Methods and Analysis; Schools, Drug Use in.

Zero Tolerance

Z

The term "zero tolerance" refers to government and private employer policies that require specific consequences or punishments for certain offenses. Most public schools now have zero-tolerance policies for firearms, weapons other than firearms, alcohol, drugs, and tobacco. Generally, zero-tolerance policies are rigid, requiring harsh punishments for any level of improper behavior, with no room for explanations or excuses. The courts have endorsed drug-testing programs that allow employers to enforce zero-tolerance policies.

Zero tolerance is also a general attitude toward drug use. According to this perspective, the use of any amount of illegal drugs is harmful to the individual and society, and the goal of drug policy should be to prohibit any and all illegal drug use. A contrasting viewpoint holds that not all drug use is equally harmful. According to this view, occasional use of drugs should be viewed as something different from and less serious than consistent, problem drug use. People who take this view argue that, although the absence of all drug use is desirable, the resources of government would be used more efficiently if they targeted problem users as well as the causes of illegal drug use.

Zero Tolerance and U.S. Drug Control Policy

Originally, zero tolerance was a federal drug policy begun during the War on Drugs campaign of the Reagan and Bush administrations (1981–1993). This policy was designed to prohibit the transfer of illicit drugs across U.S. borders. No possession, import, or export of illegal drugs was to be tolerated, and possession of any measurable amount of illegal drugs was subject to all available civil and criminal punishments. Zero tolerance was an example of a criminal justice approach to drug control. In this approach, the criminal justice system is responsible for the control of drugs, and the use of drugs is regarded as a criminal act.

Under the zero-tolerance policy, law-enforcement agents target users of illegal drugs rather than dealers or transporters. Zero-tolerance advocates argue that users create the demand for drugs and are therefore the root cause of the drug problem. A zero-tolerance policy is based on the idea that, if demand for drugs can be curbed by harshly punishing users, the supply of drugs flowing into the country will decrease.

The U.S. Customs Service, together with the U.S. Attorney's office in San Diego, California, initiated the zero-tolerance policy as part of an effort to stop drug trafficking across the U.S.-Mexican border. Individuals in possession of illegal drugs were arrested and charged with both a **misdemeanor** and a **felony** offense. Customs Service officials believed the policy was successful at reducing the flow of drugs across the border and recommended that it be put to use nationwide. Subsequently, the National Drug Policy Board, together with the White House Conference on a Drug-Free America, had all federal drug-enforcement agencies adopt the zero-tolerance policy in 1988, at all points of entry into the United States.

The policy did not require that new laws or regulations be enacted. Instead, it required strict interpretation and enforcement of existing laws. In practice, it meant that if any amount of drugs was found on any type of vehicle, including bicycles, transfer trucks, and yachts, the vehicle would be seized and the passengers arrested. The U.S. Coast Guard and the U.S. Customs Service began to crack down on all cases of drug possession on the water and at all borders. If, during the course of their regular patrols and inspections, Coast Guard personnel boarded a vessel and found one marijuana cigarette, or even the remnants of a marijuana cigarette, they arrested the individual and seized the boat. Previously, the Coast Guard had either looked the other way or issued fines when personal-use quantities of illegal substances were discovered.

Many criticized zero tolerance because it used up the resources of federal agencies to identify individual drug users rather than to stop the flow of major quantities of drugs into the country for sale on the streets. The policy of seizing boats upon the discovery of trace amounts of drugs was also controversial. Some believed the policy to be an unfair and unusually harsh punishment. In this view, seizing a commercial boat that is the sole source of income for an individual or family is too severe a penalty for possession of one marijuana cigarette. In some highly publicized cases, commercial fishing boats were seized on scant evidence that the boat owner was responsible for the illegal drugs found on board.

In the Workplace and Schools

Zero tolerance is widely applied in many workplaces and schools around the country. A zero-tolerance approach typically requires that employees undergo drug testing. In the late 1970s, employees challenged these policies in the courts. However, in 1979 the U.S. Supreme Court, in *New York City Transit Authority v. Beazer*, ruled that a city agency did not violate the U.S. Constitution by refusing

misdemeanor crime that is treated in the courts as a less serious crime than a felony

felony a very serious crime that usually warrants a more severe punishment than misdemeanor crimes

to employ people who regularly used narcotic drugs. This zero-tolerance decision has been extended to various employment situations. By 2000, many employers routinely required a drug test as part of the employee hiring process. Applicants who fail the test usually are not hired because of zero tolerance.

Zero tolerance has become a standard part of U.S. public schools. After the rash of school shootings in the 1990s, public interest grew in zero-tolerance weapons policies. Zero-tolerance drug polices are also part of school rules. Zero tolerance has widespread public support, as it requires high standards and signals a tough attitude toward drugs and school violence.

Nevertheless, zero tolerance has many critics. Critics compare zero tolerance to mandatory minimum sentencing in the criminal justice system. Under both schemes, there are no exceptions made for individual circumstances. This results in punishments that appear excessive, such as a student suspension for bringing aspirin to school without permission. SEE ALSO Law and Policy: Controls on Drug Trafficking; Law and Policy: Drug Legalization Debate; Law and Policy: Modern Enforcement, Prosecution, and Sentencing; Schools, Drug Use in; Workplace, Drug Use in.

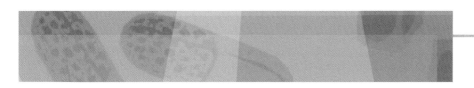

Photo and Illustration Credits

The illustrations and tables featured in *Drugs, Alcohol, and Tobacco: Learning About Addictive Behavior* were created by GGS Information Services. The images appearing in the text were reproduced by permission of the following sources:

Volume 1

AP/Wide World Photos, Inc.: **2, 26, 29, 70, 154, 214;** Custom Medical Stock Photo: **5, 80, 95, 101, 142;** The Advertising Archive Ltd.: **21;** © Prof. P. Motta/Dept. of Anatomy/University of "La Sapienza," Rome/Science Photo Library, National Audubon Society Collection/ Photo Researchers: **37;** © Roger Wood/ Corbis: **44;** © Francis G. Mayer/Corbis: **47;** © Pascal Goetgheluck / SPL / Photo Researchers, Inc.: **54;** Photograph by Robert J. Huffman. Field Mark Publications: **58;** © Photoedit: **60;** © Shepard Sherbell/Corbis: **63;** The Kobal Collection / Touchstone: **67;** © Photo Researchers, Inc.: **73, 163;** CNRI/SPL/ Photo Researchers, Inc.: **75;** © Sidney Moulds / SPL / Photo Researchers, Inc.: **105;** © Josh Sher/SPL/ Photo Researchers, Inc.: **109;** Image Works, Inc.: **116;** © Bettmann/Corbis: **121;** © Lowell Georgia/Corbis: **124;** Photograph by Secchi-Lecague/Roussel-UCLAF/CNRI/ Science Photo Library. © National Audubon Society Collection/Photo Researchers, Inc.: **133;** © Jim Varney / SPL / Photo Researchers, Inc.: **140, 196;**

NLM: **158;** © Bobbie Kingsley/SPL/ Photo Researchers, Inc.: **159;** The Library of Congress: **165;** © 1993 Peter Berndt M.D., P.A. Custom Medical Stock Photo, Inc.: **169;** © Photograph by Ken Settle: **189;** © Photo Researchers: **199;** Photograph by Robert J. Huffman. © Field Mark Publications: **207.**

Volume 2

AP/Wide World Photos, Inc.: **2, 18, 22, 45, 91, 121, 127, 134, 157, 208;** © AFP/Corbis: **26;** © Jacques M. Chenet/Corbis: **28;** © Earl and Nazima Kowall/Corbis: **31;** © Christophe Loviny/ Corbis: **33, 113;** Photo Researchers, Inc.: **43;** Custom Medical Stock Photo: **51;** © Bettmann/Corbis: **63;** Photograph by David H. Wells. © Corbis: **77;** © Sterling K. Clarren: **79;** © Phil Schermeister/ Corbis: **81;** The Kobal Collection / Columbia: **89;** UPI/Corbis Bettmann: **96;** Photograph by Will & Deni McIntyre. © Photo Researchers, Inc.: **101;** Custom Medical Stock Photo: **105, 185;** Photograph by Robert J. Huffman. © Field Mark Publications: **111;** © Reuters NewMedia Inc./Corbis.: **115, 165;** SAGA/Archive Photos, Inc.: **119;** © Scott Camazine & Sue Trainor/Photo Researchers, Inc.: **133;** Science Photo Library: **137;** © Daudier, Jerrican / Photo Researchers, Inc.: **141;** © Galen Rowell/Corbis: **146;** © Corbis: **170;** © Richard Hutchings/Corbis: **179;** © CNRI/Phototake NYC: **181;** © Lester V.

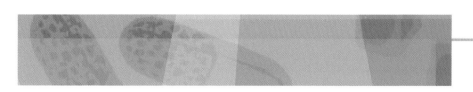

Organizations of Interest

Adult Children of Alcoholics (ACOA)
ACA WSO
PO Box 3216
Torrance, CA 90510
310-534-1815 (message only)
<http://www.adultchildren.org>
meetinginfo@adultchildren.org

African American Parents for Drug Prevention (AAPDP)
4025 Red Bud Avenue
Cincinnati, OH 45229
513-961-4158
513-961-6719 (fax)

AIDS Hotline
American Social Health Association
PO Box 13827
Research Triangle Park, NC 27713
800-342-AIDS
<http://www.ashastd.org/nah>
hivnet@ashastd.org

AIDS National Information Clearinghouse
CDC NPIN
PO Box 6003
Rockville, MD 20849-6003
800-458-5231
<http://www.cdcnpin.org>
info@cdcnpin.org (reference services)
webmaster@cdcnpin.org (web site)

Alcohol Treatment Referral Hotline
107 Lincoln Street
Worcester, MA 01605
800-ALCOHOL
508-798-9446
<http://www.adcare.com>
info@adcare.com

Alcoholics Anonymous (AA)
General Service Office
PO Box 459
New York, NY 10163
212-870-3400
<http://www.alcoholics-anonymous.org>

American Council for Drug Education
164 West 74th Street
New York, NY 10023
800-488-3784
<http://www.acde.org>
acde@phoenixhouse.org

BACCHUS Peer Education Network and GAMMA
PO Box 100043
Denver, CO 80250
303-871-3068
<http://www.bacchusgamma.org>
bacgam@aol.com

Bureau of Alcohol, Tobacco, and Firearms
Office of Liaison and Public Information
650 Massachusetts Avenue, NW
Room 8290
Washington, DC 20226
202-927-8500
<http://www.atf.treas.gov/index.htm>
ATFMail@atfhq.atf.treas.gov

Clearinghouse of the National Criminal Justice Reference System
Bureau of Justice Assistance
PO Box 6000
Rockville, MD 20849
800-688-4252
<http://www.ncjrs.org>

Bureau of Justice Statistics
810 7th Street, NW
Washington, DC 20531
202-307-0765
800-732-3277
<http://www.ojp.usdoj.gov/bjs>
askbjs@ojp.usdoj.gov

**Center for Mental Health Services
Knowledge Exchange Network**
PO Box 42490
Washington, DC 20015
800-789-2647
<http://www.mentalhealth.org>
ken@mentalhealth.org

**Center for Substance Abuse
Prevention**
5600 Fishers Lane
Rockwall II Building, Suite 800
Rockville, MD 20857
301-443-8956
<http://www.samhsa.gov/centers/csap/csap
.html>
info@samhsa.gov

Center for Substance Abuse Treatment
National Treatment Hotline
1-800-662-HELP
<http://www.samhsa.gov/centers/csat2002/
csat_frame.html>

**Centers for Disease Control and
Prevention**
Office on Smoking and Health
4770 Buford Highway, NE, MS-K50
Atlanta, GA 30341-3724
800-CDC-1311
<http://www.cdc.gov/tobacco>
tobaccoinfo@cdc.gov

Child Help USA
Childhelp USA National Headquarters
15757 N. 78th Street
Scottsdale, Arizona 85260
800-4-A-CHILD
<http://www.childhelpusa.org>

CoAnon Family Groups
PO Box 12722
Tucson, AZ 85732
800-898-9985 (Leave your name, number,
and a brief message and someone will call
you back.)
<http://www.co-anon.org>

Cocaine Anonymous (CA)
3740 Overland Ave., Suite C
Los Angeles, CA 90034
310-559-5833
<http://www.ca.org>
cawso@ca.org

DARE America
PO Box 512090
Los Angeles, CA 90051-0090
800-223-3273
<http://www.dare.com>

**Drug Enforcement Administration
(DEA)**
Information Services Section
2401 Jefferson Davis Highway
Alexandria, VA 22301
202-307-1000
<http://www.dea.gov>

**Employee Assistance Professional
Administration**
2101 Wilson Blvd., Suite 500
Arlington, VA 22201
703-387-1000
<http://www.eap-association.com>
info@eap-association.org

Families Anonymous
PO Box 3475
Culver City, CA 90231-3475
800-736-9805
<http://www.familiesanonymous.org>
famanon@FamiliesAnonymous.org

Food and Drug Administration (FDA)
5600 Fishers Lane
Rockville, Maryland 20857
888-463-6332
<http://www.fda.gov>

Gamblers Anonymous
International Service Office
PO Box 17173
Los Angeles, CA 90017
213-386-8789
<http://www.gamblersanonymous.org>
isomain@gamblersanonymous.org

Girls and Boys Town National Hotline
13943 Gutowski Road
Boystown, NE 68010
800-448-3000 (English and *Español*)

<http://www.girlsandboystown.org>
hotline@boystown.org

Higher Education Center for Alcohol and Other Drug Prevention
55 Chapel Street
Newton, MA 02458-1060
800-676-1730
617-928-1537
<http://www.edc.org/hec>

Indian Health Service
The Reyes Building
801 Thompson Avenue, Suite 400
Rockville, MD 20852-1627
301-443-2038
<http.//www.ihs.gov>
feedback@ihs.gov

Institute for Social Research
University of Michigan
426 Thompson Street
PO Box 1248
Ann Arbor, MI 48106
734-764-8354
<http://www.isr.umich.edu>
MTFinfo@isr.umich.edu

Juvenile Justice Clearinghouse
PO Box 6000
Rockville, MD 20849
800-638-8736
<http://virlib.ncjrs.org/JuvenileJustice
.asp>
askncjrs@ncjrs.org

March of Dimes
1275 Mamaroneck Avenue
White Plains, NY 10605
914-428-7100
<http://www.modimes.org>

Marijuana Anonymous
PO Box 2912
Van Nuys, CA 91404
800-766-6779
<http://www.marijuana-anonymous.org>
office@marijuana-anonymous.org

Mediascope
12711 Ventura Boulevard, Suite 440
Studio City, CA 91604
818-508-2080
<http://www.mediascope.org>
facts@mediascope.org

Mothers Against Drunk Driving (MADD)
National Headquarters
PO Box 541688
Dallas, TX 75354
800-438-6233
<http://www.madd.org>

Nar-anon Family
World Service Office
PO Box 2562
Palos Verdes, CA 90274
310-547-5800

Narcotics Anonymous (NA)
PO Box 9999
Van Nuys, CA 91409
818-773-9999
<http://www.na.org>

National Alliance for Hispanic Health
1501 Sixteenth Street, NW
Washington, DC 20036
800-725-8312
<http://www.hispanichealth.org>

National Alliance for the Mentally Ill
Colonial Place Three
2107 Wilson Boulevard, Suite 300
Arlington, VA 22201
703-524-7600
<http://www.nami.org>

National Association for Children of Alcoholics
11426 Rockville Pike
Suite 100
Rockville, MD 20852
888-554-2627
<http://www.nacoa.org>
nacoa@erols.com

National Association for Native American Children of Alcoholics (NANACOA)
1402 Third Avenue
Suite 1110
Seattle, WA 98101
800-322-5601
nanacoa@nanacoa.org

National Association of Alcoholism and Drug Abuse Counselors
1911 North Fort Myer Drive
Suite 900

Arlington, VA 22201
800-548-0497
<http://www.naadac.org>
naadc@naadc.org

**National Association of Anorexia
Nervosa and Associated Disorders**
PO Box 7
Highland Park, IL 60035
847-831-3438
<http://www.anad.org>
anad20@aol.com

**National Association of State Alcohol
and Drug Abuse Directors**
808 17th Street NW
Suite 410
Washington, DC 20006
202-293-0090
<http://www.nasadad.org>
dcoffice@nasadad.org

**National Center for Victims
of Crime**
2111 Wilson Boulevard
Suite 300
Arlington, VA 22201
800-211-7996
<http://www.ncvc.org>

**National Clearinghouse on Child Abuse
and Neglect Information**
330 C Street, SW
Washington, DC 20447
800-394-3366
<http://www.calib.com/nccanch>
nccanch@calib.com

**National Council on Alcoholism and
Drug Dependence, Inc.**
20 Exchange Place
Suite 2902
New York, NY 10005
800-NCA-CALL
<http://www.ncadd.org>
national@ncadd.org

**The National Council on Problem
Gambling, Inc.**
208 G Street, NE
Washington, DC 20002
800-522-4700 (hotline)
<http://www.ncpgambling.org>
ncpg@ncpgambling.org

**National Crime Prevention Council
Online Resource Center**
1000 Connecticut Avenue, NW
13th floor
Washington, DC 20036
202-466-6272
<http://www.ncpc.org>

National Domestic Violence Hotline
PO Box 161810
Austin, TX 78716
800-787-3224
<http://www.ndvh.org>
ndvh@ndvh.org

National Eating Disorders Association
603 Stewart St., Suite 803
Seattle, WA 98101
206-382-3587
<http://www.NationalEatingDisorders.org>
info@NationalEatingDisorders.org

National Health Information Center
PO Box 1133
Washington, DC 20013
800-336-4797
<http://www.health.gov/nhic>
nhicinfo@health.org

**National Inhalant Prevention
Coalition**
2904 Kerbey Lane
Austin, TX 78703
800-269-4237
<http://www.inhalants.org>
nipc@io.com

**National Institute of Mental Health
(NIMH)**
NIMH Public Inquiries
6001 Executive Boulevard, Rm. 8184,
MSC 9663
Bethesda, MD 20892-9663
301-443-4513
<http://www.nimh.nih.gov>
nimhinfo@nih.gov

**National Institute on Alcohol Abuse and
Alcoholism**
6000 Executive Boulevard
Willco Building
Bethesda, MD 20892
301-443-3860
<http://www.niaaa.nih.gov>

National Institute on Drug Abuse (NIDA)
6001 Executive Boulevard
Room 5213
Bethesda, MD 20892
301-443-1124
<http://www.drugabuse.gov>
information@lists.nida.nih.gov

National Institutes of Health (NIH)
9000 Rockville Pike
Bethesda, MD 20892
301-496-4143
<http://www.nih.gov>

National Maternal and Child Health Clearinghouse
Health Resources and Services
Administration
U.S. Department of Health and Human
Services
Parklawn Building
5600 Fishers Lane
Rockville, MD 20857
<http://www.ask.hrsa.gov>
ask@hrsa.gov

National Organization on Fetal Alcohol Syndrome
216 G Street, NE
Washington, DC 20002
800-666-6327
<http://www.nofas.org>
information@nofas.org

National Resource Center on Homelessness and Mental Illness
Policy Research Associates, Inc.
345 Delaware Avenue
Delmar, NY 12054
800-444-7415
<http://www.nrchmi.com/>
nrc@prainc.com

National Safety Council
1121 Spring Lake Drive
Itasca, IL 60143
800-621-7615
<http://www.nsc.org>

National Women's Health Information Center
8550 Arlington Boulevard
Suite 300
Fairfax, VA 22031

800-994-9662
<http://www.4woman.org>

Office for Victims of Crime Resource Center
Department of Justice
810 7th Street, NW
Washington, DC 20531
800-627-6872
<http:/www.ojp.usdoj.gov/ovc>

Office of Minority Health Resource Center
PO Box 37337
Washington, DC 20013
800-444-6472
<http://www.omhrc.gov>

Office of National Drug Control Policy (ONDCP)
Executive Office of the President
750 17th Street, NW
Washington DC 20503
202-395-6700
<http://www.whitehousedrugpolicy.gov>
ondcp@ncjrs.org

Office on Smoking and Health (see Centers for Disease Control and Prevention)

ONDCP's Drug Policy Information Clearinghouse
PO Box 6000
Rockville, MD 20849
800-666-3332
<http://www.whitehousedrugpolicy.gov/publications/index.html>

Overeaters Anonymous
PO Box 44020
Rio Rancho, NM 87124-4020
505-891-2664
<http://www.overeatersanonymous.org>
info@overeatersanonymous.org

Partnership for a Drug-Free America
405 Lexington Avenue
Suite 1601
New York, NY 10174
212-922-1560
<http://www.drugfreeamerica.org>

PRIDE
4684 S. Evergreen
Newaygo, MI 49337

800-668-9277
<http://www.prideyouthprograms.org>
prideyouth@ncats.net

Psychomedics, Inc
5832 Uplander Way
Culver City, CA 90230
800-522-7424

Rational Recovery
PO Box 800
Lotus, CA 95651
800-303-2873
<http://www.rational.org>
home@rational.org

Safe and Drug-Free Schools
Department of Education
Federal Building No. 6
400 Maryland Avenue, SW
Washington, DC 20202
202-260-3954 for information on grant
applications
800-624-0100 for drug prevention materials
202-260-3954
<http://www.ed.gov>
customerservice@inet.ed.gov

Secular Organizations for Sobriety
SOS Clearinghouse
5521 Grosvenor Boulevard
Los Angeles, CA 90066
310-821-8430
<http://www.secularsobriety.org>

**Self-Help and Information Exchange
Network (SHINE)**
c/o Voluntary Action Center
Suite 420

538 Spruce Street
Scranton, PA 18509
570-961-1234
570-347-5616
<http://www.vacnepa.org>

Skyshapers University
157 Chambers Street
10th floor
New York, NY 10007
800-759-9675
800-SKYSHAPERS
<http://www.skyshapers.com>
webmaster@skyshapers.com

**Students Against Destructive Decisions
(SADD)**
Box 800
Marlboro, MA 01752
800-787-5777
<http://www.saddonline.com>

**Substance Abuse and Mental Health
Services Administration (SAMHSA)**
5600 Fishers Lane
Rockville, MD 20857
301-443-6315
<http://www.samhsa.gov>

**Working Partners for an Alcohol- and
Drug-Free Workplace**
Department of Labor
Office of Public Affairs
200 Constitution Ave., NW, Room
S-1032
Washington, DC 20210
202-693-4650
<http://www.dol.gov/dol/workingpartners
.htm>

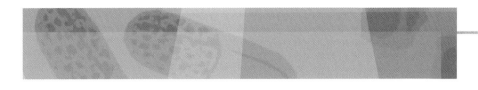

Selected Bibliography

General Texts About Alcohol and Drug Abuse

Alcohol and drug abuse take a terrible toll on teenagers. Unfortunately, studies show that more and more teenagers are using drugs and alcohol and suffering the consequences of that use. Substance abuse puts teenagers at a much greater risk for a wide variety of problems, including:

- school problems
- criminal behavior
- traffic accidents
- sexual activity at a young age
- depression and other psychiatric conditions
- victimization
- death by suicide, murder, drowning, fire

Articles and Nonfiction Books

"Alcohol: How It Affects You." *Current Health* 1, vol. 21, no. 5 (Jan. 1998).

Drug Dangers Series (Berkeley Heights, NJ: Enslow Publishers, 2001), including:

Alcohol Drug Dangers

Amphetamine Drug Dangers

Crack and Cocaine Drug Dangers

Diet Pill Drug Dangers

Ecstasy and Other Designer Drugs Drug Dangers

Herbal Drugs Drug Dangers

Heroin Drug Dangers

Inhalant Drug Dangers

LSD, PCP, Hallucinogen Drug Dangers

Marijuana Drug Dangers

Speed and Methamphetamine Drug Dangers

Steroid Drug Dangers

Tobacco and Nicotine Drug Dangers

Tranquilizer, Barbiturate, and Downer Drug Dangers

Gofen, E. "Alcohol in the Life of a Teen." Current Health 2, vol. 17, no. 2 (Oct. 1990).

"Illicit Drug Use by Teens Rising." *Alcoholism Report* 22, no. 2 (Feb./Mar. 1994).

Kuhn, Cynthia, et al. *Buzzed: The Straight Facts About the Most Used and Abused Drugs from Alcohol to Ecstasy.* New York: Norton, 1998.

Roza, Greg, ed. *Encyclopedia of Drugs and Alcohol.* New York: Franklin Watts, 2001.

Schuckit, Marc Alan. *Educating Yourself About Alcohol and Drugs: A People's Primer.* New York: Plenum Press, 1998.

"Survey Illustrates Wide Reach of Drugs in Teens' Lives." *Alcoholism and Drug Abuse Weekly* 10, no. 26 (June 29, 1998).

"Teens' Steroid Use Linked to Their Use of Other Drugs." *Addiction Letter* 11, no. 11 (Nov. 1995).

"Teens Who Do Not Try Drugs Are Better-Adjusted, Study Says." *Alcoholism and Drug Abuse Weekly* 8, no. 21 (May 20, 1996).

"Withdrawal Symptoms May be Worse for Teens." *Addiction Letter* 12, no. 1 (Jan. 1996).

"Young Teens and Drugs Use." *Current Health* 1, vol. 17, no. 2 (Oct. 1993).

Fiction of Interest

Anonymous. *Go Ask Alice.* Minneapolis: Econo-Clad Books, 1998.

Childress, Alice. *A Hero Ain't Nothin' but a Sandwich.* New York: Avon, 1995.

Draper, Sharon M. *Tears of a Tiger*. New York: Simon and Schuster, 1996.

Glovach, Linda. *Beauty Queen*. New York: Harper-Collins, 1998.

Greene, Shep. *The Boy Who Drank Too Much*. New York: Bantam Doubleday Dell, 1981.

Keizer, Garrett. *God of Beer*. New York: HarperCollins, 2002.

Web Sites

"For Tweens and Teens." National Center on Addiction and Substance Abuse at Columbia University.

<http://www.casacolumbia.org/info-url1940/info-url_list.htm?section=For%20Tweens%20%26%20Teens>.

"Mind Over Matter: The Brain's Response to Marijuana, Opiates, Inhalants, Hallucinogens, Methamphetamine, Nicotine, Stimulants, Steroids." National Institute on Drug Abuse, National Institutes of Health. Last updated September 14, 2001. <http://www.nida.nih.gov/MOM/MOMIndex.html>.

Overcoming Substance Abuse

Many substance users think they will never get addicted. But once substance abuse becomes a stranglehold, it can be exceedingly difficult for the user to struggle free. Although a wide variety of treatments are available, researchers are constantly searching for ways to help users break their addiction and to help former addicts avoid slipping back into substance abuse.

Articles and Nonfiction Books

"Alcohol and Drug Interventions for Teens Should Consider Peer Use, Peer Pressure." *DATA: The Brown University Digest of Addiction Theory and Application* 14, no. 5 (May 1995).

"Alcohol Interventions for Teens Should Address Social Factors." *DATA: The Brown University Digest of Addiction Theory and Application* 14, no. 7 (July 1995).

Chiu, Christina. *Teen Guide to Staying Sober*. New York: Rosen Publishing Group, 1995.

"Gender-Specific Substance Abuse Treatment Promising." *DATA: The Brown University Digest of Addiction Theory and Application* 20, no. 7 (July 2001).

Landau, Elaine. *Hooked: Talking About Addiction*. Brookfield, CT: Millbrook Press, 1995.

Moe, Barbara A. *Drug Abuse Relapse: Helping Teens to Get Clean Again*. Drug Abuse Prevention Library. New York: Rosen Publishing Group, 2000.

Roos, Stephen. *A Young Person's Guide to the Twelve Steps*. Center City, MN: Hazelden Information and Educational Services, 1993.

"Youth Treatment Study Shows Good Results, Parallels Findings for Adult Outcomes." *Alcoholism and Drug Abuse Weekly* 13, no. 27 (July 16, 2001).

Web Site

"Principles of Drug Abuse Treatment: A Research-Based Guide." National Institute on Drug Abuse, National Institutes of Health.

<http://www.nida.nih.gov/PODAT/PODAT1.html>.

When Parents Abuse Alcohol or Drugs

Most studies show that having a substance-abusing parent can affect children from birth on into adulthood. Babies of substance abusers can be born addicted to drugs or suffering from fetal alcohol syndrome. Children living in a home with substance-abusing parents are more likely to suffer from anxiety, depression, and behavior problems. Rates of child abuse and neglect are higher in homes with substance-abusing parents. Teenage children of substance abusers have a higher risk of themselves turning to drugs or alcohol. Adults from alcoholic homes or homes where drugs were used have more problems with anxiety and depression, greater difficulties with relationships, and a high risk of becoming addicted to alcohol or drugs.

Articles and Nonfiction Books

"Depression in Children Linked to Parents' Alcoholism." *Alcoholism and Drug Abuse Weekly* 8, no. 27 (July 1, 1996).

Emshoff, James G., and Ann W. Price. "Prevention and Intervention Strategies With Children of Alcoholics" (part 2 of 2). *Pediatrics* 103, no. 5 (May 1999).

Foltz-Gray, Dorothy. "An Alcoholic in the Family." *Health* 11, no. 5 (July/Aug. 1997).

Hornik-Beer, Edith Lynn. *For Teenagers Living with a Parent Who Abuses Alcohol/Drugs.* iUniverse.com, 2001.

Johnson, Jeannette L., and Michelle Left. "Children of Substance Abusers: Overview of Research Findings" (part 2 of 2). *Pediatrics* 103, no. 5 (May 1999).

Leite, Evelyn, and Pamela Espeland. *Different Like Me: A Book for Teenagers Who Worry about Their Parents' Use of Alcohol/Drugs.* Center City, MN: Hazelden Information and Educational Services, 1989.

Price, Ann W., and James G. Emshoff. "Breaking the Cycle of Addiction: Prevention and Intervention With Children of Alcoholics." *Alcohol Health and Research World* 21, no. 3 (1997).

Shuker, Nancy. *Everything You Need to Know About an Alcoholic Parent.* New York: Rosen Publishing Group, 1998.

"Substance Abuse Programs for Parents." *Brown University Child and Adolescent Behavior Letter* 11, no. 2 (Feb. 1995).

Tomori, Martina. "Personality Characteristics of Adolescents with Alcoholic Parents." *Adolescence* 29, no. 116 (winter 1994).

Ullman, Albert D., and Alan Orenstein. "Why Some Children of Alcoholics Become Alcoholics: Emulation of the Drinker." *Adolescence* 29, no. 113 (spring 1994).

Fiction of Interest

Bauer, Joan. *Rules of the Road.* New York: Putnam, 1998.

Gantos, Jack. *Joey Pigza Loses Control.* New York: HarperTrophy, 2002.

Web Sites

"Alateen: Hope and Help for Young People Who Are the Relatives and Friends of a Problem Drinker."

<http://www.al-anon.org/alateen.html>.

National Association for Children of Alcoholics.

<http://www.nacoa.org/kidspage.htm>.

Alcohol and Drug Policy, Drug Trafficking, and Crime

The United States and other concerned countries work to rewrite policy and law in an effort to regulate alcohol and tobacco use, to decrease drug production and drug trafficking, and to cut down on drug-related crime. The dangerous consequences of drug use range from its effects on individuals (increased risk of murder, suicide, and motor vehicle accidents) to its effects on entire nations. In recent years, many events have brought the link between drug trafficking, money laundering, and terrorism to the world's attention.

Articles and Nonfiction Books

"Alcohol Most Common 'Date-Rape' Drug: Study." *Alcoholism Report* 26, no. 3 (March 1998).

Grosslander, Janet. *Drugs and Driving.* New York: Rosen Publishing Group, 2001.

Hyde, Margaret O. *Drug Wars.* New York: Walker and Company, 2000.

"Let's Redefine U.S. Drug Policy to One of Harm Reduction." *DATA: The Brown University Digest of Addiction Theory and Application* 16, no. 2 (Feb. 1997 supplement).

Levine, Herbert M. *The Drug Problem: American Issues Debated.* New York: Raintree/Steck Vaughn, 1997.

Leviton, Susan, and Marc A. Schindler. "Drug Trafficking and the Justice System" (part 2 of 2). *Pediatrics* 93, no. 6 (June 1994).

"SAMHSA Study Links Treatment to Drops in Drug Use, Crime." *Alcoholism and Drug Abuse Weekly* 8, no. 36 (Sept. 16, 1996).

Stewart, Gail B. *Drug Trafficking.* Detroit: Gale Group, 1990.

"Study of Probationers Reveals High Drug Use." *Alcoholism and Drug Abuse Weekly* 10, no. 15 (April 13, 1998).

Fiction of Interest

Kehret, Peg. *Cages.* New York: Pocket Books, 1993.

Smith, Roland. *Zach's Lie.* New York: Hyperion Books, 2001.

Web Sites

Drug Enforcement Administration.

<http://www.dea.gov>.

Office of National Drug Control Policy.

<http://www.whitehousedrugpolicy.gov>.

Smoking

It has been known for years that smoking is deadly. Studies show that if the current rate of tobacco use holds steady, five million U.S. children who were aged 18 or under in 2000 will die prematurely as adults due to complications of the smoking habit they started during their teen years.

Articles and Nonfiction Books

"African-American Teens at High Risk from Smoking." *Alcoholism and Drug Abuse Weekly* 13, no. 10 (Mar. 5, 2001).

Hyde, Margaret O. *Know About Smoking.* New York: Walker and Company, 1995.

Kowalski, Kathiann M. "Tobacco's Toll on Teens." *Current Health* 2, vol. 23, no. 6 (Feb. 1997).

McMillan, Daniel. *Teen Smoking: Understanding the Risk.* Berkeley Heights, NJ: Enslow Publishers, 1996.

"Restricting the Movies Teens Watch May Impact Tobacco Use." *Brown University Child and Adolescent Behavior Letter* 18, no. 5 (May 2002).

"Study: Parents and Peers Influence Smoking, Drinking." *Alcoholism and Drug Abuse Weekly* 13, no. 6 (Feb. 5, 2001).

"Teens: Smoking Isn't Good. Quitting Isn't Easy." *Current Health* 2, vol. 20, no. 8 (Apr. 1994).

"Teen Smoking May Hint at Other Risky Behavior." *Health Letter on the CDC,* December 22–December 29, 1997.

"Teens Who Exhibit Problems More Likely to Smoke." *Alcoholism and Drug Abuse Weekly* 14, no. 10 (Mar. 11, 2002).

Williams, Mary E. *Teens and Smoking.* Detroit: Gale Group, 2000.

Fiction of Interest

Cossi, Olga. *The Magic Box.* New York: Pelican, 1989.

Web Sites

Campaign for Tobacco Free Kids.

<http://www.tobaccofreekids.org>.

"The Surgeon General's Report for Kids About Smoking." National Center for Chronic Disease Prevention and Health Promotion, Centers for Disease Control and Prevention.

<http://www.cdc.gov/tobacco/sgr/sgr4kids/sgrmenu.htm>.

Gambling

Gambling is spreading among younger teens and even children, mainly because of the ever-increasing number of online gambling web sites. For those people who are susceptible to becoming addicted to gambling, the ease of gambling online is a particular danger. The social costs of gambling problems among adults include increased rates of crime, financial downfall leading to bankruptcy, higher divorce rates, and a greatly increased chance of becoming addicted to alcohol or drugs.

Articles and Nonfiction Books

Cozick, Charles P., and Paul A. Winters. *Gambling.* Detroit: Greenhaven Press, 1995.

Dolan, Edward F. *Teenagers and Compulsive Gambling.* New York: Franklin Watts, 1994.

"Gambling Common Among Marijuana-Smoking Teens." *Brown University Child and Adolescent Behavior Letter* 17, no. 12 (Dec. 2001).

Haddock, Patricia. *Teens and Gambling: Who Wins?* Berkeley Heights, NJ: Enslow Publishers, 1996.

Rafenstein, Mark. "Why Teens Are Becoming Compulsive about Gambling." *Current Health* 2, vol. 26, no. 8 (Apr./May 2000).

"Teens and Gambling." *Current Health* 2, vol. 26, no. 8 (Apr./May 2000 teacher's edition).

Fiction of Interest

Hautman, Pete. *Stone Cold.* New York: Simon and Schuster, 1998.

Web Sites

"Questions and Answers About the Problem of Compulsive Gambling and the Gamblers Anonymous Recovery Program." Gamblers Anonymous.

<http://www.gamblersanonymous.org/qna.html>.

"Youth Problem Gambling." International Centre for Youth Gambling Problems and High-Risk Behaviors, McGill University, Montreal, Canada.

<http://www.education.mcgill.ca/gambling/en/problemg.htm>.

Other Conditions That May Influence Substance Abuse

A number of other psychiatric conditions may occur along with substance abuse, including depression, bipolar disorder, obsessive-compulsive disorder, eating disorders, cutting (self-harm or self-mutilation), anxiety, and conduct disorders. Why are these conditions associated with each other? Is there something similar genetically about people with substance abuse and other psychiatric problems? Is there something about the brain structure or the brain chemistry of some individuals that makes them more susceptible to these disorders, as well as to substance abuse? Do people begin using alcohol or taking drugs in order to treat the symptoms of other psychiatric illnesses?

Articles and Nonfiction Books

Cobain, Bev, et al. *When Nothing Matters Anymore: A Survival Guide for Depressed Teens.* Minneapolis: Free Spirit Publishing, 1998.

Costin, Carolyn. *The Eating Disorder Sourcebook: A Comprehensive Guide to the Causes, Treatments, and Prevention of Eating Disorders.* New York: McGraw Hill, 1999.

Farley, Dixie. "On the Teen Scene: Overcoming the Deficit of Attention." *FDA Consumer* 31, no. 5 (July/Aug. 1997).

Hallowell, Edward M., and John J. Ratey. *Driven to Distraction: Recognizing and Coping With Attention Deficit Disorder from Childhood Through Adolescence.* New York: Simon and Schuster, 1995.

Levonkron, Steven. *Cutting: Understanding and Overcoming Self-Mutilation.* New York: Norton, 1999.

McLellan, Tom, and Alicia Bragg. *Escape from Anxiety and Stress.* Broomall, PA: Chelsea House Publishing, 1988.

Normandi, Carol Emery, and Lauralee Roark. *Over It: A Teen's Guide to Getting Beyond Obsession With Food and Weight.* Novato, CA: New World Publishing, 2001.

Rapoport, Judith L. *The Boy Who Couldn't Stop Washing: The Experience and Treatment of Obsessive Compulsive Disorder.* New York: New American Library, 1997.

"Study Finds Co-morbid Eating Disorders among Women Who Abuse Substances." *DATA: The Brown University Digest of Addiction Theory and Application* 20, no. 1 (Jan. 2001).

"Study: Use of Ritalin for ADHD Reduces Substance Abuse Risk." *Children's Services Report* 3, no. 16 (Aug. 23, 1999).

"Teens with Depression Gravitate to Smoking." *Mental Health Weekly* 7, no. 1 (Jan. 6, 1997).

Fiction of Interest

Gantos, Jack. *Joey Pigza Swallowed the Key.* New York: Farrar Straus Giroux, 1998. (Concerns ADHD.)

Hesser, Terry Spencer. *Kissing Doorknobs.* New York: Bantam Books, 1999. (Concerns obsessive-compulsive disorder.)

Jenkins, A. M. *Damage.* New York: HarperCollins, 2001. (Concerns depression.)

Levonkron, Steven. *The Best Little Girl in the World.* New York: Warner Books, 1979. (Concerns eating disorders.)

Levonkron, Steven. *The Luckiest Girl in the World.* New York: Penguin, 1998. (Concerns cutting.)

McCormick, Patricia. *Cut.* New York: Scholastic, 2002. (Concerns cutting.)

Newman, Leslie. *Fat Chance.* New York: Putnam, 1996. (Concerns eating disorders.)

Willey, Margaret. *Saving Lenny.* New York: Bantam Books, 1991. (Concerns depression, codependence.)

Web Sites

"Attention Deficit Hyperactivity Disorder." National Institute of Mental Health, National Institutes of Health.

<http://www.nimh.nih.gov/publicat/adhd.cfm>.

"Eating Disorders: Facts about Eating Disorders and the Search for Solutions." National Institute of Mental Health, National Institutes of Health.

<http://www.nimh.nih.gov/publicat/eatingdisorder.cfm>.

"Let's Talk about Depression," National Institute of Mental Health, National Institutes of Health.

<http://www.nimh.nih.gov/publicat/letstalk.cfm>.

Prevention of Alcohol or Drug Abuse

The issue of preventing substance abuse is as complicated as it is important. Effective prevention seems to involve helping young people learn how to manage peer pressure and develop a strong and confident sense of self.

Articles and Nonfiction Books

Alexander, Ruth Bell. *Changing Bodies, Changing Lives: A Book for Teens on Sex and Relationships.* New York: Times Books, 1998.

Benson, Peter L., et al. *What Teens Need to Succeed: Proven, Practical Ways to Shape Your Own Future.* Minneapolis: Free Spirit Publishing, 1998.

Covey, Sean. *Seven Habits of Highly Effective Teens: The Ultimate Teenage Success Guide.* New York: Simon and Schuster, 1998.

"Improving Substance Abuse Prevention, Assessment, and Treatment Financing for Children and Adolescents." *Pediatrics* 108, no. 4 (Oct. 2001).

Palmer, Pat, and Melissa Alberti Froehner. *Teen Esteem: A Self-Direction Manual for Young Adults.* Atascadero, CA: Impact Publishers, 2000.

Scott, Sharon. *How to Say No and Keep Your Friends: Peer Pressure Reversal for Teens and Preteens.* Amherst, MA: Human Resource Development Press, 1997.

Web Sites

"CASA's Tips for Staying Drug-Free." National Center on Addiction and Substance Abuse at Columbia University.

<http://www.casacolumbia.org/info-url1940/info-url_show.htm?doc_id=20812>.

"A Guide for Teens: Does Your Friend Have an Alcohol or Drug Problem?" National Clearinghouse for Alcohol and Drug Information, Substance Abuse and Mental Health Services Administration, Department of Health and Human Services.

<http://www.health.org/govpubs/phd688>.

For Parents and Teachers

Parents have a lot of influence over their children. While parents cannot fully control their children's behavior, studies have shown that close-knit families provide some protection against alcohol and drug abuse in children. It is also clear that the use or abuse of substances by a child's parent or parents can increase that child's risk of beginning to use or abuse substances. Still, some children who come from warm, supportive homes and whose parents do not themselves abuse substances may stumble into alcohol or drug use. How can parents (and teachers) identify such problems and get their child the help he or she so desperately needs?

Articles and Nonfiction Books

Babbit, Nikki. *Adolescent Drug and Alcohol Abuse: How to Spot It, Stop It, and Get Help for Your Family.* Sebastopol, CA: Patient-Centered Guides, 2000.

Biederman, Joseph, et al. "Patterns of Alcohol and Drug Use in Adolescents Can Be Predicted by Parental Substance Use Disorders." *Pediatrics* 106, no. 4 (Oct. 2000).

Cappello, Dominic, and Xenia G. Becher. *Ten Talks Parents Must Have with Their Children about Drugs and Choices.* New York: Hyperion, 2001.

"Does Your Child Have a Gambling Problem?" *Brown University Child and Adolescent Behavior Letter* 12, no. 3 (Mar. 1996).

"'Hands-On' Parenting Reduces Teens' Substance Abuse Risk." *Nation's Health* 31, no. 4 (May 2001).

Kuhn, Cynthia. *Just Say Know: Talking with Kids about Drugs and Alcohol.* New York: Norton, 2002.

Nolen, Billy James. *Parents, Teens, and Drugs.* Baltimore: American Literary Press, 2000.

"Parents Can Influence When, How Teens Use Alcohol and Marijuana." *DATA: The Brown University Digest of Addiction Theory and Application* 19, no. 6 (June 2000).

"Program Helps Parents Cope with Substance-Abusing Teens." *DATA: The Brown University Digest of Addiction Theory and Application* 20, no. 7 (July 2001).

Wood, Barbara. *Raising Healthy Children in an Alcoholic Home.* New York: Crossroad/Herder and Herder, 1992.

Web Sites

Mothers Against Drunk Driving (MADD).

<http://www.madd.org/under21/0,1056,1108,00.html>.

Safe and Drug-Free Schools Program, U.S. Department of Education.

<http://www.ed.gov/offices/OESE/SDFS>.

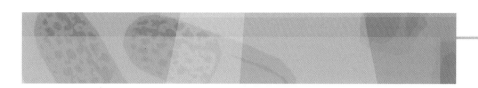

Glossary

abstinence complete avoidance of something, such as the use of drugs or alcoholic beverages

abstinent to completely avoid something, such as drug or alcohol use

abuse related to drug use, describes taking drugs that are illegal, or using prescription drugs in a way for which they were not prescribed; related to alcohol use, describes drinking in a fashion that is damaging to the drinker or to others

abuse potential chance, or likelihood, that a drug will be abused

acute having a sudden onset and lasting a short time

addiction state in which the body requires the presence of a particular substance to function normally; without the substance, the individual will begin to experience predictable withdrawal symptoms

advocate to support or defend a cause or a proposal

aesthete one who has a deep appreciation for beauty, especially in the arts or nature

aggression hostile and destructive behavior, especially caused by frustration; may include violence or physical threat or injury directed toward another

aggressive hostile and destructive behavior

agonist chemical that can bind to a particular cell and cause a specific reaction

AIDS stands for acquired immunodeficiency syndrome, the disease caused by the human immunodeficiency virus (HIV); in severe cases, it is characterized by the profound weakening of the body's immune system

alcoholism disease of the body and mind in which an individual compulsively drinks alcohol, despite its harmful effects on the person's career, relationships, and/or health; leads to dependence on alcohol, and the presence of withdrawal symptoms when alcohol use is stopped; can be progressive and fatal; research indicates the disease runs in families, and may be genetically inherited

alkaline similar in chemical composition to the alkali chemicals; possessing a pH greater than 7

amino acids organic molecules that make up proteins

amphetamine central nervous system stimulant, used in medicine to treat attention-deficit/hyperactivity disorder (ADHD), narcolepsy (a sleep disorder), and as an appetite suppressant

analgesic broad drug classification that includes acetaminophen, aspirin, ibuprofen, and addictive agents such as opiates

analog a different form of a chemical or drug structurally related to a parent chemical or drug

androgenic effects effects on the growth of the male reproductive tract and the development of male secondary sexual characteristics

anesthetic an agent or event that causes anesthesia, or the loss of sensation and/or consciousness

anorectic a substance that decreases a person's appetite

anorexia nervosa eating disorder characterized by an intense and irrational fear of gaining weight, resulting in abnormal and unhealthy eating patterns, malnutrition, and severe weight loss

antagonist an agent that counteracts or blocks the effects of another drug

anticonvulsant drug that relieves or prevents seizures

antidepressant medication used for the treatment and prevention of depression

antipsychotic drugs drugs that reduce psychotic behavior, but often have negative long-term side effects

antisocial personality disorder a condition in which people disregard the rights of others and violate these rights by acting in immoral, unethical, aggressive, or even criminal ways

antitrust relating to laws that prevent unfair business practicies, such as monopolies

anxiety disorder condition in which a person feels uncontrollable angst and worry, often without any specific cause

archaeological relating to the scientific study of material remains from past human life and activities

attention-deficit/hyperactivity disorder ADHD is a long-term condition characterized by excessive, ongoing hyperactivity (overactivity, restlessness, fidgeting), distractibility, and impulsivity; distractibility refers to heightened sensitivity to irrelevant sights and sounds, making some simple tasks difficult to complete

autopsy examination of a body after a person has died, to determine the cause of death or to explore the results of a disease

ayahuasca an intoxicating beverage made from *Banisteriopsis caapi* plants, which contain dimethyltriptamine or DMT

barbiturate highly habit-forming sedative drugs that decrease the activity of the central nervous system

behavioral therapy form of therapy whose main focus is to change certain behaviors instead of uncovering unconscious conflicts or problems

benign harmless; also, noncancerous

benzodiazepine drug developed in the 1960s as a safer alternative to barbiturates. Most frequently used as a sleeping pill or as an anti-anxiety medication

binge relatively brief period of excessive behavior, such as eating an usually large amount of food

binge drinker a man who consumes 5 or more drinks on a single occasion; or a woman who consumes 4 or more drinks on a single occasion

biopsy procedure in which a body tissue, cells, or fluids are removed for examination in a laboratory

black market sale and purchase of goods that are illegal, such as drugs like heroin

blood alcohol concentration (BAC) amount of alcohol in the bloodstream, expressed as the grams of alcohol per deciliter of blood; as BAC goes up, the drinker experiences more psychological and physical effects

borderline personality disorder condition in which a person consistently has unstable personal relationships, negative self-image, unclear self-identity, recurring impulsivity, and problems with mood

bulimia nervosa literally means "ox hunger"; eating disorder characterized by compulsive overeating and then efforts to purge the body of the excess food, through self-induced vomiting, laxative abuse, or the use of diuretic medicines (pills to rid the body of water)

buprenorphine new medication that has proven to reduce cravings associated with heroin withdrawal, and may also be helpful in treating cocaine addiction

cannabis plants and/or drug forms of the Indian hemp plant, *Cannabis sativa*, also known as marijuana

carcinogen substance or agent that causes cancer

cartel group that controls production and/or price of a good such as diamonds, oil, or illegal drugs

catatonia psychomotor disturbance characterized by muscular rigidity, excitement, or stupor

central nervous system comprised of brain and spinal cord in humans

cerebellum a large part of the brain, which helps with muscle coordination and balance

cerebral cortex surface layer of gray matter in the front part of the brain that helps in coordinating the senses and motor functions

chronic continuing for a long period of time

cirrhosis chronic, scarring liver disease that can be caused by alcohol abuse, toxins, nutritional deficiency, or infection

civil libertarian person who believes in the right to unrestricted freedom of thought and action

cleft palate congenital (present at birth) cleft or separation in the roof of the mouth

clinical trial scientific experiment that uses humans, as opposed to animals, to test the efficacy of a new drug, medical or surgical technique, or method of diagnosis or prevention

clitoris small erectile organ in females at front part of the vulva

club drug group of drugs commonly reported to be used by young people at clubs or "raves" to increase stamina and energy and/or extend the euphoric effects of alcohol

codependence situation in which someone (often a family member) has an unhealthy dependence on an individual with an addiction; the dependent relationship allows the addicted individual to be manipulative, and is often characterized as "enabling" the addict to continue his or her addiction

codependent person who has an unhealthy dependence on another person with an addiction

coma state of very deep and sometimes prolonged unconsciousness

comorbid two or more disorders that occur at the same time in a person

compensation an amount of money or something else given to pay for loss, damage or work done

completed suicide suicide attempt that actually ends in death

compound pure substance that is made up of two or more elements, but possesses new chemical properties different from the original elements

compulsion irresistible drive to perform a particular action; some compulsions are performed in order to reduce stress and anxiety brought on by obsessive thoughts

condom covering worn over the penis, used as a barrier method of birth control and disease prevention

conduct disorder condition in which a child or adolescent exhibits behavioral and emotional problems, often finding it difficult to follow rules and behaving in a manner that violates the rights of others and society

convulsion intense, repetitive muscle contraction

correlate to link in a way that can be measured and predicted

correlation relation of two or more things in a way that can be measured and predicted

corroborate to independently find proof or support

corticosteroid medication that is prescribed to reduce inflammation and sometimes to suppress the body's immune responses

crack cocaine a freebase cocaine, or a cocaine that is specially processed to remove impurities; crack cocaine is smoked and is highly addictive

craving a powerful, often uncontrollable desire

debilitating something that interferes with or lessens normal strength and functioning

deficiency having too little of a necessary vitamin or mineral

deflect to cause somebody to change from what he or she usually does or plans to do

dehydration a state in which there is an abnormally low amount of fluid in the body

delirium mental disturbance marked by confusion, disordered speech, and sometimes hallucinations

delusion unshakable false belief that a person holds onto even when facts should convince the individual otherwise

dementia type of disease characterized by progressive loss of memory and the ability to learn and think

denial psychological state in which a person ignores obvious facts and continues to deny the existence of a particular problem or situation

dental dam piece of latex used to protect the mouth; can be used in dentistry, or can be used to prevent the oral transmission of sexually transmitted diseases

dependence psychological compulsion to use a substance for emotional and/or physical reasons

dependent someone who has a psychological compulsion to use a substance for emotional and/or physical reasons

depletion state of being used up or emptied

depressant chemical that slows down or decreases functioning; often used to describe agents that slow down the functioning of the central nervous system; such agents are sometimes used to relieve insomnia, anxiety, irritability, and tension

depressed someone who feels intensely sad and hopeless

depression state in which an individual feels intensely sad and hopeless, may have trouble eating, sleeping, and concentrating, and is no longer able to feel pleasure from previously enjoyable activities; in extreme cases, it may lead an individual to think about or attempt suicide

deprivation situation of lacking the basic necessities of life, such as food or emotional security

detoxification process of removing a poisonous, intoxicating, or addictive substance from the body

dietary supplement product used to supplement an individual's normal diet, by adding a specific vitamin, mineral, herb, or amino acid, or by increasing the general caloric intake; often available without a prescription; usually not subjected to rigorous clinical testing

dilution process of making something thinner, weaker, or less concentrated, typically by adding a diluting material (often a liquid such as water); can also refer to the result of diluting, a weakened solution

disordered state characterized by chaotic, disorganized, or confused functioning; may refer to problems with a person's individual thought processes or problems within a system, such as a family

distillation process that separates alcohol from fermenting juices

diuretic drug that increases urine output; sometimes called "water pill"

divine relating to or proceeding from God or a god

Down syndrome form of mental retardation due to an extra chromosome present at birth often accompanied by physical characteristics, such as sloped eyes

downers slang term for drugs that act as depressants on the central nervous system, such as barbiturates

drug traffickers people or groups who transport illegal drugs

drug trafficking act of transporting illegal drugs

dysphoria depressed and unhappy mood state

ecstasy designer drug and amphetamine derivative that is a commonly abused street drug

efficacy ability to produce desired results

endocrine system cells, tissues, and organs of the body that are active in regulating bodily functions, such as growth and metabolism

enthusiast supporter

enzyme protein produced by cells that causes or speeds up biological reactions, such as those that break down food into smaller parts

epidemic rapid spreading of a disease to many people in a given area or community at the same time

euphoria state of intense, giddy happiness and well-being, sometimes occurring baselessly and at odds with an individual's life situation

euphoric someone who experiences a state of intense, giddy happiness and well-being, sometimes occurring baselessly and out of sync

excise tax tax that a government puts on the manufacture, sale, or use of a domestic product

expertise expert advice or opinions expressed by a person with recognized skill or knowledge in a particular area

exploitation condition in which one uses another person for one's own selfish advantage

export to send merchandise to another country as part of commercial business

expulsion act of forcing somebody out of a group or institution, such as a school or club

felony very serious crime that usually warrants a more severe punishment than those crimes considered misdemeanors

gastrointestinal tract entire length of the digestive system, running from the stomach, through the small intestine, large intestine, and out the rectum

half-life amount of time it takes for one-half of a substance to undergo a process, such as to be broken down or eliminated

hallucination seeing, hearing, feeling, tasting, or smelling something that is not actually there, like a vision of devils, hearing voices, or feeling bugs crawl over the skin; may occur due to mental illness or as a side effect of some drugs

hallucinogen a drug, such as LSD, that causes hallucinations, or seeing, hearing, or feeling things that are not there

hallucinogenic describing a substance that can cause hallucinations, or seeing, hearing, or feeling things that aren't there

heritable trait that is passed on from parents to offspring

homicide murder

hormone chemical substance, produced by a gland, that travels through the blood or other body fluids to another part of the body where it causes a physiological activity to occur

hyperactivity overly active behavior

hypersensitivity state of extreme sensitivity to something

hypnotic drug that induces sleep by depressing the central nervous system

illicit something illegal or something used in an illegal manner

immune system human body's system of protecting itself against foreign substances, germs, and other infectious agents; protects the body against illness

impair to make worse or to damage, especially by lessening or reducing in some way

impotence inability to get or maintain an erection

impotency condition in which one is unable to get or maintain an erection

impulsive acting before thinking through the consequences of the action

impulsivity state in which someone acts before thinking through the consequences of their actions

incentive something, such as a reward, that encourages a specific action or behavior

induce to bring about or stimulate a particular reaction

induction process of formally admitting somebody into a position or organization

infertility inability to have children

ingenuity inventive skill or imagination

inhalant legal product that evaporates easily, producing chemical vapors; abusers inhale concentrated amounts of these vapors to alter their consciousness

inpatient person who stays overnight in a facility to get treatment

interpret to explain the meaning of or make a judgment about technical information or data

interpretation judgment or explanation about technical information

intervention act of intervening or positioning oneself between two things; when referring to substance abuse, the term means an attempt to help an addict admit to his or her addiction, recognize the ill effects the addiction has had on the addict and on his or her relationships, and get help to conquer the addiction

intoxicant food or drink capable of diminishing physical or mental control

intoxicated someone whose physical or mental control has been diminished

intoxicating a food or drink capable of diminishing physical or mental control

intoxication loss of physical or mental control because of the effects of a substance

invasive in the context of medical actions, describing a procedure in which a part of the body is entered; relating to an infection or a cancer, describing a disease that has spread from its original site in the body

LAAM (Levo-Alpha-Acetylmethadol) a synthetic opiate used to treat heroin addiction by blunting the symptoms of withdrawal for up to 72 hours

laxative product that promotes bowel movements

legitimate meeting or conforming to legal or recognized standards

lethargy state of being slowed down, sluggish, very drowsy, lacking all energy or drive

liable responsible

licit legal; permitted by law

lobbying activities aimed at influencing public officials, especially members of the legislature

logo an identifying symbol (as for advertising) that a company uses as a way of gaining recognition

LSD lysergic acid diethylamide, known for its hallucinogenic properties

lucrative something with the potential to make a lot of money

malaria disease caused by a parasite in the red blood cells, passed to humans through the bite of mosquitoes

malnutrition unhealthy condition of the body caused by not getting enough food or enough of the right foods or by an inability of the body to appropriately break down the food or utilize the nutrients

marijuana dried leaves and flowers of female *Cannabis sativa* plants, smoked or eaten for its intoxicating effect

market share percentage of the total sales of a product that is controlled by a company

media means of mass communication, such as newspapers, magazines, radio or television

mescaline hallucinogenic drug that is the main active agent found in mescal buttons of the peyote plant

metabolic describing or related to the chemical processes through which the cells of the body breakdown substances to produce energy

metabolism chemical processes through which the cells of the body break down various substances to produce energy and allow the body to function

methadone potent synthetic narcotic, used in heroin recovery programs as a non-intoxicating opiate that blunts symptoms of withdrawal

misdemeanor crime that is treated in the courts as a less serious crime than a felony

money laundering activity in which a person or group hides the source of money that has been illegally obtained

monopoly situation that exists when only one person or company sells a good or service in a given area

morphine primary alkaloid chemical in opium, used as a drug to treat severe, acute, and chronic pain

narcotic addictive substance that relieves pain and induces sleep or causes sedation; prescription narcotics includes morphine and codeine; can refer to a drug of abuse, such as heroin, cocaine, or marijuana

neuroleptic one of a class of antipsychotic drugs, including major tranquilizers, used in the treatment of psychoses like schizophrenia

neurological relating to the nervous system

neuron nerve cell that releases neurotransmitters

neuropathic relating to a disease of the nerves

neurotransmitter chemical messenger used by nerve cells to communicate with other nerve cells

nicotine alkaloid derived from the tobacco plant that is responsible for smoking's addictive effects

noninvasive not involving penetration of the skin

norm behavior, custom, or attitude that is considered normal, or expected, within a certain social group

obscene morally offensive; describes something meant to degrade or corrupt

obsessed someone who experiences repeated thoughts, impulses, or mental images that are irrational and that the person cannot control

obsession repeating thoughts, impulses, or mental images that are irrational and that an individual cannot control

obsessive-compulsive disorder anxiety disorder in which a person cannot prevent dwelling on unwanted thoughts, accting on urges, or repeating rituals

opiate drug derived directly from opium and used in its natural state, without chemical modification; examples of opiates are morphine, codeine, thebaine, noscapine, and papaverine

opioid substance that acts in a way similar to opiate narcotic drugs, but is not actually produced from the opium poppy

oppositional defiant disorder psychiatric condition in which a person repeatedly shows a pattern of negative, hostile, disobedient, and/or defiant behavior, without serious violation of the rights of others

optimism a positive outlook

outpatient person who receives treatment at a doctor's office or hospital but does not stay overnight

overdose excessively high dose of a drug, which can be toxic or even life-threatening

paranoia excessive or irrational suspicion, illogical mistrust

paranoid someone who is excessively or irrationally suspicious

paranoid psychosis symptom of mental illness characterized by changes in personality, a distorted sense of reality, and feelings of excessive and irrational suspicion; may include hallucinations (seeing, hearing, feeling, smelling, or tasting something that is not truly there)

paraphernalia equipment that enables drug users to take the drugs, such as syringes and needles

periodic occuring at regular intervals or periods

peyote a cactus that can be used to make a stimulant drug

pharmaceuticals legal drugs that are usually used for medical reasons

pharmacology branch of science concerned with drugs and how they affect bodily and mental processes

philanthrophy acts performed with the desire to improve humanity, especially through charitable activities

physical dependence condition that may occur after prolonged use of a particular drug or alcohol, in which the user's body cannot function normally without the presence of the substance; when the substance is not used, or when the dose is decreased, the user experiences uncomfortable physical symptoms

physically dependent someone who takes drugs for relief of uncomfortable physical symptoms, rather than for emotional or psychological relief

physiological relating to the functions and activities of life on a biological level

physiology branch of science that focuses on the functions of the body

placebo effect improvement in an individual's symptoms that is not due to the specific treatment offered; for example, a patient may report that his or her pain has improved after taking a sugar pill, which contains no active medicinal ingredients

placenta in most mammals, the organ that is attached to the mother's uterus and to the fetus's umbilical cord; it is responsible for passing nutrients and oxygen from the mother to the developing fetus

predispose to be prone or vulnerable to something

predisposition condition in which one is vulnerable or prone to something

prenatal existing or occurring before birth; refers also to the care a woman receives while pregnant

problem drinking when a person's drinking disrupts life and relationships, causing difficulties for the drinker

productivity quality of yielding results or benefits

prohibit to forbid

promiscuity having many sexual partners

proportional properly related in size; corresponding

prostate gland located near the bladder and urethra in men, it secretes the fluid that contains sperm

psychedelic substance that can cause hallucinations and/or make its user lose touch with reality

psychiatric relating to the branch of medicine that deals with the study, treatment, and prevention of mental illness

psychiatry branch of medicine that deals with the study, treatment, and prevention of mental illness

psychoactive drugs that affect the mind or mental processes by altering consciousness, perception, or mood

psychology scientific study of mental processes and behaviors

psychometric relating to the technique of measuring mental abilities

psychomotor referring to processess of muscular movement directly influenced by mental processes

psychosis mental disorder in which an individual loses contact with reality and may have delusions (unshakable false beliefs) or hallucinations (the experience of seeing, hearing, feeling, smelling, or tasting things that are not actually present)

psychosocial relates to both life experiences as well as mental processes

psychostimulant medication that is prescribed to control hyperative and impulsive behaviors

psychotherapeutic drugs drugs used to relieve the symptoms of mental illness such as depression, anxiety and psychosis

psychotherapy treatment of a mental or emotional condition during which a person talks to a qualified therapist in order to understand his or her problems and change problem behaviors

psychotropic substance that affects mental function

quinine substance used to treat malaria

rave organized gathering of young people that includes loud, pulsing "house" music and flashing lights

receptor specialized part of a cell that can bind a specific substance; for example, a neuron has special receptors that receive and bind neurotransmitters

recidivism tendency to relapse into previous criminal behavior

recreational drug use casual and infrequent use of a substance, often in social situations, for its pleasurable effects

regulate to bring under the control of law or authorized agency

rehabilitate to restore or improve someone to a condition of health or useful activity

rehabilitation process of restoring a person to a condition of health or useful activity

reinforced to make something stronger by repeating an activity or by adding extra support

relapse term used in substance abuse treatment and recovery that refers to an addict's return to substance use and abuse following a period of abstinence or sobriety

repeal to revoke or cancel

repression the effort of the mind to block unpleasant or painful thoughts or desires; or, an act in which one person or group keeps another group in a lower, less advantageous position

resent to feel anger, bitterness or ill will towards someone or something

residue the quantity of some substance or material left over at the end of a process; a remainder of something

resuscitation revival from unconsciousness; restoring energy, vitality

risk an increased probability of something negative happening

Rohypnol medication that causes sleep, banned in the United States but used illegally as a club drug; also known as a "date rape" drug

sanction punishment imposed as a result of breaking a law or rule

schizophrenia psychotic disorder in which people lose the ability to function normally, suffer from severe personality changes, and suffer from a variety of symptoms, including confusion, disordered thinking, paranoia, hallucinations, emotional numbness, and speech problems

sedated describing someone who took a medication that reduced excitement

sedation process of calming someone by administering a medication that reduces excitement, often called a tranquilizer

sedative a medication that reduces excitement, often called a tranquilizer

sedative-hypnotic drug that has a calming and relaxing effect; "hypnotics" induce sleep

self-harm repeated dangerous behaviors, such as cutting the skin, head-banging, or taking pills

self-medicate when a person treats an ailment, mental or physical, with alcohol or drugs rather than see a physician or mental health professiona

serotonin neurotransmitter associated with the regulation of mood, appetite, sleep, memory, and learning

shamanism religion whose leaders perform rituals of magic, divination, and healing and act as intermediaries between reality and the spirit world

skeletal system the bones and related parts that serve as a framework for the body

sober in relation to drugs and alcohol, refers to abstaining from alcoholic beverages or intoxicants; describes a state in which someone is not under the influence of drugs or alcohol

sociologist someone who studies society, social relationships, and social institutions

sophisticated knowledgeable about the ways of the world, self-confident

specimen a sample, as of tissue, blood, or urine, used for analysis and diagnosis

spina bifida one of the more common birth defects in which the backbone never closes or its coverings stick out through the opening

sterility condition in which one is unable to conceive a child

steroid specific chemical compound; certain types of steroids are produced naturally by the body (such as sex and stress hormones); other types of steroids are laboratory-produced drugs used to treat a variety of illnesses and to reduce swelling

stigma the shame or disgrace attached to something regarded as socially unacceptable

stimulant drug that increases activity temporarily; often used to describe drugs that excite the brain and central nervous system

stimuli things that excite the body or part of the body to produce specific responses

stimulus anything that excites the body or part of the body to produce a specific response

stupor state of greatly dulled interest in the surrounding environment; may include relative unconsciousness

synapse the gap between communicating nerve cells through which impulses pass from one nerve cell to another

synthesize to produce artificially or chemically

testimonial statement that backs up a claim or support a fact

testosterone hormone produced in higher amounts in males that is responsible for male characteristics such as muscle-building and maintaining sexual organs, and during puberty causes hair growth and a deepening voice

tetanus rare but often fatal disease that affects the brain and spinal column

therapeutic healing or curing

tic repetitive, involuntary spasm that increases in severity when it is purposefully surpressed; may be motor (such as muscle contractions or eye blinking) or vocal (such as an unintended yelp or use of an expletive)

tolerance condition in which higher and higher doses of a drug or alcohol are needed to produce the effect or "high" experienced from the original dose

Tourette's syndrome chronic tic disorder involving multiple motor and/or vocal tics that cause distress or significant impairment in social, occupational, or other important areas of functioning

toxic something that is poisonous or dangerous to people

toxicity condition of being poisonous or dangerous to people

toxicology study of the nature, effects, and detection of poisons and the treatment of poisoning

trance state of partial consciousness

tranquilizer drug that decreases anxiety and tension

trauma injury or damage, either to the body or to the mind

trivialize to treat something as less important or valuable than it really is

Twelve Steps program for remaining sober developed by Alcoholics Anonymous; adopted by many other groups, such as Narotics Anonymous

ulcer irritated pit in the surface of a tissue, often on the stomach lining

unethical something that is morally questionable

uppers slang term for amphetamines, drugs that act as stimulants of the central nervous system

variable something that can change or fluctuate

vascular relating to the transport of fluids (such as blood or lymph fluid) through tubes in the body; frequently used to refer to the system of blood vessels

vulnerable at greater risk

withdrawal group of physical and psychological symptoms that may occur when a person suddenly stops the use of a substance or reduces the dose of an addictive substance

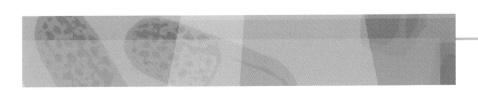

List of Authors

Darrell R. Abernethy
  Division of Clinical
  Pharmacology
  Roger Williams General
  Hospital
  Providence, RI
  Nonabused Drugs
  Withdrawal

Alfonso Acampora
  Walden House, Inc.
  San Francisco, CA
  Treatment Programs,
  Centers, and Organizations:
  A Historical Perspective

Manuella Adrian
  Addiction Research
  Foundation
  Toronto, Canada
  Cancer, Drugs, and Alcohol

Marlene Aldo-Benson
  Indiana University and
  Methodist Hospital of
  Indiana
  Indianapolis, IN
  Allergies to Alcohol and
  Drugs

Peter Andreas
  Brown University
  Providence, RI
  Law and Policy: Controls on
  Drug Trafficking

Linda Wasmer Andrews
  Albuquerque, NM
  Drug Producers
  Drug Trafficking
  Terrorism and Drugs
  Tobacco: Dependence
  Tobacco: Policies, Laws, and
  Regulations

Christopher B. Anthony
  Sparks, MD
  Users

Thomas F. Babor
  Alcohol Research Center
  Department of Psychiatry
  University of Connecticut
  Health Center
  Farmington, CT
  Diagnosis of Drug and
  Alcohol Abuse: An Overview
  Diagnostic and Statistical
  Manual (DSM)

Samuel A. Ball
  Yale University
  New Haven, CT
  Personality Disorder

Robert Balster
  Virginia Commonwealth
  University
  Richmond, CA
  Ketamine
  PCP

Jim Baumohl
  Graduate School of Social
  Work and Social
  Research
  Bryn Mawr College
  Bryn Mawr, PA
  Alcohol- and Drug-Free
  Housing
  Halfway Houses
  Homelessness
  Treatment, History of, in the
  United States

Jan Bays
  The Zen Community of
  Portland, OR
  Child Abuse and Drugs

Neil L. Benowitz
  Division of Clinical
  Pharmacology
  San Francisco General
  Hospital
  San Francisco, CA
  Nicotine
  Tobacco: History of

Michael J. Bohn
  Department of Psychiatry
  University of Wisconsin
  Hospitals
  Madison, WI
  Suicide and Substance Abuse

Joseph V. Brady
  Johns Hopkins University
  School of Medicine
  Baltimore, MD
  Drug Testing in Humans:
  Studying Potential for Abuse

Robert M. Bray
  Research Triangle
  Institute
  Triangle Park, NC
  Military, Drug and Alcohol
  Abuse in the United States

Gregory W. Brock
  Department of Family
  Studies
  University of Kentucky
  Lexington, KY
  Toughlove

Judith S. Brook
  Psychiatry and Behavioral
  Sciences
  New York Medical
  College
  Valhalla, NY
  Childhood Behavior and
  Later Drug Use

Kirk J. Brower
Department of Michigan
Alcohol Research Center
Ann Arbor, MI
Anabolic Steroids

Kathleen K. Bucholz
Department of Psychiatry
Washington University
School of Medicine
St. Louis, MO
Antisocial Personality

Alan J. Budney
Department of Psychiatry
University of Vermont
Burlington, VT
*Cocaine Treatment:
Behavioral Approaches*

Ellen Burke
Department of Family
Studies
Berea College
Berea, KY
Toughlove

Amy Buttery
Lansing, MI
*Drug Testing in Animals:
Studying Potential for Abuse
Schools, Drug Use In*

Howard D. Cappell
Addiction Research
Foundation
Toronto, Canada
*Tolerance and Physical
Dependence*

Kate B. Carey
Syracuse University
Syracuse, NY
Binge Drinking

Jerome F. X. Carroll
Project Return
Foundation, Inc.
New York, NY
*Treatment Programs,
Centers, and Organizations:
A Historical Perspective*

Jonathan Caulkins
Heinz School of Public
Policy and Management
Carnegie Mellon
University
Pittsburgh, PA
*Law and Policy: The Drug
Legalization Debate*

Timmen L. Cermak
San Francisco, CA
Codependence

Cheryl J. Cherpitel
Alcohol Research Group
Berkeley, CA
*Accidents and Injuries from
Alcohol*

Domenic A. Ciraulo
Psychiatry Service
VA Outpatient Clinic
Boston, MA
Benzodiazepines

Patricia Cohen
New York State
Psychiatric Institute
Columbia University
College of Physicians and
Surgeons
Columbia University
School of Public Health
New York, NY
*Childhood Behavior and
Later Drug Use*

Allan Cobb
La Grange, TX
*Drug Use Around the World
Opiate and Opioid Drug
Abuse*

David D. Cole
Georgetown University
Law School
Washington, DC
Racial Profiling

Shirley Coletti
Operation PAR
St. Petersburg, FL
*Treatment Programs,
Centers, and Organizations:
A Historical Perspective*

Philip J. Cook
Duke University
Durham, NC
Tax Laws and Alcohol

Valerie Curran
University College
London, England
*Sedative and Sedative-
Hypnotic Drugs*

Anne Davidson
New York, NY
*Alcohol Treatment:
Behavioral Approaches*

Valina Dawson
Molecular Neurobiology
Laboratory, Addiction
Research Center
National Institute on Drug
Abuse
Baltimore, MD
*Antidepressant
Antipsychotic
Neuroleptic*

David A. Deitch
Department of Psychiatry,
School of Medicine
University of California
San Diego, CA
*Treatment Programs,
Centers, and Organizations:
A Historical Perspective*

Nicholas DeMartinis
Department of Pyschiatry
University of Connecticut
Health Center
Farmington, CT
*Psychoactive Drug
Psychopharmacology
Sedative and Sedative-
Hypnotic Drugs*

Paolo DePetrillo
Division of Clinical
Pharmacology
Roger Williams General
Hospital
Providence, RI
*Nonabused Drugs
Withdrawal*

Don C. Des Jarlais
Chemical Dependency
Unit
Beth Israel Medical Center
New York, NY
Needle Exchange Programs

Peter Drotman
Division of Chemical
Research
National Institute on Drug
Abuse
Rockville, MD
Substance Abuse and AIDS

Linda Dykstra
Department of Psychology
University of North
Carolina
Chapel Hill, NC
Effects of Drugs on

Sensation, Perception, and Memory

Margaret E. Ensminger
Department of Health Policy and Management
Johns Hopkins School of Public Health
Baltimore, MD
Poverty and Drug Use

Nancy Faerber
Canton, MI
Beers and Brews

Theodora Fine, MA, ABD
Substance Abuse and Mental Health Services Administration
Rockville, MD
U.S. Government Agencies

Loretta P. Finnegan
Women's Health Institute
National Institute of Health
Bethesda, MD
Babies, Addicted and Drug-Exposed

Michael P. Finnegan
Alcohol, Drug Abuse, and Mental Health Administration
Division of State Assistant Office of Treatment Improvement
Rockville, MD
Babies, Addicted and Drug-Exposed

Marian W. Fischman
College of Physicians and Surgeons
Columbia University
New York, NY
Amphetamine
Coca Plant
Cocaine
Crack
Methamphetamine
Ritalin

Alice B. Fredericks
Division of Clinical Pharmocology
San Francisco General Hospital
San Francisco, CA
Nicotine
Tobacco: History of

Daniel X. Freedman
Department of Pharmacology
Louisiana State University Medical Center
New Orleans, LA
Ecstasy
Hallucinogens
Lysergic Acid Diethylamide (LSD) and Psychedelics
Peyote

Roberta Friedman
Santa Cruz, CA
Brain Chemistry
Brain Structures
Research

William A. Frosch
Department of Psychiatry
Cornell University Medical School
New York, NY
Addictive Personality

Richard K. Fuller
National Institute on Alcoholism and Alcohol Abuse
Rockville, MD
Alcohol Treatment: Medications

Jessica Gerson
Columbia University
Department of Psychiatry
C.U.N.Y–John Jay College
Department of Psychology
New York State Psychiatric Institute
Department of Neuroscience
New York, NY
Cutting and Self-Harm

Elbert Glover
Department of Psychiatry
University of West Virginia Medical School
Morgantown, WV
Tobacco: Smokeless

Penny N. Glover
Department of Psychiatry
University of West Virginia Medical School
Morgantown, WV
Tobacco: Smokeless

Nick E. Goeders
Department of Pharmacology
Louisiana State University Medical Center
Shreveport, LA
Aphrodisiac
Designer Drugs
Drugs of Abuse

Ronald Goldstock
Kroll Associates
Larchmont, NY
Crime and Drugs

Enoch Gordis
National Institute on Alcoholism and Alcohol Abuse
Rockville, MD
U.S. Government Agencies

David A. Gorelick
Addiction Research Center
National Institute on Drug Abuse
Baltimore, MD
Naltrexone

Roland R. Griffiths
Department of Psychiatry and Behavioral Science
Johns Hopkins School of Medicine
Baltimore, MD
Caffeine
Coffee
Tea

Frederick K. Grittner
St. Paul, MN
Driving, Alcohol, and Drugs
Law and Policy: Foreign Policy and Drugs
Law and Policy: Modern Enforcement, Prosecution, and Sentencing

Angela S. Guarda
Johns Hopkins University
Baltimore, MD
Eating Disorders

Becky Ham
Falls Church, VA
Gangs and Drugs
Herbal Supplements
Media Representations of Drinking, Drug Use, and Smoking

Thomas E. Hanlon
Human Behavior
Associates, Inc.
Annapolis, MD
Crime and Drugs

Dorothy Hatsukami
Department of Psychiatry
University of Minnesota
Minneapolis, MN
*Tobacco Treatment:
Behavioral Approaches*

Harry W. Haverkos
Division of Chemical
Research
National Institute of Drug
Abuse
Rockville, MD
Substance Abuse and AIDS

Dwight B. Heath
Department of
Anthropology
Brown University
Providence, RI
Alcohol: History of Drinking

Daniel S. Heit
Justice Works YouthCare
Pittsburgh, PA
*Treatment Programs,
Centers, and Organizations:
A Historical Perspective*

Jack E. Henningfield
Johns Hopkins University
School of Medicine
Baltimore, MD
Pinney Associates
Bethesda, MD
*Tobacco Treatment:
Medications*

Stephen T. Higgins
Department of Psychiatry
University of Vermont
Burlington, VT
*Cocaine Treatment:
Behavioral Approaches*

Leo E. Hollister
Veterans Administration
Medical Center
Palo Alto, CA
Stanford University School
of Medicine
Stanford, CA
*Bhang
Cannabis sativa
Hashish*

*Hemp
Marijuana*

Andrew J. Homburg
Farmington Hills, MI
*Alcohol: History of Drinking
Costs of Substance Abuse
and Dependence,
Economic*

Richard G. Hunter
Neurosciences Division
Yerkes Research Center
Atlanta, GA
*Club Drugs
Rave
Rohypnol*

M. S. Irwanto
Department of Child
Development and Family
Studies
Purdue University
West Lafayette, IN
Families and Drug Use

Ivan Izquierdo
Center of Neurobiology of
Learning
University of California
Irvine, CA
*Effects of Drugs on
Sensation, Perception, and
Memory*

James B. Jacobs
New York University Law
School
New York, NY
Driving, Alcohol, and Drugs

Nora Jacobson
School of Public Health
Johns Hopkins University
Baltimore, MD
Poverty and Drug Use

Faith K. Jaffe
Towson, MD
*Treatment Programs,
Centers, and Organizations:
A Historical Perspective*

Jerome H. Jaffe
School of Medicine
University of Maryland
Baltimore, MD
*Ayahuasca
Betel Nut
Halfway Houses
Prohibition of Alcohol*

*Tobacco: Medical
Complications
Treatment, History of, in
the United States
Treatment Programs,
Centers, and
Organizations: A
Historical Perspective*

Elaine Johnson
Substance Abuse and
Mental Health Services
Administration
Rockville, MD
U.S. Government Agencies

Eric O. Johnson
Drug Dependence
Epidemiology
National Institute on Drug
Abuse
Rockville, MD
*Dropouts and Substance
Abuse*

A. W. Jones
Department of Alcohol
Toxicology
National Laboratory of
Forensic Chemistry
University Hospital
Linkoping, Sweden
Blood Alcohol Concentration

Harold Kalant
Department of
Pharmacology
University of Toronto,
Canada
*Addiction: Concepts and
Definitions*

Peter Kalix
Department of
Pharmacology
University of Geneva
Switzerland
Khat

George A. Kanuck
Malvern Preparatory
School
Malvern, PA
*Babies, Addicted and Drug-
Exposed*

Bhushan M. Kapur
Department of Clinical
Biochemistry
University of Toronto,
Canada

CRTI Addiction Research
Foundation
Toronto, Canada
Alcohol: Chemistry

Jat M. Khanna
Department of
Pharmacology
University of Toronto,
Canada
Barbiturates

Michael Kidorf
Behavioral Pharmacology
Research Unit, Johns
Hopkins University School
of Medicine, Baltimore,
MD
Southeast Baltimore Drug
Treatment Program,
Hopkins Bayview Medical
Center
Baltimore, MD
*Heroin Treatment:
Behavioral Approaches*

Timothy W. Kinlock
Human Behavior
Associates, Inc.
Annapolis, MD
Crime and Drugs

Michael Klitzner
Litzner & Associates
Vienna, VA
*Students Against Destructive
Decisions (SADD)*

Clifford Knapp
Department of
Pharmacology and
Experimental Therapeutics
Tufts University School
Medicine
Boston, MA
Benzodiazepines

Madhu R. Korrapati
Research Service
Veterans Administration
Medical Center
Boise, ID
*Drug and Alcohol Use
Among the Elderly*

Lynn T. Kozlowski
Department of Health and
Human Development
Pennsylvania State
University
University Park, PA

*Tobacco Treatment: An
Overview*

Thomas R. Kosten
Substance Abuse
Treatment Unit
Yale University School of
Medicine
New Haven, CT
*Cocaine Treatment:
Medications*
Cocaine: Withdrawal

Michael J. Kuhar
Division of Neuroscience,
Department of
Pharmacology
Emory University
Atlanta, GA
Antidote
Chocolate
Cola

Karol L. Kumpfer
Center for Substance
Abuse Prevention
Substance Abuse and
Mental Health Services
Administration
Rockville, MD
Child Abuse and Drugs

Malcolm H. Lader
Institute of Psychiatry
University of London,
England
Benzodiazepines
Prescription Drug Abuse

Robin A. LaDue
Native American Center
for Excellence
University of Washington
Seattle, WA
*Fetal Alcohol Syndrome
(FAS)*

Phyllis A. Langton
Department of Sociology
George Washington
University
Washington, DC
Temperance Movement

J. Clark Laundergan
Center for Addiction
Studies
Duluth, MN
*Treatment Programs,
Centers, and Organizations:
A Historical Perspective*

Jill Lectka
New York, NY
Prescription Drug Abuse

Alan. I. Leshner
National Institute on Drug
Abuse
Bethesda, MD
U.S. Government Agencies

Carl G. Leukefeld
Center on Drug and
Alcohol Research
University of Kentucky
Lexington, KY
*Complications from Injecting
Drugs*
*Law and Policy: Court-
Ordered Treatment*

R. L. Lewis
Department of Family
Studies
Purdue University
West Lafayette, IN
Families and Drug Use

Barbara Lex
Harvard Medical School
McLean Hospital
Belmont, MA
Families and Drug Use

Richard Lingeman
New York, NY
Slang and Jargon

Arlene R. Lissner
Abraxas Group
Philadelphia, PA
*Treatment Programs,
Centers, and Organizations:
A Historical Perspective*

Raye Z. Litten
National Institute on
Alcoholism and Alcohol
Abuse
Rockville, MD
*Alcohol Treatment:
Medications*

Edythe D. London
Intramural Research
Program
National Institute on Drug
Abuse
Rockville, MD
*Imaging Techniques:
Visualizing the Living
Brain*

Chris Lopez
Farmington Hills, MI
*Diagnosis of Drug and
Alcohol Abuse: An Overview*

Arnold M. Ludwig
Department of Psychiatry
University of Kentucky
College of Medicine
Lexington, KY
Creativity and Drugs

Scott E. Lukas
Harvard Medical School
McLean Hospital
Belmont, MA
*Barbiturates
Beers and Brews
Alcohol: Chemistry
Fermentation
Moonshine
Quaaludes
Sedative and Sedative-
Hypnotic Drugs
Sleeping Pills*

Doris Layton Mackenzie
Department of Criminal
Justice
University of Maryland
College Park, MD
*Boot Camps and Shock
Incarceration*

David J. Mactas
Center for Substance
Abuse Treatment
Rockville, MD
*Treatment Programs,
Centers, and Organizations:
A Historical Perspective*

Rebecca Marlow-Ferguson
Farmington Hills, MI
*Effects of Drugs on
Sensation, Perception, and
Memory
Naltrexone*

Jill Max
Trumbull, CT
*Medical Emergencies and
Death from Drug Abuse
Violence and Drug and
Alcohol Use*

Thomas S. May
Toronto, Canada
*Attention-
Deficit/Hyperactivity
Disorder (ADHD)*

*Adolescents, Drug and
Alcohol Use
Diagnosis of Drug and
Alcohol Abuse: An
Overview
Ethnic, Cultural, and
Religious Issues in Drug
Use and Treatment
Prevention
Prevention Programs
Risk Factors for Substance
Abuse
Treatment Types: An
Overview*

Kevin McEneaney
Phoenix House
New York, NY
*Treatment Programs,
Centers, and Organizations:
A Historical Perspective*

James L. McGaugh
Center for Neurobiology
of Learning
University of California
Irvine, CA
*Effects of Drugs on
Sensation, Perception, and
Memory*

James R. McKay
University of Pennsylvania
Philadelphia, PA
Relapse

Ada C. Mezzich
Western Psychiatric
Institute
University of Pittsburgh
School of Medicine
Pittsburgh, PA
*Attention-
Deficit/Hyperactivity
Disorder (ADHD)
Conduct Disorder*

Tom Mieczkowski
University of South
Florida
Tampa, FL
*Drug Testing Methods and
Analysis*

William R. Miller
Department of Psychology
University of New Mexico
Albuquerque, NM
*Alcohol Treatment:
Behavioral Approaches*

Richard A. Millstein
National Institute on Drug
Abuse
Rockville, MD
U.S. Government Agencies

Marc Mooney
Transdisciplinary Tobacco
Use Research Center
University of Minnesota
Minneapolis, MN
*Tobacco Treatment:
Behavioral Approaches*

Timothy H. Moran
Department of Psychiatry
Johns Hopkins University
Baltimore, MD
Anorectic

Herbert Moskowitz
Encino, CA
*Driving, Alcohol, and
Drugs*

Ethan Nebelkopf
Director, Family and
Child Guidance Clinic
Native American Health
Center
San Francisco, CA
*Treatment Programs,
Centers, and Organizations:
A Historical Perspective*

Carl A. Newcombe
U.S. Customs Service
Canine Enforcement
Training Center
Front Royal, VA
Dogs in Drug Detection

John Newmeyer
Haight-Ashbury Free
Clinics Inc.
San Francisco, CA
*Treatment Programs,
Centers, and Organizations:
A Historical Perspective*

David N. Nurco
Human Behavior
Associates, Inc.
Annapolis, MD
Crime and Drugs

Donald A. Overton
Department of Psychology
Temple University
Philadelphia, PA
Effects of Drugs on

*Sensation, Perception, and
Memory*

Denise Paone
Chemical Dependency
Unit
Beth Israel Medical Center
New York, NY
Needle Exchange Programs

Karen Parker
Addiction Research
Foundation
Toronto, Canada
*Anxiety
Breathalyzer
Conduct Disorder
Driving, Alcohol, and
Drugs*

Gavril W. Pasternak
Department of Neurology
Memorial Sloan Kettering
Cancer Center
New York, NY
*Analgesic
Codeine
Heroin
Morphine
Naltrexone
Narcotic
Opium*

J. Thomas Payte
School of Medicine
University of California
San Francisco, CA
*Methadone Maintenance
Programs*

R. N. Pechnick
Department of
Pharmacology
Louisiana State University
Medical Center
New Orleans, LA
*Ecstasy
Hallucinogens
Lysergic Acid
Diethylamide (LSD) and
Psychedelics
Peyote*

Stanton Peele
Lindesmith Center
New York, NY
*Alcohol: Abstinence versus
Controlled Drinking*

Anthony G. Phillips
Department of Psychology

University of British
Columbia
Vancouver, Canada
Anhedonia

Beny J. Primm
Addiction Research and
Treatment Corporation
Brooklyn, NY
U.S. Government Agencies

Peter Reuter
Rand Corporation
Washington, DC
Street Value

Dorothy P. Rice
Institute for Health and
Aging
University of California
San Francisco, CA
*Costs of Substance Abuse and
Dependence, Economic*

Cynthia Robbins
Department of Sociology
University of Delaware
Newark, DE
*Gender and Substance
Abuse*

Heather Roberto
Center on Drug and
Alcohol Research
University of Kentucky
Lexington, KY
*Complications from Injecting
Drugs*

Ian Rockett
Department of
Community Medicine
West Virginia University
Morgantown, WV
*Accidents and Injuries from
Drugs*

Roger A. Roffman
School of Social Work
University of Washington
Seattle, WA
Marijuana Treatment

Myroslava Romach
University of Toronto,
Canada
*Anxiety
Breathalyzer
Conduct Disorder
Driving, Alcohol, and
Drugs*

Charles M. Rongey
Orlando, FL
*Advertising and the Alcohol
Industry
Advertising and the
Tobacco Industry*

Marc Rosen
Department of Psychiatry
VA Connecticut
Healthcare System
West Haven, CT
*Heroin Treatment:
Medications*

Carl Salzman
Massachusetts Mental
Health Center
Harvard Medical School
Boston, MA
Benzodiazepine Withdrawal

Herman H. Sampson
Department of Physiology
and Pharmacology
School of Medicine
Wake Forest University
Winston-Salem, NC
*Alcohol: Psychological
Consequences of Chronic
Abuse*

Sally L. Satel
Substance Abuse
Treatment Unit
Yale University School of
Medicine
New Haven, CT
Cocaine: Withdrawal

Joyce F. Schneiderman
Addiction Research
Foundation
Toronto, Canada
*Babies, Addicted and Drug-
Exposed*

Marc A. Schuckit
Department of Psychiatry
Veterans of Administration
Medical Center
San Diego, CA
*Adult Children of Alcoholics
(ACOA)
Betel Nut*

Leslie M. Schuh
National Institute on Drug
Abuse
Addiction Research Center
Baltimore, MD

Tobacco Treatment:
Medications

Richard B. Seymour
Haight-Ashbury Free
Clinics Inc.
San Francisco, CA
Treatment Programs,
Centers, and Organizations:
A Historical Perspective

Sidney Shankman
Second Genesis, Inc.
Bethesda, MD
Treatment Programs,
Centers, and Organizations:
A Historical Perspective

Donald R. Shopland
Smoking and Tobacco
Control Program
National Cancer
Institute
Bethesda, MD
Tobacco: Medical
Complications

Dianne Shuntich
Department of Mental
Health
Cabinet for Human
Resources
Frankfort, KY
Mothers Against Drunk
Driving (MADD)

Kenneth Silverman
Department of Mental
Health
Cabinet for Human
Resources
Frankfort, KY
Caffeine
Coffee
Tea

John Slade
University of Medicine
and Dentistry of New
Jersey
New Brunswick, NJ
Tobacco: Industry

David E. Smith
Haight-Ashbury Free
Clinics Inc.
San Francisco, CA
Treatment Programs,
Centers, and Organizations:
A Historical Perspective

Joseph Spillane
University of Florida
Gainesville, FL
Law and Policy: History of,
in the United States

Robin Solit
Department of Psychology
University of California
San Diego, CA
Treatment Programs,
Centers, and Organizations:
A Historical Perspective

June M. Stapleton
Addiction Research Center
National Institute on Drug
Abuse
Baltimore, MD
Imaging Techniques:
Visualizing the Living Brain

Marvin Steinberg
Connecticut Council on
Problem Gambling
Guilford, CT
Gambling

Robert S. Stephens
Department of Psychology
Virginia Polytechnic
Institute
Blacksburg, VA
Marijuana Treatment

Maxine L. Stitzer
Behavioral Pharmacology
Research Unit
Francis Scott Key Medical
Center
Baltimore, MD
Heroin Treatment:
Behavioral Approaches

Carla L. Storr
Department of Mental
Hygiene
Johns Hopkins School of
Public Health
Baltimore, MD
Adolescents, Drug and
Alcohol Use

John T. Sullivan
Center for Chemical
Dependence
Francis Scott Key Medical
Center
Baltimore, MD
Alcohol: Withdrawal

Nancy L. Sutherland
Alcohol and Drug Abuse
Institute
University of Washington
Seattle, WA
Alcohol: Psychological
Consequences of Chronic
Abuse

Neil Swan
ROW Sciences
Rockville, MD
Inhalants

Ralph E. Tarter
Western Psychiatric
Institute
University of Pittsburgh
School of Medicine
Pittsburgh, PA
Attention-
Deficit/Hyperactivity
Disorder (ADHD)
Conduct Disorder

Beti Thompson
Fred Hutchinson Cancer
Research Center
Seattle, WA
Nicotine Withdrawal

Michele Staton Tindall
Center on Drug and
Alcohol Research
University of Kentucky
Lexington, KY
Law and Policy: Court-
Ordered Treatment

Harrison M. Trice
Department of
Organizational Behavior
New York School of
Industry and Labor
Relations
Cornell University
Ithaca, NY
Al-Anon
Alateen
Alcoholics Anonymous
(AA)
Narcotics Anonymous
(NA)

Alison M. Trinkoff
School of Nursing
University of Maryland
Baltimore, MD
Adolescents, Drug and
Alcohol Use

George R. Uhl
Molecular Neurobiology
Laboratory, Addiction
Research Center
National Institute on Drug
Abuse
Baltimore, MD
*Antidepressant
Antipsychotic
Neuroleptic*

Jane Velez
Project Return
Foundation, Inc.
New York, NY
*Treatment Programs,
Centers, and Organizations:
A Historical Perspective*

Robert E. Vestal
Clinical Pharmacology and
Gerontology Research
Unit
Veterans Administration
Medical Center
Boise, ID
*Drug and Alcohol Use in the
Elderly*

Alexander C. Wagenaar
School of Public Health,
Division of Epidemiology
University of Minnesota
Minneapolis, MN
Drinking Age

Michael Walsh
The Walsh Group
Bethesda, MD
Workplace, Drug Use in the

Ronald R. Watson
College of Public Health
and School of Medicine
University of Arizona
Tucson, AZ
*Alcohol: Complications
Treatment Programs,
Centers, and
Organizations: A
Historical Perspective*

Amy Windham
Department of Mental
Hygiene
Johns Hopkins School of
Hygiene and Mental
Health
Baltimore, MD
Zero Tolerance

Michael Winkelman
Department of
Anthropology
Arizona State University
Tempe, AZ
Drugs Used in Rituals

Friedner D. Wittman
KLEW Associates
Berkeley, CA
*Alcohol- and Drug-Free
Housing*

William L. Woolverton,
Ph.D.
University of Mississippi
Medical Center
Department of Psychiatry
Jackson, MS
*Drug Testing in Animals:
Studying Potential for Abuse*

Ronald W. Wood
New York University
Medical Center
Tuxedo Park, NY
Inhalants

Jill Anne Yeagley
University of New Mexico
Albuquerque, NM
Alcohol Poisoning

Robert Zaczek
Du Pont Merck
Pharmaceuticals
Wilmington, DE
*Jimsonweed
Kava*

Joan Ellen Zweben
School of Medicine
University of California at
San Francisco
San Francisco, CA
Clinic and Medical Group
and East Bay Community
Recovery Project
Oakland, CA
*Methadone Maintenance
Programs*

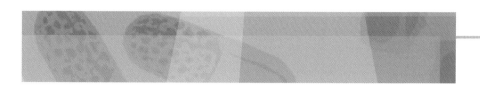

Cumulative Index

In this cumulative index, the boldface number before the colon indicates the volume number. Page numbers in boldface type indicate article titles, and italics indicate an image. Numbers followed by a "t" indicate the presence of a table; "f" indicates an illustration.

A

AA. *See* Alcoholics Anonymous

AAEFP (African-American Extended Family Program), **2**:64

Aaron, Hank, **3**:150

Abraxas Foundation, **3**:181

Absolut vodka, advertising of, **1**:*21*

Abstinence
   vs. controlled drinking, **1**:71–72
   defined, **1**:12, **2**:16, **3**:6
   incentives for, **2**:119
   Temperance Movement and, **3**:109–113

Abstinence syndrome. *See* Withdrawal syndrome

Abuse. *See* Child abuse; Drug abuse

Abuse potential
   defined, **3**:17
   of new drugs, **2**:9–15

Academic achievement, drug abuse and, **2**:2–3, **2**:73–74, **3**:203

Acceptance, in twelve-step program, **1**:69

Accidents
   from alcohol, **1**:1–4, **1**:*1f*, **2**:96
   from drug abuse, **2**:96
   from drugs, **1**:4–7
   with elderly and alcohol, **2**:3
   vs. injuries, **1**:6–7
   from ketamine abuse, **2**:143
   See also Motor vehicle accidents

Acetaldehyde, as carcinogen, **1**:146

Acetaminophen, **1**:83

Acetylcholine, nicotine and, **3**:13

"Acid culture," **2**:182

Acne, from anabolic steroids, **1**:82

ACOA. *See* Adult Children of Alcoholics

Acquired immune deficiency syndrome. *See* AIDS

Acting out, **1**:89–90

Acton, James, **3**:79

Acupuncture, to quit smoking, **3**:122

Acute, defined, **1**:8, **3**:21

Acute coronary syndrome, **1**:179

ADAM program. *See* Arrestee Drug Abuse Monitoring program

ADD. *See* Attention deficit disorder

Adderall. *See* Dextroamphetamine

Addicted by Prescription: One Woman's Triumph and Fight for Change (Gadsby), **3**:17

Addiction
   ADHD treatment and, **1**:91
   Alcoholics Anonymous and, **1**:71
   brain structure in, **1**:137–138
   chemistry of, **1**:125–132
   concepts and definitions, **1**:7–12, **1**:*7t*, **1**:*10f*
   defined, **1**:9, **1**:91, **2**:11, **3**:37
   vs. dependence, **2**:209
   federally funded treatment programs, **2**:173
   to nicotine, **3**:117–118, **3**:131, **3**:133, **3**:136
   to opioids, **3**:22–24
   physical and psychological dependence with, **3**:165
   to prescription drugs, **3**:38–39
   research, **1**:130–132, **1**:138–139, **3**:60–65, **3**:*62f*
   See also Alcoholism; Dependence; Drug abuse

Addictive gambling. *See* Pathological gambling

Addictive personality, **1**:12–13

Adenosine, caffeine and, **1**:130–131

ADHD. *See* Attention-deficit/hyperactivity disorder

Adipex. *See* Phentermine

Administration techniques, for morphine, **3**:2
   See also Intravenous injections; Smoking

Adolescent Alcohol Involvement Scale, **1**:212

Adolescent Drinking Index, **1**:212